RADIOGR/

MW01611913

Richard R. Carlton, M.S., R.T.(R)(CV)
Chairman of Radiography
Lima Technical College
Lima, Ohio

with a chapter on Test-Taking Skills contributed by

Steven B. Dowd, M.A., R.T.(R)
Lincolnland Community College
Springfield, Illinois

J.B. Lippincott Company
Philadelphia

Acquisitions Editor: Andrew Allen
Cover Designer: Tom Jackson
Printer/Binder: R. R. Donnelley & Sons

6 5 4 3 2

ISBN 0-397-54899-0

Any procedure or practice described in this book should be applied by the health-care practitioner under appropriate supervision in accordance with professional standards of care used with regard to the unique circumstances that apply in each practice situation. Care has been taken to confirm the accuracy of information presented and to describe generally accepted practices. However, the authors, editors, and publisher cannot accept any responsibility for errors or omissions or for any consequences from application of the information in this book and make no warranty, express or implied, with respect to the contents of the book.

Every effort has been made to ensure drug selections and dosages are in accordance with current recommendations and practice. Because of ongoing research, changes in government regulations, and the constant flow of information on drug therapy, reactions, and interactions, the reader is cautioned to check the package insert for each drug for indications, dosages, warnings and precautions, particularly if the drug is new or infrequently used.

to my favorite radiographer

Lynn Carlton

Examinations usually do not give an indication of the capacity for a subject, but unfortunately they are a necessary evil.

Wilhelm Konrad Röntgen

ABOUT THE AUTHOR

Richard R. Carlton is Chairman and Assistant Professor of Radiography at Lima Technical College in Lima, Ohio. He is ARRT certified in radiography and cardiovascular-interventional technology, has taught radiography for 14 years and, with Arlene Adler, is the author of *Principles of Radiographic Imaging.* His other Lippincott books are *Cardiovascular-Interventional Technology Exam Review*, with Deborah Phlipot and *Mammography Exam Review* with Deborah Phlipot, Judy McLaughlin, and Pat Miller. Rick has written thousands of items for simulated examinations and state quiz competitions; conducted review seminars; written textbooks, workbooks, instructor's guides, and journal articles; and designed instructional computer programs. He has published several series of guides to examination reviews in radiologic technology newsweekly magazines.

Camera-ready copy produced by Linda Benson, Word Processing Specialist, Lima Technical College, Lima, Ohio.

TABLE OF CONTENTS

[1] Table of contents categories copyrighted 1988 The American Registry of Radiologic Technologists. Reprinted by permission.

PREFACE

This Radiography Examination Review is designed to assist persons preparing for the Examination in Radiography of the American Registry of Radiologic Technologists (ARRT) in anticipation of gaining the Registered Technologist (Radiographer) credential of R.T.(R)(ARRT). The review is a useful tool in evaluating the validity of knowledge, pinpointing weak areas for further study, and as a guide to appropriate references for in-depth investigation. The content is also appropriate for students who wish to review a particular subject area during academic coursework, as a continuing education or remediation activity for registered technologists, an evaluation guide for planning re-entry study, and as a review of diagnostic imaging for students in radiation oncology, nuclear medicine, and ultrasonography.

The American Registry of Radiologic Technologists does not review, evaluate, or endorse publications. Permission to reproduce ARRT copyrighted materials within this publication should not be construed as an endorsement of the publication by the ARRT. Any implication of ARRT approval of this book violates the policies of the ARRT. I have never served as a member of an ARRT examination committee to review question items, nor have I had any questions accepted for consideration for the examination in radiography. The questions in this book have not to my knowledge been used for any ARRT examination in radiography.

Every attempt has been made to provide questions that require problem-solving skills from the entire radiography curriculum consistent with subject information in the most popular textbooks in current use. Because of the rapid changes that are always occurring in the radiologic sciences, especially radiography, special effort has been made to create questions that will assure students have been exposed to recent advances in the profession. However, the vast majority of the questions are based on the traditional radiography content areas.

Questions 1-1400 are categorized according to the ARRT Table of Specifications for the Examination in Radiography. This permits review by specific content areas congruent with the examination. There is also a 200 question simulated examination that can be used as a post-test following the review activities. This examination is also weighted according to the ARRT specifications. Explanations of the correct answers with suggested references for in-depth study are provided in a separate section. Index keywords to locate the information in the references also are provided.

ACKNOWLEDGMENTS

This was a project that had been in the back of my mind since the 1970s until it was received with enthusiasm by Andrew Allen at Lippincott. Thanks to both Andrew and Miriam Benert for their kindness and support throughout.

Although my family always takes priority, without the infinite patience of my wife, Lynn, this book would not have been written. My children, Michelle, Kristöfer, Ærik, Edward, and Michael have not only been understanding, but have been my motivation to continue when it seemed impossible to write ten more questions.

Numerous professional friends have made significant contributions to this work. I am indebted to Steven Dowd for the generous contribution of his manuscript on test-taking skills which forms a complete chapter. In addition to serving as a primary reviewer for this work, his long friendship and willingness to provide criticism and

1

contributions are greatly appreciated. I owe a special thanks to Dennis Spragg, Assistant Professor of Radiography at Lima Technical College, who not only contributed questions and always constructive criticism, but throughout the years has made it possible for me to become an author by making sure our program was running smoothly at all times, especially when deadlines were looming. Thanks are due my frequent co-author Deborah Phlipot and also Andrew Shappell, both Lima Tech faculty members, for taking the time to review and comment on many of these questions. All of my students throughout the years, who have demonstrated their professionalism as they never hesitated to point out my errors and shortcomings in a positive manner, have made this a better work.

I am indebted to Bruce Long of Indiana University in Indianapolis and Wanda Weslowski of the Community College of Philadelphia, who provided a meticulous critical review of the entire manuscript. The changes made as a result of their commentary have increased the value of this book immeasurably.

Linda Benson, through her skills as a word-processing specialist, produced camera-ready text copy for the final printing. Without her willingness to take on one more extra project, and without the support of her husband Brian, it is unlikely this book would ever have been completed. Consideration is also due Linda as well as Beverly Thomas, who tolerate abuses beyond the call of duty and still produce hundreds of pages of laser print and a half dozen letters before the 4:00 PM mail. Finally, the consistent support of my authoring efforts by Sam Bassitt, our Vice President of Instruction at Lima Technical College, has given me the necessary motivation to complete this project.

Rick Carlton
Lima, Ohio

TERMINOLOGY

It is the policy of the ARRT that new terminology and concepts are used on examination questions only after they achieve general usage throughout the profession. This means that at any given time, the ARRT is engaged in the process of preparing to use new information as schools begin to teach and the profession begins to assimilate new changes. Because students are often taught new information that is not yet appearing on the examinations, it is helpful to review the current stand of the ARRT in these areas as part of the review process.

The ARRT maintains a list of approved terminology, abbreviations, and formats in a document known as the *Conventions Specific to the Radiography Examination*. The purpose of the document is to assure that questions on the examination in radiography are consistent. The most critical information from this document is "Standard Terminology for Positioning and Projection," which is reproduced in the front of each examination booklet for reference by examinees. (This document is reproduced by permission of the ARRT as Figure A in this book.) The more important conventions are listed below to permit students to acquaint themselves with them in advance and avoid time memorizing terms that will not appear on the examination.

It should be recognized that the ARRT board publishes notices of changes in conventions in the *ARRT Newsletter* which is published twice a year and sent to all CAHEA-accredited programs. Students should check with their program director to bring the information given below up to date. This is easily accomplished by checking each issue of the *ARRT Newsletter* since a year prior to the publication date on the back of the title page of this book.

CONVENTIONS USED IN THE ARRT EXAMINATION IN RADIOGRAPHY

TERM CURRENTLY IN USE	TERM NOT IN USE
ANATOMIC SCIENCES	
acanthiomeatal	acanthomeatal
AP	anteroposterior
LAO	left anterior oblique
LPO	left posterior oblique
PA	posteroanterior
RAO	right anterior oblique
RPO	right posterior oblique

TERM CURRENTLY IN USE	TERM NOT IN USE
PHYSICAL SCIENCES	
automatic exposure control	phototimer, phototiming
automatic collimation	automatic positive beam limitation
average photon energy	wavelength [except when comparing form of electromagnetic radiation (such as x and gamma rays)]
blur	penumbra (when due to patient motion)
bucky grid	moving grid
contrast, higher or shorter	increased contrast
contrast, lower or longer	decreased contrast
detail screens	slow screens
exit radiation	remnant radiation
FFD	focal-film distance, or source to image receptor distance (SID), or target to film distance (TFD), or anode to film distance (AFD)
focus to object distance (FOD)	source to object distance (SOD), or target to object distance (TOD)
geometrically recorded detail	geometric sharpness
grid focusing distance	grid radius
Hertz (Hz)	cycles per second (cps)
high speed screens	fast screens
image forming radiation	remnant radiation
MPD	maximum permissible dose
motion	penumbra (when due to patient motion)
OFD	object-film distance, or part-film distance, or object to image receptor distance (OID)
reciprocating grid	moving grid

TERM CURRENTLY IN USE	TERM NOT IN USE
recorded detail	sharpness, or sharpness of detail, or definition or detail
scale contrast	scale of contrast
scattered radiation	scatter radiation
tomography	body section radiography
unsharpness of recorded detail	penumbra (when due to focal spot or intensifying screen)

Radiation Measurement

As of the publication of this book, the ARRT had not yet implemented either dose equivalent limits in place of the outdated maximum permissible dose (MPD) or the SI radiation measurement units in place of the old British system units. Because the profession appears to be moving gently toward the new usage, and because the ARRT advised schools to begin teaching effective dose equivalents in 1988, the effective dose equivalent limits are used in some questions in this book, while the old MPDs are used in others. Questions with both old radiation units (roentgen, rad, rem) and new SI units (coulomb/kilogram, gray, sievert) have been used as well. In addition, there are some questions on the conversions between the conventional and SI system units, also in anticipation of this change. Appendix B provides both the important Dose Equivalent Limits and Maximum Permissible Doses. Appendix C provides information on the SI Radiation Units.

Official status was given Le Systeme International d'Unites (the SI units) at the Eleventh General Conference on Weights and Measures in 1960. The NCRP recommended the replacement of maximum permissible doses with dose equivalency limits in 1987 in *NCRP Report No. 91: Recommendations on Limits for Exposure to Ionizing Radiation*.

Radiation protection standards as announced in the 1989 *NCRP Report #102: Medical X-Ray, Electron Beam, and Gamma-Ray Protection for Energies Up To 50 MeV (Equipment Design, Performance, and Use)* have been used for the radiation protection questions in this book.

Intensifying Screen Speeds

Descriptions of intensifying screen speeds are stated with the screen speed number (the relative speed number). The older generic names are no longer used when screen speed comparisons are being made: for example, "50" instead of "detail." The relative screen speed numbers are described as shown below.

INTENSIFYING SCREEN RELATIVE SPEED NUMBER AND GENERIC NAME

RELATIVE SCREEN SPEED NUMBER	GENERIC NAME
<100	detail
100	medium speed
>100	high speed

Copyrighted by The American Registry of Radiologic Technologists. Reprinted by permission.

The relationship of older and newer generic names that have been replaced by the relative screen speed numbers.

INTENSIFYING SCREEN GENERIC NAMES

NEWER NAME	OLDER TERM
detail	slow
medium speed	par speed
high speed	fast

Copyrighted by The American Registry of Radiologic Technologists. Reprinted by permission.

Grid Technique Conversion

The ARRT does not specify exact grid technique conversion factors. Published sources, all of which are included in the references section of this book, are used as guidelines. The lowest and highest mAs conversion ranges from all sources is shown below. Because the ranges are so wide, especially for the high ratio grids, most grid problems can be expected to be concerned with the lower ratio grids or to be dramatic comparisons.

GRID TECHNIQUE mAs CONVERSION MINIMUM AND MAXIMUM RANGES

FROM NO GRID TO:	MINIMUM	MAXIMUM
5:1	1.5 X	3 X
6:1	2 X	3 X
8:1	2.5 X	4.25 X
10:1	3 X	3.5 X
12:1	3.5 X	6.25 X
16:1	4 X	8 X

Anatomy
Anatomic descriptions of radiographic positions are used in place of the proper names of individuals who developed the procedures. The exceptions to this rule are descriptions of cranial positions, for which proper names continue to be used to describe specific methods in parenthesis after the anatomic description. These conventions have been used throughout this book. For example, the Waters position of the facial bones is described as the parietoacanthial position (Waters method), while the term PA axial is used instead of the Holmblad position.

The Twelfth International Congress of Anatomists in 1985 adopted substantial alterations of anatomic nomenclature that were subsequently published in the sixth edition of *Nomina Anatomica* in 1989. Although these alterations have very recently begun to appear in radiologic literature, they were not used in this book as it will probably be some time before either the profession or the ARRT adopts them.

To assist students in understanding the relationship between view, position, and projection plus positioning terminology such as supine, decubitus, the obliques, etc. the ARRT has published Figure A. This illustration is provided as part of each examination booklet. In this format, it is available for reference by each examinee during the examination.

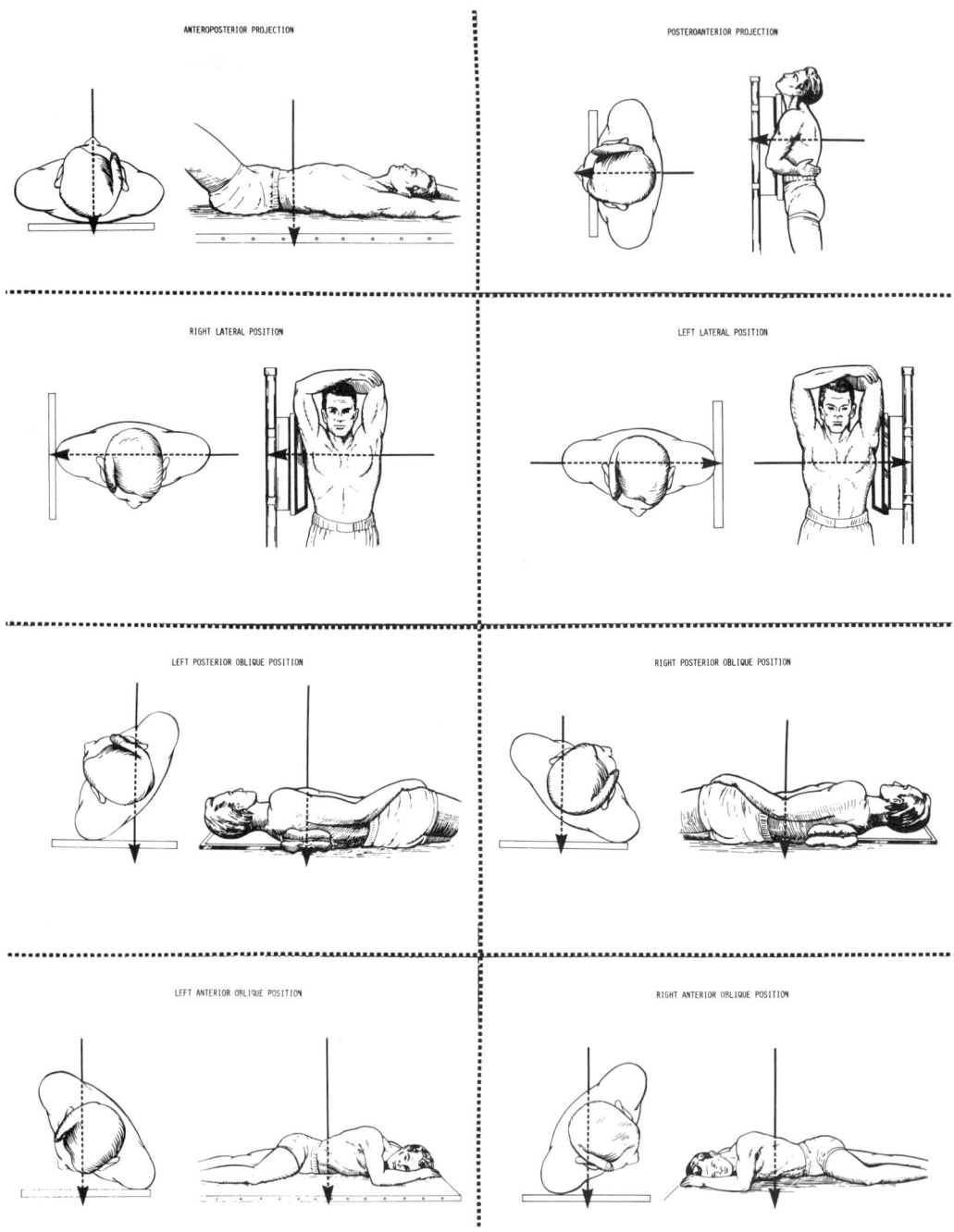

ANTEROPOSTERIOR PROJECTION

POSTEROANTERIOR PROJECTION

RIGHT LATERAL POSITION

LEFT LATERAL POSITION

LEFT POSTERIOR OBLIQUE POSITION

RIGHT POSTERIOR OBLIQUE POSITION

LEFT ANTERIOR OBLIQUE POSITION

RIGHT ANTERIOR OBLIQUE POSITION

S–2

Figure A. (copyrighted by The American Registry of Radiologic Technologists; reprinted by permission)

Definitions

Following are critical definitions that are used in the examination.

DEFINITIONS USED IN THE ARRT EXAMINATION IN RADIOGRAPHY

TERM	DEFINITION
ANATOMIC SCIENCES	
anterior position	facing the film
decubitus	lying down with a horizontal x-ray beam
oblique, left anterior	erect or upright, facing the film, body rotated with the left anterior portion closest to the film
oblique, left posterior	erect or upright, facing the radiographic tube, body rotated with the left posterior portion closest to the film
oblique, right anterior	erect or upright, facing the film, body rotated with the right anterior portion closest to the film
oblique, right posterior	erect or upright, facing the radiographic tube, body rotated with the right posterior portion closest to the film
position	restricted to discussion of the patient's specific physical body position (i.e., supine, erect, Trendelenburg)
posterior position	facing the radiographic tube
projection	restricted to discussion of the path of the central ray
prone	lying face downward
recumbent	lying down in any position
supine	lying on the back
view	restricted to discussion of a radiograph or image when describing a body part as seen by the recording media

TERM	DEFINITION

PHYSICAL SCIENCES

blur	loss of recorded detail due to patient motion
contrast	visible differences between any two selected areas of density levels within the radiographic image
contrast, film	inherent ability of the film emulsion to react to radiation and record a range of densities as determined from the sensitometric properties of the characteristic H and D curve
contrast, scale	number of densities (or shades of gray) visible in the radiographic image
contrast, scale (long)	when slight differences between densities are present (low contrast) but the total number of densities is increased
contrast, scale (short)	when considerable or major differences between densities are present (high contrast) but the total number of densities is decreased
contrast, subject	difference in the quantity of radiation transmitted by a particular part as a result of the different absorption characteristics of the tissues and structures making up that part
density	degree of blackening or opacity of an area in a radiography due to the accumulation of black metallic silver following exposure and processing of a film

$$\text{density} = \text{Log} \frac{\text{incident light intensity}}{\text{transmitted light intensity}}$$

distortion	misrepresentation of the size or shape of a structure recorded in the radiographic image (see size and shape distortion)
elongation	see shape distortion
foreshortening	see shape distortion
latitude, film	inherent ability of the film to record a long range of density levels on the radiograph as determined from the sensitometric properties of the characteristic H and D curve

TERM	DEFINITION
magnification	see size distortion
recorded detail	sharpness of the structural lines as recorded in the radiographic image
shape distortion	also known as elongation **and** foreshortening, the misrepresentation of the shape of the structure recorded as compared to the actual shape of the structure
size distortion	also known as magnification, the enlargement of the recorded image as compared to the actual size of the structure

Copyrighted by The American Registry of Radiologic Technologists. Reprinted by permission.

Exposure Factors
The ARRT has published a flow chart to assist students in understanding the relationship between recorded detail, distortion, density, and contrast. The chart is reproduced by permission of the ARRT as Figure B below.

STANDARD DEFINITIONS FOR RADIOGRAPHY EXAMINATION

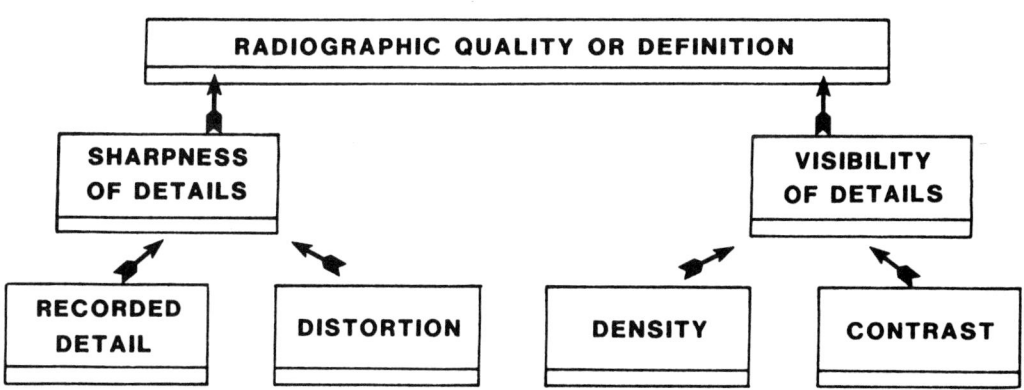

Figure B. (copyrighted by The American Registry of Radiologic Technologists; reprinted by permission)

Content Not Used
Over the years, the ARRT ceased to ask questions in extremely controversial areas or in areas no longer considered to be a universal part of the profession. These areas are listed below.

CONTENT NOT USED IN THE ARRT EXAMINATION IN RADIOGRAPHY

PHYSICAL SCIENCES

capacitor discharge units
cast versus no cast, or wet versus dry cast
contrast and screen speed
direct exposure film
edge gradient
impulse timer
manual processing
mechanical timers
non-screen technique
par speed
stereoradiography

All information on the ARRT examination in radiography conventions is copyrighted by The American Registry of Radiologic Technologists and reprinted by permission.

USING THIS REVIEW TO BEST ADVANTAGE

This review is designed to be used as a helpful tool in reminding students of content that was learned some time ago, diagnosing weak areas for further study, and adding a strong measure of confidence to those subject areas in which both academic and clinical success already have been proven.

This review is not a substitute for two or more years of study in a radiography program. It is not possible to prepare for a major national certification examination by studying from questions. Instead, it is critical to engage in the careful study of appropriate textbooks in radiography, such as those listed in the reference appendix.

To use this review to best advantage, it is suggested that study begin 2-3 months prior to the examination. This review can be used to good advantage by answering questions from each content category section as a pre-test to determine which sections need more review, reviewing reference books, trying additional questions from the same content area, and finally using the post-test as a double check or final assessment of progress.

Each question includes the answer, a short explanation, and references for further information. Answers to questions appear at the edge of the page beneath the question and in the answer section with the explanation and reference at the end of the book.

Explanations and References
Short explanations are located at the end of the book to keep the question pages uncluttered. The explanation is followed by a reference if further review or study is needed. The short phrases are the index words that should be used to locate more information in the index of any text. Several references that have information on the topic are then provided. The full citations for each reference are included in the reference appendix.

Answers
Answers are located on the page beneath the question. When the book is open, answers to questions on the left side will be found by lifting the page to see the far-left side of the previous page. Answers to questions on the right side are found by lifting the page to see the far-right side of the next page. In this manner, each question can be studied without the answer, yet the answer is easily seen without turning pages to the end of the book or attempting to locate the answer among tight columns of numbers in an answer key.

Studying From References
It is a good strategy to scan your favorite textbook in each major subject area, skimming headers, bold or italicized words, and figure captions. Most authors emphasize important content by using these devices to bring attention to a content area. Figures are expensive to produce and are used only when important ideas need to be explained carefully. Reading the figure captions is a good way to catch all the high points of a particular text. When something is not remembered, either because it has been forgotten or was never taught or learned previously, stop and study the section. If the entire textbook is reviewed in this manner, few of the "nationally recognized" content areas will be overlooked. The following list illustrates common subject areas for which textbooks should be obtained for this approach to preparing for a certification examination.

COMMON SUBJECT AREAS FOR TEXTBOOK REVIEW
with recommended references
   (full citations at end of book)

ANATOMY, PHYSIOLOGY, AND PATHOLOGY
   Anthony
   Ballinger
   Bontrager
   Eisenberg POSITIONING
   Eisenberg PATHOLOGY
   Hole

RADIOGRAPHIC POSITIONING
   Ballinger
   Bontrager
   Eisenberg POSITIONING

RADIOGRAPHIC PHYSICS AND IMAGING EQUIPMENT
   Bushong
   Carlton
   Carroll
   Curry
   Cullinan
   Seeram
   Selman

RADIATION PROTECTION AND RADIOBIOLOGY
   Bushong
   Carlton
   Hall
   NCRP Reports
   Noz
   Travis
   Selman

PATIENT CARE
   Ehrlich
   Gurley
   Torres

SPECIAL PROCEDURES
   Snopek
   Tortoricci

QUALITY ASSURANCE
   Bushong
   Carlton
   Carroll
   Gray
   Jenkins

PRINCIPLES OF EXPOSURE (TECHNIQUE)
Bushong
Carlton
Carroll
Curry
Cullinan
Donohue
Jenkins
Selman

Appendices
The appendices tables are designed to facilitate study, provide information that is often memorized, and assist in locating state licensing agencies. The appendices are: **References, Dose Equivalent Limits and Maximum Permissible Doses, SI Radiation Units, Table of Common Abbreviations and Symbols,** and **State Licensing Agencies.**

IMPROVING STUDY AND TEST-TAKING SKILLS
by Steven B. Dowd, M.A., R.T.(R)

The ARRT Examination in Radiography focuses strongly on basic skills, but also relates content to the clinical setting. Thus, there is a need for examinees to be able to understand how to apply knowledge and definitions to the work environment - something that has been called "critical thinking skills." In past years, the examination was very strongly "definition-based"; that is, there was a greater concern that students could understand and repeat back information than apply it. It tested what were considered to be primarily "lower-level" thinking skills as well.

Beginning the Goal-Setting Process
The obvious goal of anyone using this book is to pass the examination in radiography. The goal of this book is to help you in expressing and meeting this goal.

Many people feel that simply expressing a goal is enough to permit the "real work" towards meeting the goal to begin. However, businesses know that, to succeed, they must first analyze their goals. One means of doing this is a "**WOTS UP**" analysis, a look at **W**eaknesses, **O**pportunities, **T**hreats, and **S**trengths that culminates in a long-range strategic plan. At the end of this book, you should have your own study plan.

One author has noted that the phrase "forewarned is forearmed" has never been more apt than when applied to examinations, especially standardized examinations. The first thing you should do is list all the relevant information shown below to begin your journey towards passage of the examination in radiography.

1. Purpose of the examination.

2. Scope of the examination.

3. Minimum educational and professional requirements.

4. Date and place of the examination.

5. Total time allowed for the examination.

6. Weight and passing score of the examination.

7. Subjects to be tested.

8. Weight for each subject.

9. Total time allowed for each subject.

10. Forms and types of questions.

11. Equipment needed and allowed.

12. Application and deadlines.

This information may seem obvious, but it is your foundation. For example, you might say that of course you know what subjects are to be tested. But which area of your physics background will match the examination's Equipment Operation and Maintenance section? It is strongly recommended that every student obtain a copy of the *Content Specifications for the Examination in Radiography*, which is available from the ARRT at 1255 Northland Drive, Mendota Heights, Minnesota 55120, phone 612-687-0048, for use as a study guide. This document subdivides the number of questions in each content category by subject. This permits students to concentrate on reviewing information in heavily weighted areas to gain maximum advantage from the probability of the content expected on the examination. The entire content specifications are not included in the *Examinee Handbook* that contains the application that is submitted by each student. Most radiography educators keep a copy of the complete specifications on file, and it may be easier to obtain a copy from a radiography program director than it is to write the ARRT.

The end of section assessments in this chapter are designed to actively involve the student in the development of a personal study plan. The questions in these sections should be answered and then reviewed again after finishing this chapter to complete the personal study plan.

Study Self-Diagnosis Test
The goal of this test is to help you identify potential weak areas that you may want to focus on before you begin to study for the examination. Obviously, you cannot remediate years of bad habits in the space of a few months. However, you can learn how to improve weak spots within the time remaining and emphasize your strengths. Answer each of the questions with a "yes" or "no."

YES NO

— — 1. Do you usually study every day in the same place?

— — 2. Do you usually know in the morning how you are going to spend your day?

— — 3. Does your study area have anything in or on it that would distract you from your work?

— — 4. When studying, do you frequently skip graphs and tables in the book?

— — 5. Do you make your own charts and graphs to illustrate points in notes and readings?

— — 6. Do you look up words you don't know in the text?

— — 7. Do you usually skim a chapter <u>before</u> you do the reading?

— — 8. Do you look at paragraph headings before you do the reading?

— — 9. Do you usually read the summary at the end of a chapter before you do the reading?

— — 10. Do you keep you notes for each subject together?

— — 11. Do you take lecture notes in outline form?

— — 12. Do you take reading notes in outline form?

— — 13. Do you try to summarize readings into a short paragraph?

— — 14. Do you sit up late at night routinely studying for tests?

— — 15. Do you try to memorize the text to prepare for an exam?

— — 16. Do you try to do all of your memorizing at one time?

— — 17. Do you sometimes "stop-out" to reflect on your weak areas?

— — 18. Do you consciously try to use facts learned from one course in another?

Good students usually answer as follows:	Your Answer Agreed	Your Answer Disagreed
1. Yes	——	——
2. Yes	——	——
3. No	——	——
4. No	——	——
5. Yes	——	——
6. Yes	——	——
7. Yes	——	——
8. Yes	——	——
9. Yes	——	——
10. Yes	——	——
11. Yes	——	——
12. Yes	——	——
13. Yes	——	——
14. No	——	——
15. No	——	——
16. No	——	——
17. Yes	——	——
18. Yes	——	——

This is not a test that allows for so many "yes" or "no" responses and then classifies you as a good or poor student. It intended to let you identify some of your study weaknesses to allow you to focus on them in preparation for the examination in radiography.

Preparing for the Examination in Radiography
This text assumes that you have 2 to 3 months to prepare for the examination. You should make room for at least one hour per night, five days per week. It should take you, on a self-paced basis, about 2-3 weeks to get through this book and identify your various action plans. At that time, you should know how to study as well as your major content weaknesses. This is achieved through the assessments at the end of each section.

The following contains a sample study plan developed after using the principles in this book. After that, you will find the first assessment. These are a very important component of this section because they are a self-analysis that will translate into a workable study plan. This self-analysis should be similar to the business planning procedure discussed earlier. First, the goal to be achieved is identified and discussed. Then weaknesses (for example, your poor areas in school), opportunities (your current support, for example), threats (such as test anxiety), and strengths (usually your strong study areas) are analyzed. Then a personal plan is developed.

Study Plan

Goal: Pass the ARRT Examination in Radiography.

Objectives	Activities	Date
1. Establish a positive self attitude.	1. Develop study plan. 2. Work with fellow grads in study group. 3. Attend review seminar at state convention.	Ongoing May 4
2. Decrease test anxiety.	1. Learn relaxation techniques.	Ongoing
3. Review basic concepts of all areas.	1. Review notes and write summaries. 2. Use strategic reading principles for review.	June 5 Ongoing
4. Achieve an 85% on review questions.	1. Pay attention to my test-taking type. 2. Look at test items and underline key terms.	Ongoing Ongoing

End of Section Assessment

In this section, I:

1. Outlined, in a list, relevant points to consider before I begin the goal-setting and study process:

2. Identified some of my strengths and weaknesses as a student:

3. Plan to use my study strengths as follows:

4. Plan to work on the following weaknesses through the next chapters:

Mastering Content
The steps listed below show you how to develop content mastery. Although some points are self-evident, a brief review may be helpful. First, you need to know and attack your weaknesses, especially before a test such as the Examination in Radiography. Some radiography students don't like physics and will try to overcompensate by studying more of what they prefer, such as anatomy or positioning. A basic skills yet comprehensive test such as the ARRT examination may prove extremely difficult to pass with such a strategy. A 100% on anatomy and positioning (which comprises about 50% of the examination) combined with a 20% on the other half still translates into failure. Combining an average score of 80% in anatomy and positioning with a 70% knowledge of the other areas on the examination would produce a passing score.

CONTENT MASTERY

1. Review content and identify weaknesses.

2. Review your time constraints.

3. Develop a study plan.

4. Remove distractions.

5. Avoid getting hung up on details.

6. Select a very few resources.

Be honest in dealing with time constraints. Don't over plan and produce a study plan based on 10 hours per week of study time when you only have 5 hours available. Also, it is better to study for 15 minutes with no distractions than for one hour with multiple distractions.

Getting caught up in details can cause problems. It is better to know the basics well, especially definitions, than to only partly understand many areas. There is a value to slight over learning of relevant points, that is, some review once you understand the points well, but little value can be attached to trying to learn everything about a topic at this point.

Finally, don't try to read every book. Choose one from each subject, or even more ideally, just two or three books. Ballinger's *Merrill's Atlas* has a nice radiation protection chapter, for example. Nearly all libraries participate in interlibrary loan agreements and can obtain a text that better suits your needs.

Guide to More Effective Use of Textbooks
To make more effective use of texts, plan the purpose of your reading. Then preview by planning what sections of a given text to use before beginning to read. This enables you to become familiar with the structure or plan of the material to be read before studying it in depth.

The preview method includes, in order:

1. Title

2. Preface (highlights the author's purpose and the intended use of the book)

3. Table of Contents (outlines the book and shows how its parts relate to one another)

4. Appendix

In each chapter you should read, in order:

1. Title and all subheadings

2. Subheadings, margin notes, and italicized words (all of which can be turned into questions as a review)

3. Charts, graphs, tables, and illustrations

4. End of chapter questions or review suggestions

Another useful method of reviewing a book is skimming by allowing the eyes to travel quickly over a page, stopping here and there to gain an idea. This technique is useful to:

1. get an overall point

2. get main idea

3. find out how difficult material might be

4. discover if you need to read more

5. reviewing

The skimming method includes:

1. reading the title or caption

2. reading the first paragraph

3. reading subheadings and first sentences of other paragraphs

4. skimming the remainder while looking for:

   a. main ideas and supporting details

   b. clue words

   c. direction words, agreement or disagreement

   d. numbered sequences of ideas

5. reading the summary

Scanning is a process for finding facts quickly. It is accomplished by looking very quickly through information to find answers to a specific question. Its main uses are in research, referencing, and answering questions. It is important to let the eyes move rapidly while remembering key words or phrases.

Guidelines for marking textbooks include:

1. Use double lines under words or phrases to signify main ideas.

2. Use single lines under words or phrases to signify supporting material.

3. Mark small circled numbers near the initial word of an underlined group of words to indicate a series of arguments, facts, or ideas.

4. When three or more lines are important, use brackets in the margin instead of underlining.

5. Use one asterisk in the margin to indicate ideas of special importance.

6. Circle key words, terms, and phrases.

7. Use top and bottom margins to record important ideas.

8. Insert small sheets of paper between pages for longer summaries or ideas.

Strategic Reading
Many students have been taught summary strategies such as the SQ3R method. The five steps are survey, question, read, recite, and review. Following a brief survey of a chapter, questions are formulated based on text subheadings. Reading involves identification of key terms while re-reading passages that are difficult, looking up unfamiliar terms, and relating the new knowledge to old. Relating is an especially important concept that is designed to increase understanding of similarities between ideas. Considering each concept in isolation to others does not permit a full understanding of most content material. Reciting the content that has been studied is a form of reinforcement that should be combined with a review of the questions without using the text. The entire SQ3R method actually requires reviewing the same information five times in five different ways to assure in depth understanding.

Following is a checklist for use when reading. It is a more formal statement of the material in the previous section designed to monitor reading progress. Make an "assignment" and pre-read the material first, answering the questions. Then, while reading, ask the "reading" questions on an occasional basis. After reading, answer the "post-reading" questions to see how well the material was understood and whether re-reading or looking for the information in another text or reference work will be necessary.

READING CHECKLIST

Assignment:

Make light notes as necessary while reading, paying special attention to these questions:

Pre-Reading Questions

____ 1. What is this chapter about?

____ 2. What main ideas are found in the headings?

____ 3. In what fashion is the material organized?

____ 4. What questions should I prepare to help review later?

____ 5. How does this material relate to concepts already known?

Reading Questions

____ 1. What words are unfamiliar and must be looked up?

____ 2. Does this material make sense?

____ 3. Will further review be necessary?

____ 4. Are new questions needed?

____ 5. How does this chapter relate to information already known?

Post-Reading Questions

____ 1. Can I outline this assignment?

____ 2. Of what practical use is this information?

____ 3. Are my questions similar to expected exam questions?

____ 4. How can I clarify this material?

____ 5. Can I answer my pre-reading questions without the text?

Problem-Solving

Problem-solving is a series of procedures that establishes a method to approach difficult questions. It includes:

1. Understanding the problem.

2. Selecting and collecting the data necessary for solving the problem.

3. The selection and implementation of one or more solution strategies.

4. Answering the problem.

5. Evaluation of the answer in terms of reasonableness.

Although this section focuses on math problem-solving, these principles are useful for all types of problem-solving. It is important to apply old knowledge to new problems by "pre-solving" them. When each problem is viewed in isolation, it becomes a new experience instead of repetition of previously understood methods.

In the above method, the first three steps are actually pre-solving steps. It is important to analyze each and every component. Every problem should be broken down into as many components as possible before starting to solve it. Pre-solving is essential because it provides a framework on which to base the actual solution process.

For example, question #575 requires use of these skills. A first reading helps understand the problem as one requiring a determination of the various factors that would produce the greatest density on a radiograph. The next step is to select and collect the data necessary for solving the problem. As the answer and explanation demonstrates, converting all of the differences in this problem into mAs changes sets up a common data base. The selection and implementation of a solution strategy permits a comparison of the four choices. The next step is to solve the problem by determining which choice would produce the greatest density. Finally, a second review of the answer to be sure it is reasonable helps avoid miscalculation errors.

Question #691 is another good example where problem-solving skills can easily be applied. If all that is known is that low humidity is undesirable due to the possibility of static and that high humidity is undesirable due to the possibility of fogging, choices "a" and "d" can be eliminated. It is reasonable to assume that less than 10% or more than 90% humidity would probably produce static or fog conditions. This leaves only two choices, which now increases the odds of a correct answer from 25% to 50%. It is also reasonable to choose the wider range of humidity values (30-60%), and this is in fact the correct answer.

Making Better Use of Notes

Content areas in which weaknesses are discovered can be strengthened by reworking course lecture notes. Rewriting notes with a textbook available often helps bring back questions that can assist in re-studying old material. Making notes directly in textbook margins is recommended by many authorities. Good note writing includes:

1. Main ideas marked with Roman numerals.

2. Supporting ideas indented and marked with capitalized letters.

3. The outline is structured from general to specific.

End of Section Assessment

1. I plan to use the material in Content Mastery, page 26, as follows:

2. I plan to make better use of textbooks by use of the following principles:

3. I will improve my problem-solving ability by:

4. I feel that my course lecture notes are (adequate/inadequate). I plan to use them for review as follows:

Improving Self-Knowledge

Test Anxiety
It is important to know how to deal with tests and test anxiety. It is important to focus on taking charge of the testing situation, instead of being intimidated by the examination itself.

Test anxiety is simply worry or fear caused in anticipation of tests. Without some fear of failure (which is probably the number one cause of test anxiety), few people would be motivated to succeed. Other causes of test anxiety include pressure from self and others, previous poor experiences, and inadequate study habits. Test anxiety can be controlled by:

1. Avoiding the tendency to let emotion interfere with logic.

2. Using imagination positively (visualize being calm and in control).

3. Using relaxation techniques.

Developing a Positive Attitude
A positive attitude about success on examinations can go a long way toward not only relieving test anxiety but also toward maximizing study time. Successful and effective students exhibit several characteristics that can be copied easily to achieve better preparation for the examination in radiography. Some of these characteristics are:

1. There are specific goals related to education.

2. The reasons for reaching the goals are understood.

3. There is an optimistic hope for success.

4. The possibility of failure is acknowledged but used to motivate better study.

5. Small successes are acknowledged to enhance positive feelings of accomplishment.

6. Shortcomings are viewed as small obstacles on the road to success.

7. An awareness of both good and bad personal habits exists, with the good ones reinforced, while attempts are made to change the bad ones.

8. External problems (such as personal conflicts, financial resources, study time, etc.) are anticipated with potential methods of overcoming them considered in advance.

9. Places and people to ask for help are known, and there is no hesitation to ask for it.

10. There is a specific plan for achieving goals with regular check points used.

These characteristics can be achieved by mastering the concepts listed below. Not everyone who begins education in radiography completes it. Simply the fact that a person has graduated or will soon graduate places him or her in a very select group. Nearly everyone who has graduated from a CAHEA-approved radiography program is capable of passing the examination in radiography. Even those who have failed before can overcome that liability and change the failure into the motivation needed to study hard enough to correct the weak areas and achieve the success of becoming a Registered Technologist, Radiographer of the ARRT.

CONCEPTS OF THE SECRETS TO SUCCESS

Concept	Principle	Motivating Thought
Control	Winners set goals, establish plans, take control.	Winners have plans, losers have excuses.
Freedom	Attitude of freedom.	No one else can give it to you or take it away.
Self-Fulfilling Prophecy	Outcomes are directly related to self-image and expectations.	You can be your own master.

Self-Awareness	Success begins with knowing yourself.	The day you stop making excuses is the day you begin to succeed.
Courage and Failure	Failure is a natural consequence of courage.	True failure only occurs when self-respect and confidence are gone.
Perseverance	No goal can be achieved without perseverance.	Success is failure turned inside out.
Motivation	Motivation is the muscle of success.	Once you have done your best, wait for the results in peace.

End of Section Assessment

1. I plan to alleviate my test anxiety by:

2. I plan to develop or improve my positive attitude by:

General Suggestions for Memory Improvement
Motivation helps memory considerably, including everything that helps with motivation: positive attitudes, good study skills, clear goals, etc. It is important to remember facts and ideas as well as the sources and relationship to other information. These elements are best located from:

1. Syllabus and other printed information distributed as part of a course.

2. Lecture notes

3. Tests and quizzes.

4. Topic headings in textbooks.

5. Chapter objectives in textbooks.

6. Chapter summaries in textbooks.

7. End-of-chapter questions, laboratory, and workbook exercises.

There are several other suggestions that can be helpful when studying:

1. Study reading material paragraph by paragraph.

2. Use reference books to clarify difficult information.

3. Ask for help when information is not clear.

4. Find an easier book about the same subject (many teachers provide recommended reading lists for this purpose).

5. Work from the general to the specific.

6. Always take notes.

Self-testing is useful. A classical investigation by Spitzer in 1939 that has been repeatedly validated found that persons who immediately self-tested after learning had 100% recall three weeks after studying as opposed to 50% recall by those who tested themselves the next day. A group that did not self-test had 10% recall.

Learning Levels
Basic learning occurs at the level of recall and comprehension. Students often mistake a large quantity of information that can be recalled for knowledge. A person who can recall many facts is not necessarily smarter than someone who can recall fewer facts but can relate them properly to other information to achieve higher levels of synthesis, analysis, and evaluation. In other words, the ability to use an average amount of information to solve problems will produce a higher examination score than will a large amount of memorized but unrelated factual data.

Comprehension is a basic understanding of facts that have been memorized at the recall level. For example, if recall of the term contrast is a definition involving density differences, the difference between high and low contrast would take this information to the comprehension level. Everyone needs to work on recall and comprehension. It isn't possible to accomplish problem-solving unless the basic information is understood first. Following is a summary of some ways in which these skills can be improved.

IMPROVING RECALL AND COMPREHENSION SKILLS

Acronyms — Rad (radiation absorbed dose) is an example of an acronym. Another example is IPMAT to remember the stages of cell division.

Acrostics — Catchy phrases such as "Never Lower Tillie's Pants, Grandma Might Come Home" to recall the order of the carpal bones.

ABCs — Forming words about content into alphabetical phrases. For example:

angling the
beam
causes
distortion

Association	Connecting a name to an image, for example, a Water's projection is obtained by positioning the head so the nose would be above water.
Others	Sometimes an absurd pattern can be retained as a rhyme, song, or story sequence. For example, the 12 cranial nerves have an absurd story that goes:

On Old Olympus Towering Tops A Finn And German Vault And Hop.

Advanced learning occurs at the level of application, analysis, synthesis, and evaluation. These are the skills necessary to accomplish reasoning and problem-solving. Application is the ability to use information. For example, comprehension of high and low contrast could be applied to determine which factors need to be changed to achieve a low-contrast image. Analysis is the use of abstract and logical thought to show relationships. For example, a question that gives several sets of exposure factors and asks which would produce the greatest image density requires an analysis of each of the factors that affect density to determine the answer. Synthesis is the ability to combine several known facts to create new information. For example, the knowledge that a high ratio grid will absorb more radiation and the knowledge that less radiation reaching the film will produce less image density can be synthesized to produce new information that a high ratio grid will produce less image density. Evaluation involves the highest level of learning because it requires a complete understanding of all the other learning levels in order to make judgments about information. For example, a question that gives a number of exposure factors and then asks which would increase detail is an evaluation question because it requires that each factor be evaluated for its effect on detail. The infamous K-type items (also known as multiple multiple choice questions) as shown below are often used to test analysis relationships.

Which of the following would increase radiographic density?

1. lower ratio grid
2. increased kVp
3. decreased mAs

a. 1 and 2 only
b. 1 and 3 only
c. 2 and 3 only
d. 1, 2, & 3

To solve this type of question, it is important to determine which variables are relevant to the question. Simply discovering that "1" is correct is not sufficient to correctly answer the question because "2" is also correct. Therefore this question must be approached by carefully considering choice "a" by looking back to see if both "1" and "2" are correct and "3" is incorrect. Even when this is true, as it is in the example, it is important to continue to follow the same pattern for "b," the "c," and "d." Jumping to a conclusion before reading and considering all possible answers is a common cause of incorrect choices. Although this takes a considerable amount of time, remember that this examination is the cummulation of two or more years of education and it is certainly worth the extra effort. Some methods that can be used to improve higher level skills include:

Imagery	Imagining the performance of a procedure may assist in locking knowledge into memory that might otherwise be forgotten.
Small Groups	When they are focused and noncompetitive, study groups can be one of the best means of review.
Creating Questions	The TV game show "Jeopardy" is an excellent example because it requires contestants to work backwards from answer to question. Creating questions from answers in the book (for example, subject headings) or practice review in a small group using a Jeopardy-style format can be a useful study method.
Practice Test Questions	These are one of the best and the most easily available means of evaluating study progress. The key to using review texts and questions is to always look up question answer explanations for questions both answered correctly and those missed and then to use the results to study further in weak areas.

The Anatomy of Questioning
One of the secrets to highly successful studying is learning how to ask the right questions. It is important to understand the general types of questions that will be asked on the examination in radiography. The primary question types include:

Memory	Simple questions that involve recall of information, stated facts, and concepts.
Translation	More involved questions that require the expression of an idea in a different form: for example, changing from words to symbols or diagrams.
Interpretation	Questions that draw relationships from among facts, definitions, and generalizations.
Application	Questions involving the transfer of concepts to actual clinical problem-solving.
Analysis	Higher level questions that require extracting an understanding of information from the initial information given.
Synthesis	Higher level questions that require several pieces of information to be combined to solve a problem through the creation of new information.
Evaluation	The highest level of questioning that includes judgments measured against specific standards.

These question types demonstrate a major problem that many students encounter when study is directed at learning facts without understanding how to apply the information to clinical problem-solving. The examination in radiography continues to evolve toward more higher level questioning that measures the ability of students to use information in clinical practice instead of simply recalling basic information.

Learning how to look for application, analysis, synthesis, and evaluation while studying is probably the best method of preparing for the examination. Learning the structures that should be demonstrated on a particular projection, the centering points, appropriate exposure factors, etc., is not as valuable as learning which variations will enhance a particular pathology without increasing patient dose. For example, increasing kVp and centering at T6 instead of T4 when using an automatic exposure control for an erect PA chest will produce a longer scale image with less dose to the patient and will permit better visualization of fluid levels and the cardiac outlines.

End of Section Assessment

1.   Using general suggestions for retention, I plan to do the following:

2.   I need to improve my recall and comprehension skills by using the following strategies:

3.   I need to improve my higher level skills by using the following strategies:

4.   I plan to use the following questioning strategies to improve my study:

This is the most important test of your career. Do not underestimate your need to study for it. Most students find they require at least 3-4 months to prepare properly. A 2- or 3-week study plan is usually insufficient to permit proper coverage of the multiple content areas you must investigate in depth. Beginning more than 6 months before the examination is not advisable because your ability to maintain an effective level of concentration will be exhausted by the time you begin the critical 1-2 months prior to your test date.

Students who have completed school more than a month before beginning to study for the examination may need an additional period to get back into study habits.

Without the framework of assignments, examinations, and the end of an academic term, you must rely on your own conscience to study. Procrastination can be fatal to your performance on the examination. It is advisable to establish a written study schedule and adhere to it. Many students find that requiring double study time when a session is missed is the only way to maintain a regular schedule.

Ideally, all the books listed in the Reference section should be used in study. All these references will be found in any good medical library. Many of the major titles are commonly found in school faculty offices, hospital radiology departments, and radiologists' personal libraries.

General Habits

1. A quiet place away from distractions, such as music and talking helps with concentration.

2. Group study sessions are valuable but should be limited to 3-4 persons and should not be the only study method. Group sessions should be terminated at least 2-3 days before the examination to avoid anxiety spreading among the individuals.

3. Concentrate on a single topic area at one time (such as anatomy/positioning or physics/exposure technique).

4. Areas of difficulty should be noted for further study by reading a different textbook, consulting with an instructor, or attending a review session.

Remember that isolated data are difficult to remember. For example, the centering points for each projection are much easier to remember if each point is linked to its anatomic location and the shape of the structures that should be visualized. Try to use concepts to remember data instead of just memorizing the data.

When data must be memorized, it is often helpful to use acronyms or other mnemonic devices. For example, most students learn the mnemonic, "never lower Tillie's pants, grandmother might come home" for the carpal bones, which represents: navicular, lunate, triangular, pisiform, greater multangular, lesser multangular, capitate, and hamate. You can invent your own devices for data as well as those you have learned previously. You can only remember so much information. Be selective in what you choose to memorize so that other more important knowledge is not lost in the process.

HELPFUL HINTS FOR THE EXAMINATION IN RADIOGRAPHY

Take two calculators that are battery (not solar) powered. Include new batteries for both. Work a variety of different types of problems with both calculators to be sure you know how to use the keyboard before you leave for the examination site. Do not take a programmable calculator to the examination as you could be accused of cheating by entering formulas into the memory.

1. Always read every word of all instructions. There may be a slight change from your past experiences that could cause correct answers to be marked wrong.

2. Most questions are written with the distractors (the possible choices that are labeled a,b,c, and d) designed so there is a correct answer, a closely related choice, and two choices that are less likely. Consequently, the best method of answering all questions is:

    (a) Read the entire question and all choices before choosing an answer. Although the first choice may appear correct, the fourth choice may turn out to be a better or more comprehensive answer.

    (b) Look for keywords that target important information and don't assume information unless it is stated.

    (c) Determine which two choices are the less likely ones and eliminate them first.

    (d) Choose the best answer from the two remaining choices. When you must guess, this process improves the odds of guessing a correct answer from 25% to 50%. If you guess at 20 questions over the entire examination, this produces 10 correct answers instead of only 5. This is enough to raise your entire examination score by 2.5 percentile points.

3. Always work all mathematical calculations twice to make sure you didn't press the wrong key by mistake.

4. Do not spend a long period (more than 2-3 minutes) on a single question. You can mark it and return after you have completed the entire examination. It is normal to have numerous questions that require more than 2-3 minutes. Nearly all students will return to re-study particularly difficult questions after all the questions have been attempted once.

5. It is acceptable to skip difficult questions entirely and return to them after completing the entire examination.

6. At question number 100, remember to check the time and see how you are progressing. If you have taken longer than 1 1/2 hours to reach question 100 you must work faster. If this is the case, when you reach number 150 check the time again and, if necessary, mark in guesses for all questions on the answer card. Then continue the examination by erasing the guess and entering your answer. In this manner, if time is called while you are working you will have 25% of the questions you did not answer marked correctly just because of your guesses. These extra correct answers could make the difference between passing and failing the examination.

7. After completion, the entire examination should be read a second time to search for errors in marking answers.

8. When re-reading the examination remember that the first choice of an answer may not have the highest probability of being correct. Research has shown that students are more likely to change from wrong to right than not. A study by Jordan and Johnson found that almost all students changed answers and that 55% gained points from changing answers, 18% lost points, and the rest experienced no total score change. If it is determined that a question was not read correctly or if more information has been obtained from answering other questions, don't hesitate to change an answer.

9. Always mark an answer for all questions, even if it is a guess. With 4 distractors, 25% of all guesses will be correct, and these add to your total score. For example, if you only knew the answers to 180 of the 200 questions and you answered 145 (73%) correctly, there is a high possibility that you would not pass the examination. However, if you guessed at all 20 of the questions you did not know, it is highly likely that you would get 5 more questions right, which would raise your total score to 75%, probably pass the examination, and become a registered technologist.

TEST-TAKING REFERENCES

Alford, RL. *Tips on Testing: Strategies for Test-Taking.* Washington, DC: University Press of America, 1979.

Cassidy, VR. Response changing and student achievement on objective tests. *Nursing Education.* 26:60-62, 1987.

Charles, RI. The role of problem-solving. *Arithmetic Teacher.* 32(6):48-50, 1985.

Cooper, C, Sullivan, A, Shulman, J. *Making It in College: Strategies for Studying and Learning.* Lansing: Michigan State University, 1977.

Dickenson-Hazard, N. Making the grade as a test-taker. *Pediatric Nursing.* 15:302-304, 1989.

Dickenson-Hazard, N. Develop your thinking skills for improved test-taking. *Pediatric Nursing.* 16:480-481, 1990.

Divine, JH, Kylen, DW. *How to Beat Test Anxiety.* New York: Barrons Educational Series, Inc, 1979.

Dowd, SB. Strategic reading can simplify learning. *Advance for the Radiologic Technologist.* 3:20, 1990.

Dowd, SB. Teaching strategies to foster critical thinking. *Radiologic Technology.* 62:374-378, 1991.

Gurley, LT, Callaway, WJ. *Introduction to Radiologic Technology.* 2nd Ed. St. Louis: CV Mosby, 1986.

Honig, F. *Taking Tests and Scoring High.* New York: Arco, 1982.

Jordan, L, Johnson, D. The relationship between changing answers and performance on multiple-choice nursing examinations. *Journal of Nursing Education.* 1990.

Millman, J, Pauk, W. *How to Take Tests.* New York: 1969.

Roberts, GH. A crash course in cramming. *Radiologic Technology.* 60:431-433, 1989.

Robbins, Y. Teaching critical thinking to the respiratory care student. *AARC Times.* 12(5):23-24, 26-27, 1988.

Sides, M., Cailles, NB. *Nurse's Guide to Successful Test Taking.* Philadelphia: JB Lippincott, 1989.

Spitzer, HF. Studies in retention. *Journal of Educational Psychology.* 30:641-656, 1939.

Usova, GM. *Efficient Study Strategies.* Pacific Grove, CA: Brooks/Cole Publishing Company, 1989.

Wight, P. The test of a profession. *Radiologic Technology.* 54:78, 1984.

DIRECTIONS FOR ANSWERING THE QUESTIONS IN THIS BOOK

Select the single, best answer for each question from the four possible answers or completions.

Answers
The answer to each question is printed at the edge of the page beneath the question. Lifting the page slightly will reveal the answer. (Each answer has its question number in superscript to avoid mixups.)

Answers, Explanations, and References
The *Answers and Explanations* section at the end of the book gives the answer again with a short explanation. Each explanation is followed in bold type by the index keywords and references necessary to locate a full discussion of the content in the question. The complete library citation for each reference is listed in the *References* section at the end of the book.

Post-Test
The post-test is a simulated examination with the same number of questions with the subject content weighted in the same manner as the ARRT examination. A separate answer key permits a quick evaluation of the total score.

Radiation Protection

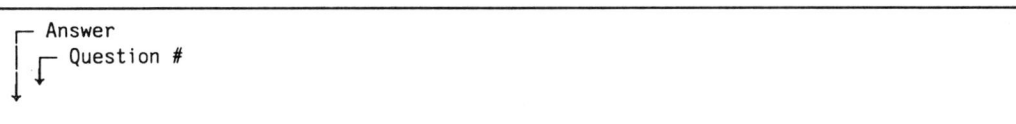

C^{11}

C^{12}

C^{13}

B^{14}

C^{15}

Question #
Answer

Patient Protection 8% (112) 1-112

1. Which of the following are acute radiation syndromes?
   1. hemopoietic
   2. gastrointestinal
   3. central nervous system
      a. 1 & 2 only
      b. 1 & 3 only
      c. 2 & 3 only
      d. 1, 2, & 3

2. Which of the following would not be considered background radiation?
      a. cosmic rays
      b. atmospheric radioisotopes
      c. radiation therapy treatments
      d. radioactive minerals in building materials

3. How many half value layers are required to reduce a beam to less than 10% of its original energy?
      a. 1
      b. 2
      c. 4
      d. 10

4. Which type of shielding is suspended from the radiographic collimator to absorb the primary beam photons before they reach the reproductive organs?
   1. contact
   2. shadow
   3. flat
      a. 1 only
      b. 2 only
      c. 3 only
      d. 1, 2, & 3

5. What term describes radiation effects which become evident in the descendants of the irradiated individuals?
      a. genetic
      b. somatic
      c. stochastic
      d. low level

Radiation Protection

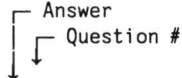
A[16]

6. Which term describes the gonad dose, which, if received by every member of the population, would be expected to produce the total genetic effect on the population as the sum of the individual doses actually received?
    a. relative biologic effect
    b. genetically significant dose
    c. linear attenuation coefficient
    d. linear energy transfer

D[17]

7. Which portion of the small bowel is most radiosensitive?
    a. duodenum
    b. ileum
    c. jejunum
    d. all are equally radiosensitive

A[18]

8. Which of the following results of irradiation of cell DNA would have the least potential for lethal consequences?
    a. base damage
    b. single-strand break
    c. double-strand break
    d. all have equal potential

C[19]

9. What is the primary reason air-gap techniques provide slightly lower patient exposure doses than equivalent grid techniques?
    a. because grids absorb more of the exit radiation
    b. the loss of scattered radiation due to the air-gap reduces patient exposure due to backscatter
    c. the increased subject to image receptor distance requires greater primary beam intensity
    d. patient motion is increased with air-gap techniques

C[20]

10. What is the primary purpose of placing a filter in the primary beam of a diagnostic radiographic unit?
    a. increasing the number of high-energy photons that reach the patient
    b. decreasing the number of high-energy photons that reach the patient
    c. increasing the number of low-energy photons that reach the patient
    d. decreasing the number of low-energy photons that reach the patient

11. Which of the following terms best describes the filtration that occurs as the primary beam passes through the glass window of the x-ray tube?
    1. added filtration
    2. total filtration
    3. inherent filtration
        a. 1 only
        b. 2 only
        c. 3 only
        d. 1, 2, & 3

D^1

12. What is the proper term for the automatic collimation systems required by the United States government on all new radiographic units?
        a. automatic collimation system
        b. primary beam limitation
        c. positive beam limitation
        d. scatter elimination system

C^2

13. Which term describes the amount of material required to reduce the intensity of the beam by 50% of its original value?
        a. $LD_{50/30}$
        b. half-life
        c. half value layer
        d. 50% rule

C^3

14. What is the primary function of a PBL mechanism?
        a. assures the accuracy of the centering light
        b. automatically limits the primary beam field size
        c. opens the collimator to maximum primary beam field size
        d. restricts access to the bucky tray

15. Which of the following sets of technical factors would most likely produce the least patient exposure?
        a. 68 kVp, 100 mA, 0.12 s
        b. 74 kVp, 100 mA, 0.12 s
        c. 74 kVp, 100 mA, 0.06 s
        d. 74 kVp, 200 mA, 0.06 s

B^4

A^5

Radiation Protection

16. Which of the following would not affect patient dose?
    a. focal spot size
    b. mAs
    c. kVp
    d. filtration

17. Which of the following intensifying screen relative speeds would produce the minimum total patient exposure?
    a. 40
    b. 100
    c. 250
    d. 400

A²⁴

18. Which of the following patients would contribute the highest genetically significant dose as a result of a colon examination?
    a. 4-year-old female
    b. 12-year-old male
    c. 65-year-old female
    d. 70-year-old male

B²⁵

19. What is the minimum source-to-skin distance for stationary fluoroscopic equipment?
    a. 12 cm (5 in)
    b. 30 cm (12 in)
    c. 38 cm (15 in)
    d. 50 cm (20 in)

D²⁶

20. What is the minimum aluminum equivalency of total filtration required for diagnostic x-ray tubes operating above 70 kVp?
    a. 0.5 mm
    b. 1.5 mm
    c. 2.5 mm
    d. 3.5 mm

21. Which of the following projections would afford the greatest radiation protection to the lens of the patient's eye?
    a. left lateral skull
    b. right lateral skull
    c. PA skull
    d. AP skull

Question # ⌐
Answer ⌐ ↓

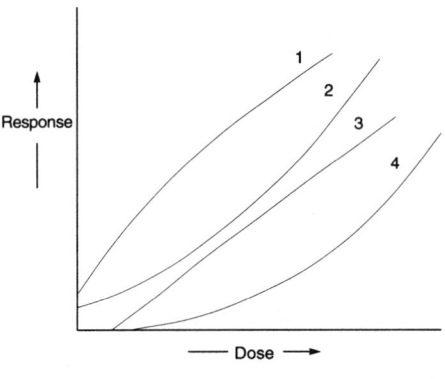

Figure 1

C^{11}

C^{12}

22. Which of the curves in Figure 1 represents a nonlinear
    nonthreshold radiation dose effect?
    a. 1
    b. 2
    c. 3
    d. 4

C^{13}

23. Which of the curves in Figure 1 represents a linear nonthreshold
    radiation dose effect?
    a. 1
    b. 2
    c. 3
    d. 4

B^{14}

C^{15}

Radiation Protection

A³²

24. How does the use of an appropriate back-up time when using an automatic exposure control permit reductions in patient exposure dose?
    1. It eliminates the possibility of the tube overload terminating an exposure.
    2. It eliminates the possibility of a repeated exposure.
    3. It backs up the penetrating ability of the beam, thus assuring sufficient density and contrast.
       a. 1 only
       b. 2 only
       c. 3 only
       d. 1, 2, & 3

D³³

25. Which of the following best encompasses the concept of nonspecific life shortening?
    a. delayed and chronic aging and disease
    b. accelerated and premature aging and disease
    c. accelerated and premature aging only
    d. accelerated and premature disease only

26. What is the primary indication of somatic effects of radiation?
    a. immediate effects are demonstrated
    b. effects are not delayed
    c. effects are not readily discernible
    d. effects are readily discernible

A³⁴

B³⁵

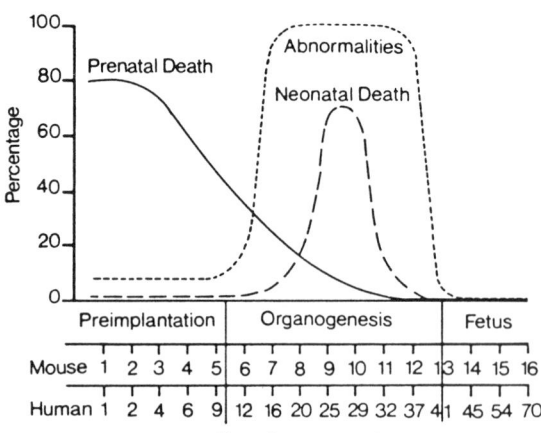

A³⁶

Figure 2 (from Journal of Cellular Physiology 1 [suppl 43]: 103, copyright © 1954; reprinted by permission of Wiley-Liss, a division of John Wiley and Sons, Inc.)

27. According to Figure 2, which of the following would be most likely as the result of a radiation dose delivered to a human embryo between 20 to 30 days postconception?
    a. spontaneous abortion
    b. bone abnormalities
    c. cancer
    d. prenatal death

28. What term describes the safety measure that assures that automatic exposure control exposures will not reach the x-ray tube limit if improper console settings are made (i.e., tube is centered to an upright bucky while table ion sensors are activated)?
    a. overexposure
    b. exposure rate
    c. backup time
    d. minimum reaction time

29. Which of the following filtrations would result in the highest entrance skin exposure to a patient?
    a. 0.5 mm Al/Eq
    b. 1.5 mm Al/Eq
    c. 2.5 mm Al/Eq
    d. 3.5 mm Al/Eq

    B^{22}

30. Which of the following x-ray generator configurations and ripple factors would produce the highest, average x-ray energy and the lowest patient exposure?
    a. single-phase, 2-pulse with 100% ripple
    b. three-phase, 6-pulse with 13% ripple
    c. three-phase, 12-pulse with 3% ripple
    d. high-frequency generator with <2% ripple

    A^{23}

31. If all other factors remain the same, which of the following would result in the lowest patient exposure dose?
    a. 10 mAs, 8:1 grid
    b. 12 mAs, 8:1 grid
    c. 10 mAs, 10:1 grid
    d. 12 mAs, 10:1 grid

┌─ Answer
│ ┌─ Question #
│ │
↓ ↓

32. Which of the following types of radiation shields are appropriate for use in protecting the breasts and gonads?
   1. contact
   2. shadow
   3. inherent
      a. 1 & 2 only
      b. 1 & 3 only
      c. 2 & 3 only
      d. 1, 2, & 3

33. Which of the following are general effects of radiation on the embryo and fetus?
   1. lethality
   2. congenital abnormalities
   3. long-term effects
      a. 1 only
      b. 2 only
      c. 3 only
      d. 1, 2, & 3

34. What term is used to describe radiation damage that increases the probability of inducing a late effect but will not increase the severity of the effect (i.e., carcinogenesis)?
      a. stochastic
      b. non-stochastic
      c. congenital
      d. chronic

C[41]

35. What term is used to describe the dose of radiation that will increase the number of mutations by a factor of two?
      a. half-life
      b. doubling dose
      c. stochastic dose
      d. congenital dose

B[42]

36. Which of the following are normally included in radiation effect discussions of the hemopoietic system?
   1. bone marrow
   2. circulating blood
   3. heart
      a. 1 & 2 only
      b. 1 & 3 only
      c. 2 & 3 only
      d. 1, 2, & 3

B[43]

Question #
Answer

37. Which of the following is part of the acute radiation syndromes?
    1. manifest illness
    2. latent period
    3. prodromal syndrome
       a. 1 only
       b. 2 only
       c. 3 only
       d. 1, 2, & 3

B[27]

38. Which of the following may be a result of red bone marrow damage due to radiation?
    1. skin erythema
    2. spinal cord myelitis
    3. anemia
       a. 1 only
       b. 2 only
       c. 3 only
       d. 1, 2, & 3

C[28]

39. Which of the following would be the most likely result of repeatedly subjecting the hands to radiation (such as the early radiologists did) or to treatment for conditions such as ringworm and acne with high doses of low-energy x-rays?
    a. bone cancer
    b. skin cancer
    c. breast cancer
    d. thyroid cancer

A[29]

40. Which of the following characterize the radiosensitivity of sperm cells?
    a. mature spermatozoa are dividing slowly and are relatively radioresistant
    b. mature spermatozoa are dividing rapidly and are relatively radiosensitive
    c. immature spermatogonia are dividing rapidly and are relatively radioresistant
    d. immature spermatogonia are dividing slowly and are relatively radiosensitive

D[30]

C[31]

Radiation Protection

A⁵⁰

B⁵¹

D⁵²

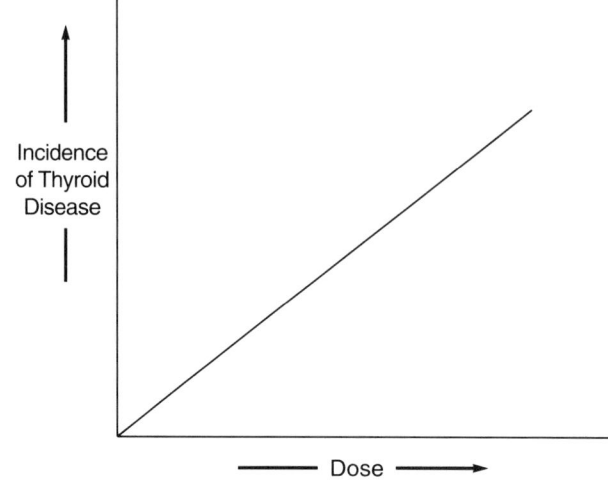

Figure 3

41. If the incidence of thyroid disease is reported to be as shown in Figure 3, which of the following best describes the relationship between radiation dose and disease?
   a. non-linear, non-threshold
   b. non-linear, threshold
   c. linear, non-threshold
   d. linear, threshold

A⁵³

42. What is the dose required to produce permanent male sterility?
   a. 2 to 3 Gy
   b. 5 to 6 Gy
   c. 8 to 10 Gy
   d. 18 to 20 Gy

B⁵⁴

43. What term describes reddening of the skin due to radiation exposure?
   1. desquamation
   2. erythema
   3. epilation
   a. 1 only
   b. 2 only
   c. 3 only
   d. 1, 2, & 3

D⁵⁵

Question #
Answer

44. During which portion of pregnancy is the embryo and fetus most radiosensitive?
    a. 1st trimester
    b. 2nd trimester
    c. 3rd trimester
    d. all trimesters are equally radiosensitive

    D^{37}

45. What is currently considered the most reasonable approach to handling the pregnant radiographer in the work place?
    a. therapeutic abortion
    b. termination of employment
    c. avoidance of high-radiation areas
    d. continued practice

46. Which* of the following patients would have the most radiosensitive tissue?
    a. 75-year-old male
    b. 40-year-old female
    c. 18-year-old male
    d. 6-year-old female

    C^{38}

47. How many half value layers of filtration must be added to the primary beam to reduce its intensity to less than 1% of its original value?
    a. 9
    b. 7
    c. 5
    d. 1

    B^{39}

48. What is the relationship between film/screen combination and patient exposure dose?
    a. faster film/screen combinations increase patient dose
    b. faster film/screen combinations decrease patient dose
    c. slower film/screen combinations increase patient dose
    d. slower film/screen combinations decrease patient dose

49. What is represented by LET in radiobiology?
    a. long-energy transmission
    b. linear energy transfer
    c. linear-enhanced transmission
    d. loss from energy transfer

    A^{40}

Answer

Question #

A⁶¹

50. Which of the following are part of the Law of Bergonie and Tribondeau?
1. highly specialized cells are less radiosensitive
2. highly mitotic cells are more radiosensitive
3. highly mitotic cells are less radiosensitive
   a. 1 & 2 only
   b. 1 & 3 only
   c. 2 & 3 only
   d. 1, 2, & 3

D⁶²

51. What is meant by the term "interphase death" in radiobiology?
   a. cells die before going into interphase
   b. cells die before leaving interphase
   c. cells die in between mitotic phases
   d. the organism dies before the average cell leaves interphase

B⁶³

52. What is represented by the acronym PBL?
   a. primary beam limiter
   b. primary beam light
   c. primary backscatter limitation
   d. positive beam limitation

A⁶⁴

53. What effect does a reciprocating grid have on the primary beam as compared to a stationary grid?
   a. absorbs a greater percentage of the beam
   b. produces more scattered radiation
   c. produces less scattered radiation
   d. reduces off-focus radiation

C⁶⁵

54. What are the purposes a of a collimator?
1. reduce secondary scattered radiation
2. filtration
3. restricting the primary beam to the area of interest
   a. 1 & 2 only
   b. 1 & 3 only
   c. 2 & 3 only
   d. 1, 2, & 3

D⁶⁶

55. Which of the following is a primary cell radiosensitizer?
   a. low dose rate
   b. low LET
   c. sulfahydryls
   d. oxygen

56. Which of the following procedures would most likely contribute a higher gonadal dose to a female than a male?
    a. AP abdomen
    b. AP knee
    c. lateral hip
    d. PA chest

    A⁴⁴

57. Which of the following sets of technical factors would most likely produce the greatest patient exposure?
    a. 80 kVp, 200 mA, 0.06 s
    b. 80 kVp, 400 mA, 0.03 s
    c. 86 kVp, 200 mA, 0.04 s
    d. 92 kVp, 400 mA, 0.01 s

    C⁴⁵

58. Which of the following projections would afford the greatest radiation protection to the breast?
    a. left lateral chest
    b. right lateral chest
    c. PA chest
    d. AP chest

    D⁴⁶

59. Which of the following best describes the effect of filtration on exposure factors?
    1. exposure factors must be increased to compensate for increased filtration; however, the filter absorbs many low-energy photons, resulting in an overall decrease in patient exposure dose
    2. the filter absorbs only the low-energy photons that would not contribute to the diagnostic image; therefore, no change in exposure factors is usually required
    3. there in an inverse relationship between filtration and the exposure factors necessary that results in less absorption of low-energy photons and a decreased patient exposure dose
    a. 1 only
    b. 2 only
    c. 3 only
    d. 1, 2, & 3

    B⁴⁷

    B⁴⁸

60. What does the term RBE represent in radiobiology?
    a. relative biological effect
    b. radiation biology effect
    c. response to biological effects
    d. relative botanical effect

    B⁴⁹

Answer

Question #

61. What term describes filtration that is part of the x-ray tube, housing, and collimator?
    a. inherent
    b. added
    c. compensating
    d. total

62. Which of the following have a major impact on patient exposure dose?
    1. film/screen combination
    2. filtration
    3. beam restriction
    a. 1 & 2 only
    b. 1 & 3 only
    c. 2 & 3 only
    d. 1, 2, & 3

63. Which of the following procedures will require gonad shielding?
    a. PA chest
    b. lateral hip
    c. lateral knee
    d. AP skull

64. Which of the following best describes off-focus radiation?
    a. x-rays produced at locations other than the tube target
    b. scattered radiation from the patient's body
    c. x-rays that have come off the focus of the tube
    d. scattered radiation absorbed by the tube and housing

A^{72}

65. Which of the radiation syndromes would be expected from an acute whole body exposure of 50 Gy?
    1. hemopoietic
    2. gastrointestinal
    3. central nervous system
    a. 1 only
    b. 2 only
    c. 3 only
    d. 1, 2, & 3

A^{73}

66. What is the carcinogenic property of radiation?
    a. ability to cause genetic mutations
    b. probability of cell death
    c. ability to destroy cancer
    d. ability to produce cancer

A^{74}

Question # ⌐
Answer ⌐ |
↓ |
↓

67. Which of the following are symptoms associated with the prodromal stage of acute radiation syndromes?
    1. nausea
    2. lethargy
    3. diarrhea
        a. 1 & 2 only
        b. 1 & 3 only
        c. 2 & 3 only
        d. 1, 2, & 3

A^{56}

68. What is the most likely result of an acute radiation exposure of 1 to 2 Gy?
        a. death
        b. recovery
        c. cataractogenesis
        d. carcinogenesis

D^{57}

69. Which of the following cells are most radiosensitive?
        a. cardiac
        b. mucosal
        c. hepatic
        d. renal

C^{58}

70. Which of the following systems is most radioresistant?
        a. circulating blood
        b. respiratory
        c. central nervous
        d. renal

71. Which of the following can occur as a result of a late effect of exposure to radiation?
    1. skin cancer
    2. leukemia
    3. diabetes
        a. 1 & 2 only
        b. 1 & 3 only
        c. 2 & 3 only
        d. 1, 2, & 3

A^{59}

A^{60}

┌ Answer
│ ┌ Question #
↓ ↓

B 80

A 81

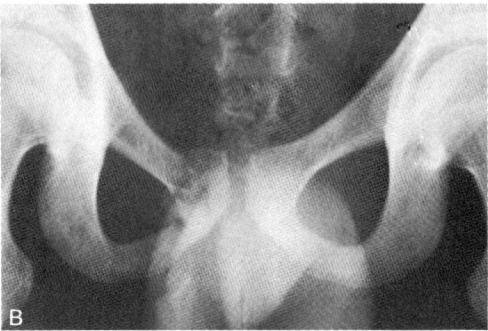

Figure 4 (from Cullinan AM: Producing Quality Radiographs. Philadelphia, JB Lippincott, 1987)

D 82

72. Which of the following is an accurate description of the procedures that were performed to produce Figures 4A and B?
   a. Figure A is not a diagnostic image for the pubic bones
   b. Figure A includes a female gonad shield
   c. Figure B is not a diagnostic image for the pubic bones
   d. Figure B includes a female gonad shield

C 83

73. If a patient's gonads lie within the distances given below from the edge of the primary beam field, which require shielding?
   1. 2 cm
   2. 4 cm
   3. 8 cm
      a. 1 & 2 only
      b. 1 & 3 only
      c. 2 & 3 only
      d. 1, 2, & 3

C 84

A 85

74. What term is used in radiobiology to describe cell damage from radiation that does not kill the cell?
   a. sublethal damage
   b. cell repair
   c. cell healing
   d. cognition

75. Which of the following conditions should be considered when determining when to use gonad shielding?
    1. potential reproductive ability of patient
    2. reduction of primary beam field size
    3. area of diagnostic interest
        a. 1 & 2 only
        b. 1 & 3 only
        c. 2 & 3 only
        d. 1, 2, and 3

D^{67}

76. What is the minimum aluminum equivalency of filtration required for diagnostic x-ray tubes operating below 50 kVp?
        a. 0.5 mm
        b. 1.5 mm
        c. 2.5 mm
        d. 3.5 mm

B^{68}

77. Which of the following procedures would most likely contribute a higher gonadal dose to a male than a female?
        a. AP abdomen
        b. AP knee
        c. lateral hip
        d. PA chest

B^{69}

78. What term is used to describe ulceration, necrosis, and loss of skin cells due to radiation exposure?
    1. desquamation
    2. erythema
    3. epilation
        a. 1 only
        b. 2 only
        c. 3 only
        d. 1, 2, & 3

C^{70}

79. Which of the following would have the highest LET?
        a. x-rays
        b. electrons
        c. neutrons
        d. alpha particles

A^{71}

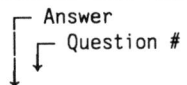

80. Which of the following primary beam field sizes would produce the greatest radiation exposure to a patient?
   a. 4" x 4"
   b. 6" x 14"
   c. 8" x 8"
   d. 8" x 10"

A[92] 81. In which of the following clinical situations is a manual technique most likely to reduce the risk of a repeated exposure?
   a. AP abdomen with considerable bowel gas
   b. AP chest with diffuse pneumonia
   c. lateral knee
   d. AP hip with intertrochanteric fracture

D[93] 82. Why is free radical formation in the human body so dangerous?
   a. scattered radiation is produced within the body
   b. all radiation shielding is penetrated
   c. carcinogenic tendencies have been proven
   d. toxic effects have been observed

A[94] 83. Which of the following structures would receive the greatest radiation exposure from a PA abdomen?
   a. liver
   b. stomach
   c. kidneys
   d. bladder

B[95] 84. Which type of beam-restricting device would eliminate the most off-focus scatter?
   a. collimator
   b. short cylinder
   c. extension cylinder
   d. aperture diaphragm

C[96] 85. Which of the following would experience the greatest reduction in radiation exposure when primary beam filtration is increased?
   a. entrance skin
   b. exit skin
   c. organ near entrance skin surface
   d. bone near exit skin surface

D[97]

Question # ⌐
Answer   ⌐|
         ↓|
          ↓

86. Which factors determine the shielding ability of a material?
    1. atomic number
    2. thickness
    3. density
       a. 1 & 2 only
       b. 1 & 3 only
       c. 2 & 3 only
       d. 1, 2, & 3

B^{75}

87. Which type of radiation exposure is of most concern to patients?
    a. chronic
    b. acute
    c. interstitial
    d. backscatter

88. Which of the following is suspected of being the prime target of
    the target theory of cell damage?
    a. cytoplasm
    b. endoplasmic reticulum
    c. deoxyribonucleic acid (DNA)
    d. nuclear membrane

A^{76}

89. Which grid ratio would reduce patient exposure dose the most if
    image density is maintained?
    a. 6:1, 80 lines per inch
    b. 8:1, 80 lines per inch
    c. 10:1, 80 lines per inch
    d. 10:1, 100 lines per inch

C^{77}

90. What is meant by an indirect effect of ionizing radiation?
    a. a genetic effect is produced
    b. ionizations in one location may produce effects at a
       distant location
    c. an organism other than the one irradiated may be effected
    d. potentially lethal metabolic disfunction is produced

A^{78}

91. What is the unit/s of measurement for LET?
    a. V/micron
    b. keV/micron
    c. Gy/volt
    d. Gy/keV

D^{79}

Radiation Protection

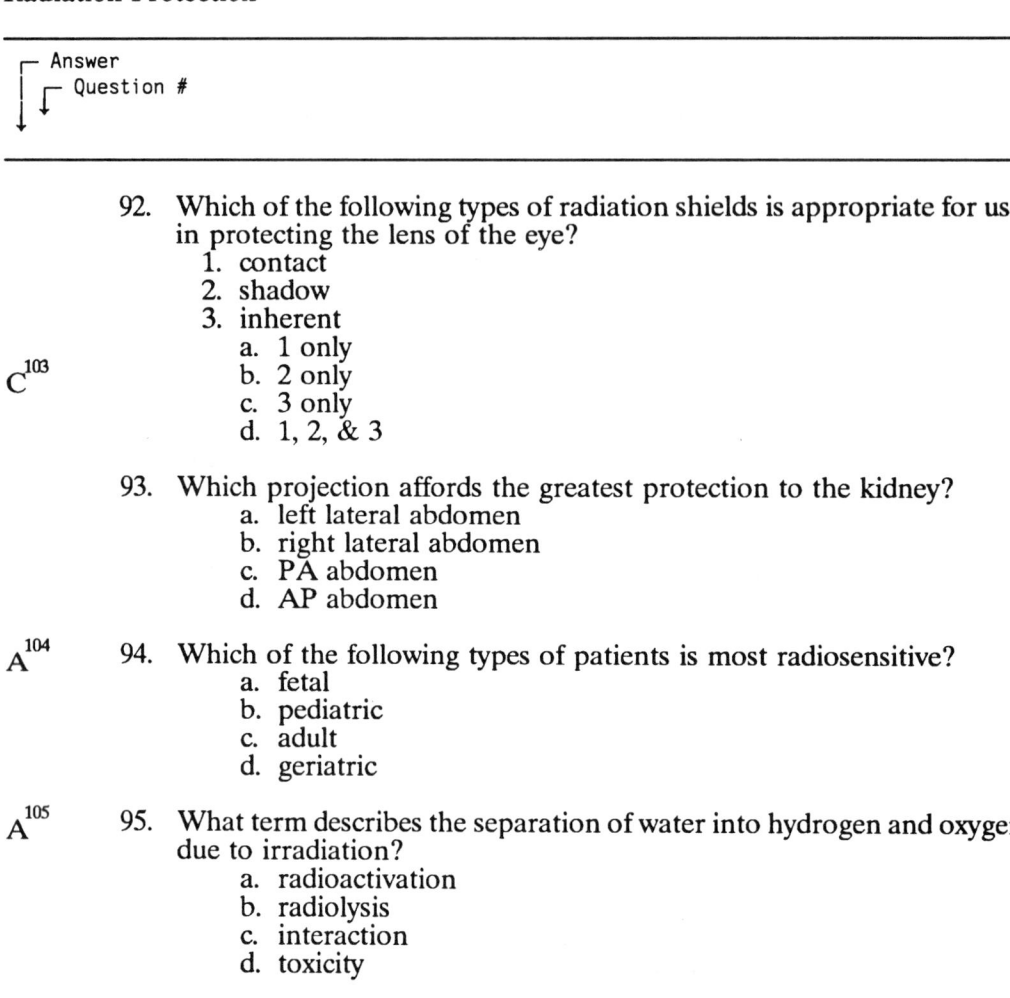

Answer
Question #

92. Which of the following types of radiation shields is appropriate for use in protecting the lens of the eye?
    1. contact
    2. shadow
    3. inherent
       a. 1 only
       b. 2 only
       c. 3 only
       d. 1, 2, & 3

C^{103}

93. Which projection affords the greatest protection to the kidney?
       a. left lateral abdomen
       b. right lateral abdomen
       c. PA abdomen
       d. AP abdomen

A^{104}

94. Which of the following types of patients is most radiosensitive?
       a. fetal
       b. pediatric
       c. adult
       d. geriatric

A^{105}

95. What term describes the separation of water into hydrogen and oxygen due to irradiation?
       a. radioactivation
       b. radiolysis
       c. interaction
       d. toxicity

B^{106}

96. Which of the following beam restriction devices provides the greatest patient protection when using edge-to-edge coverage of a square film?
       a. cylinder
       b. cone
       c. collimator
       d. circular aperture diaphragm

B^{107}

97. Which intensifying screen factors reduces patient exposure dose?
    1. thicker phosphor layer
    2. more efficient photon absorption
    3. higher conversion efficiency
       a. 1 only
       b. 2 only
       c. 3 only
       d. 1, 2, & 3

B^{108}

58

98. During attenuation of the x-ray beam in the patient, which range of photon energies contributes to the highest patient dose within the first few centimeters of tissue?
    1. high-energy
    2. moderate-energy
    3. low-energy   D[86]
        a. 1 only
        b. 2 only
        c. 3 only
        d. 1, 2, & 3

99. Which of the following technical factors would result in the lowest B[87] patient exposure dose?
        a. 120 kVp, 3   mAs, 200 relative film/screen speed
        b. 120 kVp, 1.5 mAs, 400 relative film/screen speed
        c. 102 kVp, 6   mAs, 200 relative film/screen speed
        d. 102 kVp, 3   mAs, 400 relative film/screen speed

100. Which type of mammography results in significantly lower patient C[88] exposure dose?
    1. xeroradiography
    2. film/screen and low ratio grid
    3. fluoroscopy
        a. 1 only   A[89]
        b. 2 only
        c. 3 only
        d. 1, 2, & 3

101. Which conditions would make a tissue relatively radioresistant?
        a. capillary dilation
        b. increased metabolic rate
        c. vasoconstriction   B[90]
        d. hyperventilation

102. Which grid factors are related to a reduction of patient exposure dose?
    1. ratio
    2. frequency
    3. type (focused or linear)   B[91]
        a. 1 & 2 only
        b. 1 & 3 only
        c. 2 & 3 only
        d. 1, 2, & 3

B¹¹⁴

103. What effect does the use of a carbon graphite table-top have on average patient exposure dose as compared to a plastic or plywood top?
  a. increases exposure at low kVp while decreasing exposure at high kVp
  b. decreases exposure at low kVp while increasing exposure at high kVp
  c. decreases exposure across the kVp range
  d. increases exposure across the kVp range

D¹¹⁵

104. Which of the following are related to patient exposure dose?
  1. film speed
  2. intensifying screen speed
  3. focal spot size
  a. 1 & 2 only
  b. 1 & 3 only
  c. 2 & 3 only
  d. 1, 2, & 3

B¹¹⁶

105. Which of the following would penetrate most into tissue?
  a. x-rays
  b. electrons
  c. neutrons
  d. alpha particles

D¹¹⁷

106. Which type of chemical can be produced by free hydrogen radicals?
  a. water
  b. hydrogen peroxide
  c. sulfahydryls
  d. oxygen

C¹¹⁸

107. What is the approximate dose required to produce permanent female sterility?
  a. 2 to 3 Gy
  b. 5 to 6 Gy
  c. 8 to 10 Gy
  d. 18 to 20 Gy

108. What is the minimum aluminum equivalency of filtration required for diagnostic x-ray tubes operating between 50 and 70 kVp?
  a. 0.5 mm
  b. 1.5 mm
  c. 2.5 mm
  d. 3.5 mm

109. What is the primary indication of genetic effects of radiation?
    a. demonstration of immediate effects
    b. delayed effects
    c. not readily discernible
    d. readily discernible

110. What term is used to describe loss of hair due to radiation exposure?   C[98]
    1. desquamation
    2. erythema
    3. epilation
      a. 1 only
      b. 2 only   B[99]
      c. 3 only
      d. 1, 2, & 3

111. Which of the following technical factors would result in the lowest patient exposure dose?
      a. 80 kVp, 6 mAs, 400 relative film/screen speed
      b. 80 kVp, 12 mAs, 200 relative film/screen speed
      c. 92 kVp, 3 mAs, 400 relative film/screen speed
      d. 92 kVp, 6 mAs, 200 relative film/screen speed

112. If 5.2 Gy produce a particular radiobiological response in a mouse with 250 kVp x-rays and it requires 4.0 Gy to produce the same B[100] effect with neutrons, what is the RBE of the neutrons?
      a. 0.7
      b. 1.3
      c. 9.2
      d. 20.8

                                                       C[101]

Personnel Protection 4% (56) 113-168

113. What term describes the fraction of time that a radiation beam is directed at a specific barrier?
      a. workload factor
      b. attenuation factor
      c. use factor
      d. occupancy factor   A[102]

Radiation Protection

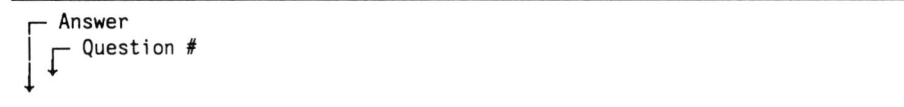

114. What is the maximum amount of leakage radiation permitted from a radiographic tube housing at a distance of one meter?
    a. 5 mR/hr
    b. 100 mR/hr
    c. 500 mR/hr
    d. 5 R/hr

D¹²⁴ 115. A radiographer receives a dose of 200 mR/wk at 100 cm; in order to reduce the dose to less than 25 mR/wk, to what distance should the person move?
    a. 25 cm
B¹²⁵   b. 50 cm
    c. 200 cm
    d. 400 cm

116. What is the total effective dose equivalent limit recommendation for the embryo-fetus once the pregnancy of an occupational worker has been diagnosed?
    a. 0.5 mSv
C¹²⁶   b. 5 mSv
    c. 50 mSv
    d. 500 mSv

117. Calculate the occupation dose for a radiographer who receives 0.7 m Sv per year while working within a controlled area, 0.4 mSv per year
C¹²⁷ from required employment health chest radiographs, and 0.8 mSv from all other environmental sources.
    a. 1.5 mSv per year
    b. 1.1 mSv per year
    c. 0.8 mSv per year
    d. 0.7 mSv per year

D¹²⁸ 118. What is the effective dose equivalent limit recommendation for the hands of an occupational worker?
    a. 5 rem
    b. 30 rem
    c. 50 rem
    d. 75 rem

C¹²⁹

119. What is/are the requirement/s for the exposure activation switch of a diagnostic radiographic unit?
    1. it cannot be located in the examination room
    2. it must be a dead-man type
    3. it must produce an audible signal and visual signal when activated
        a. 1 only
        b. 2 only
        c. 3 only
        d. 1, 2, & 3

B[109]

120. What is the annual effective dose equivalent limit recommendation for whole body exposure of occupational workers?
        a. 0.05 rem
        b. 0.5 rem
        c. 5 rem
        d. 50 rem

C[110]

121. What is the recommended thickness of the protective curtain or panel located between the fluoroscopist and the patient?
        a. 0.15 mm Pb/Eq
        b. 0.25 mm Pb/Eq
        c. 2.50 mm Al/Eq
        d. 3.50 mm Al/Eq

C[111]

122. What is the maximum thickness of the tabletop over a bucky tray?
        a. 0.15 mm Pb/Eq
        b. 0.25 mm Pb/Eq
        c. 1.00 mm Al/Eq
        d. 2.00 mm Al/Eq

B[112]

123. Which of the following are requirements for diagnostic radiography?
    1. only persons whose presence is necessary shall be in the radiographic room during exposure
    2. the radiographer shall not hold a patient during exposure
    3. the radiographer shall stand behind the barrier provided for protection during exposure
        a. 1 & 2 only
        b. 1 & 3 only
        c. 2 & 3 only
        d. 1, 2, & 3

C[113]

Answer

Question #

124. Which of the following contribute to the production of scattered radiation?
    1. photoelectric effect
    2. coherent (classical) effect
    3. Compton effect
        a. 1 & 2 only
        b. 1 & 3 only
        c. 2 & 3 only
        d. 1, 2, & 3

B[135]

125. What is the approximate range of mA used during fluoroscopy?
    a. 0.1 to 0.5 mA
    b. 1 to 5 mA
    c. 100 to 500 mA
    d. 300 to 1000 mA

A[136]

126. What is the minimum distance for mobile radiographic exposure switch cord?
    a. 1 ft
    b. 5 ft
    c. 6 ft
    d. 20 ft

A[137]

127. What is the minimum filtration required for a fluoroscopic beam?
    a. 0.5 mm Al/Eq
    b. 1.5 mm Al/Eq
    c. 2.5 mm Al/Eq
    d. 3.5 mm Al/Eq

B[138]

128. What is the effective dose equivalent limit recommendation for the lens of the eye of an occupational worker?
    a. 750 rem
    b. 75 rem
    c. 30 rem
    d. 15 rem

B[139]

129. What is the function of a bucky slot cover?
    a. keeps the bucky tray in place during fluoroscopic procedures
    b. monitors the movement of the fluoroscopic tube
    c. absorbs scattered radiation from under the x-ray table during fluoroscopy
    d. locks the bucky tray in place during radiographic procedures

A[140]

130. What is the maximum time permitted on a fluoroscopic timer before it can be reset?
    a.   2 minutes
    b.   5 minutes
    c.   10 minutes
    d.   15 minutes

131. Which of the following affect the average photon energy, thus affecting patient exposure dose?
    1. kVp
    2. mA
    3. generator phase
    a. 1 & 2 only
    b. 1 & 3 only
    c. 2 & 3 only
    d. 1, 2, & 3

D[119]

C[120]

132. Which of the following persons can be permitted in the fluoroscopic room during a procedure?
    1. radiologist
    2. respiratory therapist attending the patient
    3. hospital administrator
    a. 1 & 2 only
    b. 1 & 3 only
    c. 2 & 3 only
    d. 1, 2, & 3

A[121]

133. What is the minimum source-to-skin distance for mobile fluoroscopic equipment?
    a. 12 cm (5")
    b. 30 cm (12")
    c. 38 cm (25")
    d. 50 cm (20")

C[122]

134. What term describes the electron that is ejected from an atom during a Compton interaction?
    a. characteristic electron
    b. recoil electron
    c. photoelectron
    d. incident electron

B[123]

Radiation Protection

135. What type of barrier is designed to shield areas from scattered radiation?
    a. primary
    b. secondary
    c. lead
    d. lead equivalent

D^{147} 136. Which of the following are unlikely to contribute to scattered radiation?
    1. photoelectron
    2. recoil electron
    3. characteristic photon
        a. 1 & 2 only
C^{148} b. 1 & 3 only
        c. 2 & 3 only
        d. 1, 2, & 3

137. What is the function of a fluoroscopic automatic brightness control?
        a. maintains image density
        b. provides the highest density image possible
B^{149} c. decreases image density except in areas of interest
        d. maintains an appropriate level of light in the fluoroscopic room

138. What is the effective dose equivalent limit recommendation for the hands of an occupational worker?
        a. 750 mSv
A^{150} b. 500 mSv
        c. 300 mSv
        d. 50 mSv

139. What is the approximate dose reduction to the radiographer if the distance from the patient during fluoroscopy is doubled?
        a. 1/2
        b. 1/4
        c. 1/8
        d. 1/9

D^{151} 140. What is the minimum thickness for a bucky slot cover?
        a. 0.25 mm Pb/Eq
        b. 2.50 mm Pb/Eq
        c. 2.50 mm Al/Eq
        d. 3.50 mm Pb/Eq

141. What is the maximum fluoroscopic tabletop exposure rate?
    a. 0.1 R/mA min
    b. 2.1 R/mA min
    c. 3.2 R/mA min
    d. 10.0 R/mA min

B[130]

142. Which interaction is most likely to occur with photons above 50 keV in bone tissue?
    a. photoelectric
    b. coherent (classical) scatter
    c. Compton
    d. pair production

143. What type of barrier is designed to shield areas from the primary beam?
    a. primary
    b. secondary
    c. lead
    d. lead equivalent

B[131]

144. What is the required protective shielding of a conventional fluoroscopic barrier for operation at less than 125 kVp?
    a. 1.0 mm Pb/Eq
    b. 2.0 mm Pb/Eq
    c. 3.0 mm Pb/Eq
    d. 4.0 mm Pb/Eq

A[132]

145. Which of the following would be the best choice for an assistant when a pediatric patient must be held during exposure?
    a. student radiographer
    b. radiology department aide
    c. nurse
    d. parent

B[133]

146. Which interaction includes an annihilation reaction?
    a. photoelectric effect
    b. coherent (classical) scatter
    c. Compton effect
    d. pair production

B[134]

147. Which of the following terms describes automatic fluoroscopic image control systems?

B¹⁵⁸

1. automatic brightness control (ABC)
2. automatic dose control (ADC)
3. automatic brightness stabilization (ABS)
   a. 1 only
   b. 2 only
   c. 3 only
   d. 1, 2, & 3

148. What term describes the electron that is ejected from an atom during a photoelectric interaction?
    a. characteristic electron

A¹⁵⁹

    b. recoil electron
    c. photoelectron
    d. incident electron

149. What is the minimum thickness for fluoroscopic protective aprons?
    a. 0.15 mm Pb/Eq
    b. 0.25 mm Pb/Eq

A¹⁶⁰

    c. 2.50 mm Al/Eq
    d. 2.50 mm Pb/Eq

150. Which interaction is most likely to occur with photons below 40 keV in bone tissue?
    a. photoelectric
    b. coherent (classical) scatter

C¹⁶¹

    c. Compton
    d. pair production

151. Which of the following rules applies when patients are being held during exposure?
    1. appropriate shielding devices such as gloves and an apron must be worn

A¹⁶²

    2. no part of the holder's body can be struck by the useful primary beam
    3. the holder's body must be as far as possible from the edge of the primary beam
       a. 1 only
       b. 2 only

B¹⁶³

       c. 3 only
       d. 1, 2, & 3

152. What is the annual maximum permissible dose for the hands of an occupational worker?
    a.   0.75 rem
    b.   7.5 rem D^{141}
    c.   75 rem
    d. 750 rem

153. Which interactions between x-rays and matter does not ionize the atom?
    a. photoelectric effect
    b. coherent (classical) scatter C^{142}
    c. Compton effect
    d. pair production

154. What is the effective dose equivalent limit recommendation for the breast of an occupational worker?
    a. 5 rem
    b. 30 rem A^{143}
    c. 50 rem
    d. 75 rem

155. Which demonstrates that distance is the best radiation protection?
    a. Law of Bergonie and Tribondeau
    b. inverse square law
    c. power formula B^{144}
    d. grid conversion formula

156. Which of the following types of radiation are secondary barriers not designed to protect against?
    1. primary
    2. secondary
    3. exit D^{145}
    a. 1 & 2 only
    b. 1 & 3 only
    c. 2 & 3 only
    d. 1, 2, & 3

157. What is the minimum energy necessary to initiate a pair D^{146} production interaction?
    a. 0.51 keV
    b. 1.02 keV
    c. 0.51 MeV
    d. 1.02 MeV

Radiation Protection

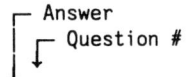

Answer
Question #

158. What is the minimum thickness for fluoroscopic protective gloves?
    a. 0.15 mm Pb/Eq
    b. 0.25 mm Pb/Eq
    c. 2.50 mm Al/Eq
    d. 2.50 mm Pb/Eq

B^166

159. What is the formula used to determine the lifetime cumulative effective dose equivalent limit recommendation for the whole body of an occupational worker?
    1. 10 mSv x age
    2. 10 rem x age
    3. 1 mSv x age
    a. 1 only
    b. 2 only
    c. 3 only
    d. 1, 2, & 3

C^167

160. What is the minimum source to tabletop distance permitted with a stationary fluoroscopic unit?
    a. 12"
    b. 15"
    c. 18"
    d. 40"

D^168

161. What is the annual maximum permissible dose for any organ, tissue, or organ system of an occupational worker?
    a.   0.15 rem
    b.   1.5 rem
    c.   15 rem
    d.   150 rem

C^169

162. Which electron shell binding energies would be most likely to be involved in a photoelectric interaction with a 35 keV incident photon?
    a. 33.2 keV
    b. 37.4 keV
    c. 69.5 keV
    d. 88.0 keV

A^170

163. What is the minimum source-to-skin distance for mobile radiographic equipment?
    a. 12 cm (5")
    b. 30 cm (12")
    c. 38 cm (25")
    d. 50 cm (20")

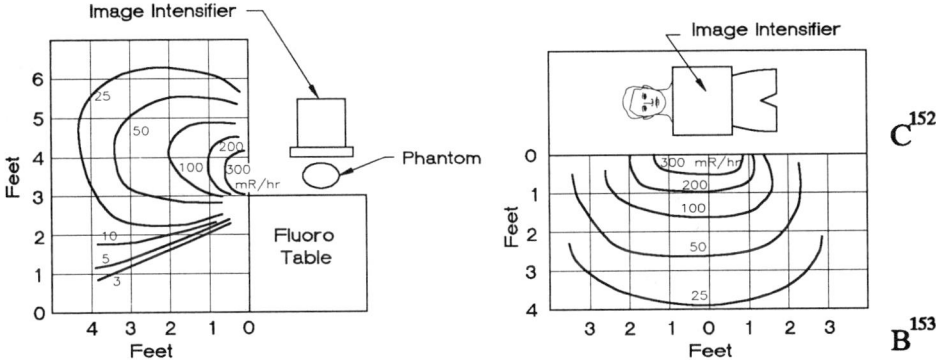

Figure 5 (reproduced by permission; Principles of Radiographic Imaging by Richard R. Carlton and Arlene McKenna Adler. Delmar Publishers Inc., Albany, NY; copyright 1992; adapted with permission from Wold GJ, Scheele RV, Agarwal SK: Evaluation of physician exposure during cardiac catheterization, *Radiology*, 99:188–190, 1971)

C[152]

B[153]

C[154]

164. According to the isodose curve shown in Figure 5, moving from a point 1 ft from the image intensifier to a point 1.5 ft away would produce the same percentage reduction in radiation exposure as moving from 1.5 ft to a point how far away?
B[155]

    a. 2.0 ft
    b. 2.5 ft
    c. 3.0 ft
    d. 4.0 ft

165. How far must the radiographer stand during a fluoroscopic examination in the room shown in Figure 5 to avoid a dose rate of 50 mR/hr?
B[156]

    a. 1 ft
    b. 2 ft
    c. 3 ft
    d. 4 ft

D[157]

Radiation Protection

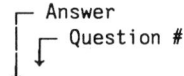

166. Approximately what dose would be received at the outside of the lead apron of a radiographer assisting a radiologist between 1 to 2 ft from the table in Figure 5 for 20 minutes?
    a.   20 mR
    b.   33 mR
    c.   100 mR
    d. 2,000 mR

B[176]

167. Which interaction is most likely to occur with photons above 30 keV in soft tissue?
    a. photoelectric
    b. coherent (classical) scatter

B[177]
    c. Compton
    d. pair production

168. What is the annual effective dose equivalent limit recommendation f or whole body exposure of occupational workers?
    a.   0.05 mSv
A[178]
    b.   0.5 mSv
    c.   5 mSv
    d. 50 mSv

Radiation Exposure and Monitoring 4% (56) 169-224

169. Which of the following is a monitoring device that records exposure to radiation by recording a silver-halide-based latent image?
    a. pocket ionization chamber
C[179]
    b. digital dosimeter
    c. film badge
    d. thermoluminescent dosimeter

A[180]
170. Which of the following can be used as personnel monitoring devices?
    1. thermoluminescent dosimeter
    2. film badge
    3. digital dosimeter
    a. 1 & 2 only
    b. 1 & 3 only
    c. 2 & 3 only
    d. 1, 2, & 3

C[181]

171. If two personnel monitoring devices are worn, which device would receive the highest dose after a month of routine diagnostic and fluoroscopic work?
    a. neck outside lead apron
    b. neck inside lead apron
    c. waist outside lead apron
    d. waist inside lead apron

172. What is the most commonly employed detecting device for scattered radiation?
    a. scintillation counter
    b. pocket dosimeter
    c. thermoluminescent dosimeter
    d. ionization chamber

173. Which of the following can be used to indicate exposure rate?
    1. R/min
    2. mrem/hr
    3. Sv/hr
    a. 1 & 2 only
    b. 1 & 3 only
    c. 2 & 3 only
    d. 1, 2, & 3

174. Which of the following is a device used for measuring the quantity of ionizing radiation?
    a. densitometer
    b. dosimeter
    c. sensitometer
    d. galvanometer

B¹⁶⁴

175. Which of the following symbols represents radiation exposure as measured in air?
    a. Gy
    b. Sv
    c. R
    d. rad

D¹⁶⁵

Radiation Protection

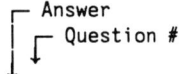
C¹⁸⁷

176. If a pocket dosimeter indicates that a radiographer received a dose of 14 mrem for a single fluoroscopic procedure when the average distance from the patient was 24", what would the approximate dose have been if the radiographer had been able to maintain an average distance of 4'?

    a.   2.4 mrem
    b.   3.5 mrem
    c.   56 mrem
    d. 504 mrem

C¹⁸⁸

177. What is the rad to rem conversion factor?

    a.   0.1
    b.   1.0
    c.   10
    d. 100

C¹⁸⁹

178. Which of the following SI units replaces the rad?

    a. Gy
    b. Sv
    c. C/kg
    d. joule

179. Which personnel monitoring system is the most accurate?

    1. pocket ionization chamber
    2. film badge
    3. thermoluminescent dosimeter
      a. 1 only
      b. 2 only
      c. 3 only
      d. 1, 2, & 3

A¹⁹⁰

180. If the intensity of the radiation beam at 40" is 1.1 R, what will be its intensity at 72"?

    a.   340 mR
    b.   611 mR
    c. 1,980 mR
    d. 3,564 mR

C¹⁹¹

181. What is the annual dose equivalent limit for the fetus of an occupational worker?

    a. 0.05 rem
    b. 0.1 rem
    c. 0.5 rem
    d. 5.0 rem

182. What is the annual cumulative whole body effective dose equivalent limit for occupational workers?
     a.   1 mSv x age
     b.   10 mSv x age
     c.   100 mSv x age   C[171]
     d. 1,000 mSv x age

183. Which of the following is equal to 1 rad?
     a. 1 gray
     b. 1 sievert
     c. 0.01 gray
     d. 0.001 sievert

184. What is the ALARA concept?   D[172]
     a. maintain exposure as low as reasonably achievable
     b. alert authorities when accidental radiation exposure hazards exist
     c. it represents the acronym, always limit all radiation alwa ys
     d. Dr. Alara discovered the biological hazard of radiation, and his concept is to limit all exposure as much as possible   D[173]

185. What is the most acceptable period for reporting film badge reports?
     a. daily
     b. weekly
     c. monthly   B[174]
     d. quarterly

186. What is the function of a control film badge?
     a. it measures the maximum exposure for a series of film badges
     b. it measures the average exposure for a series of film badges
     c. it measures the base-plus-fog level for a series of film badges   C[175]
     d. it limits fog exposure for a series of film badges

Answer
Question #

187. Which of the following personnel monitors must be read daily?
1. thermoluminescent dosimeter
2. film badge
3. pocket ionization chamber
   a. 1 only
   b. 2 only
   c. 3 only
   d. 1, 2, & 3

D¹⁹⁴

188. Which of the following personnel must wear a radiation monitor?
1. radiology department file room clerk
2. radiographer
3. administrative technologist
   a. 1 & 2 only
   b. 1 & 3 only
   c. 2 & 3 only
   d. 1, 2, & 3

A¹⁹⁵

189. What is the quality factor for alpha particles?
   a. 0.01
   b. 1
   c. 20
   d. 100

C¹⁹⁶

190. Which of the following are acceptable locations at which to place a film badge personnel monitor?
1. collar
2. waist
3. inside front pants pocket
   a. 1 & 2 only
   b. 1 & 3 only
   c. 2 & 3 only
   d. 1, 2, & 3

C¹⁹⁷

191. What would be the most appropriate action to take regarding a pregnant radiographer who received a monthly accumulative dose of 80 mrem?
   a. abort the fetus
   b. terminate the radiographer's employment
   c. assign non-radiation exposure related duties
   d. continue assignments with a warning to limit activities in radiation areas

D¹⁹⁸

Question # ┐
Answer ┐

mR/mAs CHART

source to receptor distance = 40" (100 cm)

kVp	mR/mAs
50	0.7
60	1.1
70	1.9
80	3.1
90	5.4
100	6.8
110	7.3
120	8.1

Figure 6

B 182

C 183

A 184

192. What is the approximate entrance skin exposure for a single AP abdomen exposure of 80 kVp and 22.5 mAs according to Figure 6 if the patient measured 24 cm?
    a. 3.1 mR
    b. 69.8 mR
    c. 120.8 mR
    d. 248.0 mR

C 185

193. What is the approximate total entrance skin exposure for an intravenous pyelogram consisting of four AP abdomen exposures of 70 kVp and 37 mAs and two oblique abdomen exposures of 70 kVp and 44 mAs according to Figure 6 if the patient measured 32 cm?
    a. 11.4 mR
    b. 332.8 mR
    c. 448.4 mR
    d. 969.7 mR

C 186

Radiation Protection

B²⁰⁵   194. If two personnel monitoring devices are worn, which would record the gonadal dose?
a. neck outside lead apron
b. neck inside lead apron
c. waist outside lead apron
d. waist inside lead apron

B²⁰⁶   195. Which of the radiation units is/are used to report personnel monitoring exposure to occupational workers?
1. sieverts
2. coulombs per kilogram
3. grays
a. 1 only
A²⁰⁷   b. 2 only
c. 3 only
d. 1, 2, & 3

196. Which of the following interactions between x-rays and matter result in the production of the most scattered radiation from which occupational exposure occurs?
1. photoelectric effect
B²⁰⁸   2. coherent scatter
3. Compton effect
a. 1 only
b. 2 only
c. 3 only
d. 1, 2, & 3

A²⁰⁹   197. At what point would a film badge be expected to provide the highest reading?
a. at the collar outside a lead apron
b. at the collar inside a lead apron
c. at the waist outside a lead apron
d. at the waist inside a lead apron

A²¹⁰   198. What would be the most appropriate action to take regarding a pregnant radiographer who received a monthly accumulative dose of 30 mrem?
a. abort the fetus
B²¹¹   b. terminate the radiographer's employment
c. assign non-radiation exposure related duties
d. continue assignments with a warning to limit activities in radiation areas

Question # ─┐
Answer ─┐ │
        ↓ │
          ↓

199. What is the monthly dose equivalent limit for the fetus of an occupational worker?
    a. 0.05 mSv
    b. 0.1 mSv
    c. 0.5 mSv
    d. 5.0 mSv

200. What is the annual cumulative whole body effective dose equivalent limit for occupational workers?
    a.   1 mrem x age
    b.   10 mrem x age
    c.   100 mrem x age
    d. 1,000 mrem x age

201. When is it appropriate to wear a personnel monitoring device?
    1. while assisting with a fluoroscopic procedure
    2. during a personal dental examination
    3. while having a personal chest radiograph done
    a. 1 only
    b. 2 only
    c. 3 only
    d. 1, 2, & 3

202. What is the quality factor for a rem?
    a.   0.01
    b.   1
    c.   20
    d. 100
C^{192}

203. What is the normal period for which a film badge is worn to measure occupational exposure?
    a. 1 week
    b. 1 month
    c. 3 months
    d. 1 year

204. What is the annual dose equivalent limit for a nurse working in a D^{193} cardiac catherization laboratory?
    a.   0.1 rem
    b.   0.5 rem
    c.   5.0 rem
    d. 1,000 rem

C^{218}

205. What is the quality factor for a gray?
    a.   0.01
    b.   1
    c.   20
    d. 100

206. What is the SI unit for absorbed radiation exposure?
    a. sievert
    b. gray
    c. rad
    d. coulomb per kilogram

B^{219}

207. What material is used in thermoluminescent dosimeters?
    a. lithium fluoride
    b. silver halide
    c. sodium iodide
    d. cesium iodide

208. At what exposure rate must a radiation warning sign be posted?
    a.   1 mR/hr
    b.   5 mR/hr
    c.   10 mR/hr
    d. 100 mR/hr

A^{220}

209. What is the recommended annual whole body dose equivalent limit for students under 18 years of age?
    a. 0.1 rem
    b. 0.5 rem
    c. 1.0 rem
    d. 5.0 rem

A^{221}

210. Convert 1,338 mrad to Gy.
    a. 0.01338
    b. 1.338
    c. 133.8
    d. 1,338

C^{222}

211. Which personnel monitor can be worn for up to 3 months?
    a. thermoluminescent dosimeter
    b. film badge
    c. pocket ionization chamber
    d. dosimeter

212. What is the monthly dose equivalent limit for the fetus of an occupational worker?
    a. 0.05 rem
    b. 0.1 rem
    c. 0.5 rem
    d. 5.0 rem

C^{199}

213. What is the mR/mAs at 40" if an exposure at 60 kVp and 15 mAs produces a dosimeter reading of 180.4 mR at 18"?
    a. 2.4 mR
    b. 3.0 mR
    c. 12.0 mR
    d. 36.5 mR

D^{200}

214. If a film badge report reads 0.01 millisievert, what would the total dose be in millirem?
    a. 0.01
    b. 1.0
    c. 10.0
    d. 100

A^{201}

215. If two personnel monitoring devices are worn, which would receive the lowest dose after a month of routine diagnostic and fluoroscopic work?
    a. neck outside lead apron
    b. neck inside lead apron
    c. waist outside lead apron
    d. waist inside lead apron

B^{202}

216. Convert 3.2 Gy to rad.
    a. 0.032 rad
    b. 3.2 rad
    c. 320 rad
    d. 3,200 rad

B^{203}

217. Which of the following best adheres to the ALARA concept?
    a. convincing patients not to have procedures
    b. using high kVp and low mAs exposure factors
    c. using high ratio and frequency grids
    d. developing films longer

A^{204}

Answer

Question #

218. For what type of protection are secondary barriers designed?
     a. high-energy primary beam
     b. filtered primary beam
     c. low-energy scattered radiation
     d. neutron emissions

B[228]

219. Which of the following are not acceptable storage conditions for a film badge?
     1. automobile
     2. desk drawer
     3. counter top in radiographic room
        a. 1 & 2 only
        b. 1 & 3 only
        c. 2 & 3 only
        d. 1, 2, & 3

D[229]

220. Which of the following interactions between x-rays and matter results in the highest occupational exposure?
     1. photoelectric effect
     2. coherent scatter
     3. Compton effect
        a. 1 only
        b. 2 only
        c. 3 only
        d. 1, 2, & 3

C[230]

B[231]

221. If a pocket dosimeter indicates that a radiographer received a dose of 22 mrem for a single cardiac catherization procedure when the average distance from the patient was 12", what would the approximate dose have been if the radiographer had been able to maintain an average distance of 3'?
     a.   2.4 mrem
     b.   5.5 mrem
     c.   22 mrem
     d. 352 mrem

B[232]

222. Convert 12.75 mSv to rem.
     a.   0.1275
     b.   12.75
     c.   127.5
     d. 1,275

B[233]

223. How does a film badge distinguish between different types of radiation, such as heat, light, x-ray, neutrons, etc.?
    a. different speed and contrast film chips are used
    b. different filters are used
    c. different thicknesses of plastic are used
    d. film badges cannot distinguish between radiations

A^{212}

224. What is the maximum permissible exposure for a 22-year-old radiographer who received 25 mrem when he or she were 19, 80 mrem he or she were 20, 180 mrem when he or she were 21, and has received 350 mrem during the current year?
    a.   365 mrem
    b.   650 mrem
    c. 3,365 mrem
    d. 4,650 mrem

A^{213}

Radiographic Equipment 11% (154) 225-378

225. How does the mA setting used during fluoroscopic radiography compare with diagnostic mA settings that produce the same image density?
    a. slightly lower
    b. slightly higher
    c. significantly lower
    d. significantly higher

C^{214}

226. What is the primary requirement for the production of x-rays?
    a. high-speed photons from a tungsten filament
    b. high-speed electrons striking a target
    c. electrons moving at high speed along a wire
    d. massive resistance to current flow

B^{215}

227. What is the total resistance of a circuit including three series resistances of 0.4, 0.8, and 2.4 ohms?
    a. 0.24 ohm
    b. 0.75 ohm
    c. 3.6 ohms
    d. 4.15 ohms

C^{216}

B^{217}

228. What material within the x-ray tube is most likely to cause tube failure by vaporizing and forming a layer on the inside of the tube envelope?

B²³⁹
    a. oil
    b. tungsten
    c. aluminum
    d. copper

229. Which of the following radiographic units will produce the greatest effective tube current when identical exposure factors are used?

B²⁴⁰
    a. single-phase, half-wave
    b. single-phase, full-wave
    c. three-phase, six-pulse
    d. three-phase, twelve-pulse

230. What is the most probable cause of a loud grinding noise emitting from the housing of a rotating anode x-ray tube?

B²⁴¹
    a. tube arcing
    b. improperly seated guide shoes
    c. damaged rotor bearings
    d. insufficient insulating oil

B²⁴² 231. What effect does a large-diameter conductor have on resistance?
    a. increases
    b. decreases
    c. alternately increases and decreases
    d. it has no effect

232. Which of the following factors are included in Ohm's Law?
    1. resistance
    2. capacitance
    3. current

D²⁴³
    a. 1 & 2 only
    b. 1 & 3 only
    c. 2 & 3 only
    d. 1, 2, & 3

233. What is the total resistance of a circuit including three parallel resistances of 8.6, 12, and 114 ohms?

B²⁴⁴
    a. 0.209 ohm
    b. 5.0 ohms
    c. 48.1 ohms
    d. 134.6 ohms

234. Which of the following components of a diagnostic x-ray tube have a negative charge during the production of x-rays?
    1. anode
    2. cathode
    3. filament
        a. 1 & 2 only
        b. 1 & 3 only
        c. 2 & 3 only
        d. 1, 2, & 3

B[223]

235. What is the normal rotational speed of a diagnostic x-ray tube rotating anode that is not equipped for high-speed rotation?
        a. 20,000 to 30,000 rpm
        b. 10,000 to 12,000 rpm
        c. 2,000 to 3,000 rpm
        d. 100 to 200 rpm

D[224]

236. What is the maximum voltage across an x-ray tube during an exposure of 80 kVp with a three-phase, six-pulse generator?
        a. 80,000 volts
        b. 77,600 volts
        c.   108 kilovolts
        d.   80 volts

237. Which of the magnetic classifications most strongly repels magnetic fields?
        a. nonmagnetic
        b. diamagnetic
        c. paramagnetic
        d. ferromagnetic

C[225]

238. Which of the following materials are used in diagnostic x-ray tube anode focal tracks?
    1. tungsten
    2. molybdenum
    3. rhenium
        a. 1 & 2 only
        b. 1 & 3 only
        c. 2 & 3 only
        d. 1, 2, & 3

B[226]

C[227]

239. Which of the following structures is enclosed within a diagnostic x-ray tube cathode assembly focusing cup?
A²⁵¹
    a. focal track
    b. filament
    c. rotor
    d. stator

240. What charge is on the focusing cup?
A²⁵²
    a. positive
    b. negative
    c. neutral
    d. alternating

241. What unit is used to measure potential difference?
    a. ampere
    b. volt
    c. ohm
    d. watt

242. What is the current flow in the armature of an AC generator?
D²⁵³
    a. direct
    b. alternating
    c. neutral
    d. direct during half of each turn, alternating the other half

243. Which of the following are correct differences between series and parallel circuits?
    1. resistances are added in a series circuit
    2. amperage is added in a parallel circuit
    3. voltage is added in a series circuit
B²⁵⁴
    a. 1 & 2 only
    b. 1 & 3 only
    c. 2 & 3 only
    d. 1, 2, & 3

244. What term is used to describe the process where an atom gains or loses an electron?
D²⁵⁵
    a. valence
    b. ionization
    c. electrolysis
    d. electromagnetism

245. What type of wiring configurations are used in the secondary coils of three-phase transformers?
    1. star
    2. helix
    3. delta wye
       a. 1 & 2 only C^{234}
       b. 1 & 3 only
       c. 2 & 3 only
       d. 1, 2, & 3

246. What is indicated by the direction of the middle finger in the right-hand and left-hand generator and motor rules?
       a. movement of conductor
       b. direction of magnetic lines of force C^{235}
       c. direction of current or electron flow
       d. generator force velocity

247. Which of the following units measure magnetic field strength?
    1. watt
    2. gauss
    3. tesla A^{236}
       a. 1 & 2 only
       b. 1 & 3 only
       c. 2 & 3 only
       d. 1, 2, & 3

248. What is the range of useful wavelengths for radiography?
       a. 0.001 to 0.010 angstroms D^{237}
       b. 0.1 to 0.5 angstroms
       c. 1.0 to 2.5 angstroms
       d. 1.0 to 2.5 micrometers

249. What particle moves to create electrical current?
       a. electrons
       b. protons
       c. atoms
       d. neutrons

250. Which formula solves for current? D^{238}
       a. V/I = R
       b. IV = R
       c. V/R = I
       d. R/V = I

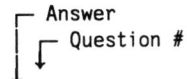

251. What is the maximum number of electrons that can occupy the K shell of an atom?

A²⁶¹

   a. 2
   b. 8
   c. 18
   d. 32

252. How many heat units are generated by a single-phase generator operating at 75 kVp, 100 mA, for 0.4 seconds?

C²⁶²

   a. 3,000
   b. 4,050
   c. 4,230
   d. 5,168

253. Which of the following are functions of the oil that surrounds the x-ray tube?
   1. heat dissipation
   2. shock prevention
   3. primary beam filtration

B²⁶³

   a. 1 and 2 only
   b. 1 and 3 only
   c. 2 and 3 only
   d. 1, 2, & 3

254. What is the primary effect observed if a conductor is moved through magnetic lines of force?
   1. magnetic field strength is increased
   2. electricity is generated
   3. x-rays are created
   a. 1 only
   b. 2 only
   c. 3 only
   d. 1, 2, & 3

255. How much power is produced by a current of 50 amperes and 10 volts?
   a. 0.2 ohms
   b. 5.0 ohms
   c. 50 watts
   d. 500 watts

256. What occurs to the magnetic field in a coil if more loops are added?
    1. it increases
    2. it decreases
    3. there will be no change
      a. 1 only
      b. 2 only
      c. 3 only
      d. 1, 2, & 3

B^{245}

257. What is the unit of frequency?
    1. Hz
    2. watt
    3. cps
      a. 1 & 2 only
      b. 1 & 3 only
      c. 2 & 3 only
      d. 1, 2, & 3

C^{246}

258. What term describes the number of electrons in the outermost shell of an atom?
      a. ionization
      b. valence
      c. atomic number
      d. atomic weight

C^{247}

259. Where in the basic x-ray circuit is the autotransformer located?
      a. between incoming line and exposure switch
      b. in filament circuit between incoming line and step-down transformer
      c. between exposure switch and step-up transformer
      d. separate circuit to stator of anode motor

B^{248}

260. How many pulses per cycle are produced by a single-phase full-wave rectified circuit?
      a. 1
      b. 2
      c. 6
      d. 12

A^{249}

C^{250}

┌─ Answer
│ ┌─ Question #
↓ ↓

261. What describes the electron cloud created by heating the filament?
     a. thermionic emission
     b. subatomic emission
     c. hysteresis
     d. saturation current

C²⁶⁹ 262. What is the primary purpose of rectification?
     a. intensify alternating current
     b. intensify direct current
     c. convert alternating to direct current
     d. convert direct to alternating current

263. Which of the following is/are step-up transformer/s?
     1. 10,000 turns on primary coil, 4,000 turns on secondary coil
     2. 20,000 turns on primary coil, 40,000 turns on secondary coil
     3. 1,000 turns on primary coil, 400 turns on secondary coil

A²⁷⁰
     a. 1 only
     b. 2 only
     c. 3 only
     d. 1, 2, & 3

B²⁷¹

B²⁷²

B²⁷³

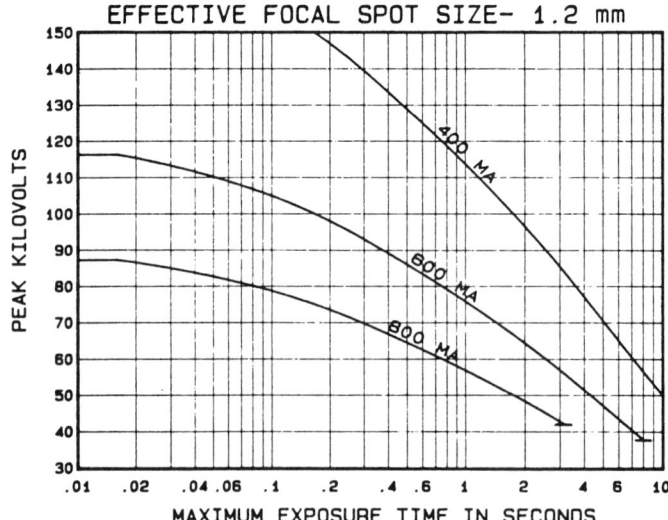

Figure 7 (courtesy of Varian Power Grid & X-ray Tube Products, Salt Lake City, Utah)

B²⁷⁴

264. According to the tube rating chart in Figure 7, which of the following technical factors would not be safe?
a. 90 kVp, 600 mA, 0.6 sec
b. 80 kVp, 600 mA, 0.6 sec
c. 70 kVp, 800 mA, 0.2 sec
d. 60 kVp, 800 mA, 0.6 sec

265. According to the tube rating chart in Figure 7, which of the following technical factors would be safe?
a. 120 kVp, 600 mA, 0.02 sec
b. 110 kVp, 600 mA, 0.02 sec
c. 90 kVp, 800 mA, 0.2 sec
d. 80 kVp, 600 mA, 1.0 sec

A [256]

266. If a transformer receives 80 volts into 10,000 turns on the primary coil and the secondary coil has 100 turns, what is the voltage in the secondary coil?
a. 0.00008 volts
b. 0.8 volts
c. 1.3 volts
d. 1.3 kilovolts

B [257]

267. Which of the following fluoroscopic image recording systems is capable of recording dynamic images?
a. 105 mm. cut film
b. 70 mm. roll film
c. radiographic cassettes
d. videotape

B [258]

268. Which of the following is characteristic of a mobile radiography unit which operates without being plugged in to a wall outlet?
1. tube leakage is a potential problem even when it is not plugged in
2. when insufficiently charged, the unit cannot produce an exposure
3. exposures are made immediately when the exposure switch is activated
a. 1 & 2 only
b. 1 & 3 only
c. 2 & 3 only
d. 1, 2, & 3

A [259]

B [260]

269. Which of the following functions are not taken over by an automatic exposure control?
    1. time
    2. mA
    3. kVp
        a. 1 & 2 only
        b. 1 & 3 only
        c. 2 & 3 only
        d. 1, 2, & 3

D^{281}

270. If the primary coil of a transformer has 2,000 turns of wire and the secondary side has 200, what will be the result on the secondary side?
    1. amperage will increase
    2. amperage will decrease
    3. voltage will increase
        a. 1 only
        b. 2 only
        c. 3 only
        d. 1, 2, & 3

A^{282}

271. What is measured by a meter wired in parallel with a resistance?
        a. current
        b. potential difference
        c. resistance
        d. radiation dose

A^{283}

272. What is indicated by the direction of the index finger in the right and left hand generator and motor rules?
        a. movement of conductor
        b. direction of magnetic lines of force
        c. direction of current or electron flow
        d. generator force velocity

A^{284}

273. Which of the magnetic classifications weakly repels all magnetic fields?
        a. nonmagnetic
        b. diamagnetic
        c. paramagnetic
        d. ferromagnetic

274. What is the approximate speed of a normal rotating anode?
        a. 100 to 200 rpm
        b. 3,000 to 3,500 rpm
        c. 10,000 to 12,000 rpm
        d. 30,000 to 50,000 rpm

C^{285}

275. What term describes the phenomena where the intensity of primary beam radiation is slightly greater at the cathode end of the x-ray tube?   A[264]
    a. line-focus principle
    b. anode-heel effect
    c. Lenz's Law
    d. the fractionation effect

276. What factor/s is/are not under the control of the radiographer during an automatic exposure control exposure with a falling load generator?   B[265]
    1. mA
    2. time
    3. kVp
        a. 1 & 2 only
        b. 1 & 3 only
        c. 2 & 3 only
        d. 1, 2, & 3

277. What conversion occurs in the image at the output phosphor of   B[266] an image intensification tube?
    a. x-rays are converted to electrons
    b. x-rays are converted to light
    c. light is converted to electrons
    d. electrons are converted to light

278. What is measured by a meter wired in series with a resistance?   D[267]
    a. current
    b. potential difference
    c. resistance
    d. radiation dose

279. What device is used to transmit alternating current from a generator?
    a. slip rings
    b. commutator ring
    c. rotor
    d. stator

280. Which types of magnets can be turned on and off at will?   C[268]
    a. lodestone
    b. permanent
    c. electromagnet
    d. superconducting magnet

```
┌─ Answer
│  ┌─ Question #
│  │
↓  ↓
```

281. What is the difference between series and parallel circuits?
    1. resistances are added in a series circuit
    2. voltage is the same through all resistances of parallel circuit
    3. amperage is added in a parallel circuit but remains the same through all resistances of a series circuit
    a. 1 & 2 only
    b. 1 & 3 only
    c. 2 & 3 only
    d. 1, 2, & 3

282. What unit is used to measure resistance?
    a. ampere
    b. volt
    c. ohm
    d. watt

283. Which of the following charts assist in avoiding damage to x-ray tubes?
    1. housing cooling
    2. anode cooling
    3. cable heating
    a. 1 & 2 only
    b. 1 & 3 only
    c. 2 & 3 only
    d. 1, 2, & 3

A^{291}

284. What are the functions of the oil between the x-ray tube and the housing?
    1. cooling of the x-ray tube
    2. insulation of the x-ray tube
B^{292} 3. filtration of the x-ray beam
    a. 1 & 2 only
    b. 1 & 3 only
    c. 2 & 3 only
    d. 1, 2, & 3

C^{293}

285. Which of the following is the difference between an ordinary and a grid-biased x-ray tube?
    a. higher kVp settings are available to penetrate high ratio grids
    b. high kilowattage ratings are possible to avoid biasing the anode grid
    c. a third wire is added to the cathode assembly to change the charge on the focusing cup
    d. the stator windings are grid-biased to permit them to rapidly slow a high speed anode disk

286. Where in the basic x-ray circuit is the mA selector located?
    a. between incoming line and exposure switch
    b. in filament circuit between incoming line and step-down transformer
    c. between exposure switch and step-up transformer B^{275}
    d. separate circuit to stator of anode motor

287. Which of the following are located on the high voltage side of the x-ray circuit?
    1. rectification circuit
    2. x-ray tube
    3. autotransformer
    a. 1 & 2 only
    b. 1 & 3 only
    c. 2 & 3 only
    d. 1, 2, & 3

288. Which of the following are possible results of failing to warm up A^{276}
an x-ray tube prior to clinical use?
    1. cracking the cold anode disk
    2. vaporizing the filament
    3. burning a hole in the anode focal track D^{277}
    a. 1 only
    b. 2 only
    c. 3 only
    d. 1, 2, & 3

289. Which of the following is a device that is capable of accumulating and storing an electrical charge?
    a. transformer A^{278}
    b. rheostat
    c. capacitor
    d. diode

290. What is the current flow in the armature of a DC generator?
    a. direct A^{279}
    b. alternating
    c. neutral
    d. direct during half of each turn, alternating the other half

C^{280}

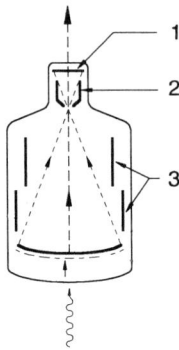

Figure 8 (reproduced by permission; Principles of Radiographic Imaging by Richard R. Carlton and Arlene McKenna Adler. Delmar Publishers Inc., Albany, NY; copyright 1992)

291. **What is #1 in Figure 8?**
C²⁹⁹
   a. output screen
   b. anode
   c. electrostatic lenses
   d. output screen

292. **What is #2 in Figure 8?**
A³⁰⁰
   a. output screen
   b. anode
   c. electrostatic lenses
   d. output screen

293. **What is #3 in Figure 8?**
B³⁰¹
   a. output screen
   b. anode
   c. electrostatic lenses
   d. output screen

D³⁰²

294. Which of the following is a correct difference/s between series and parallel circuits?
    1. voltage is added in a series circuit but is the same through all resistances of a parallel circuit
    2. voltage is the same through all resistances of a series circuit but is added in a parallel circuit
    3. amperage remains the same in all resistances of a series circuit
       a. 1 & 2 only
       b. 1 & 3 only
       c. 2 & 3 only
       d. 1, 2, & 3

B[286]

295. What effect does a high temperature have on resistance?
    a. increases
    b. decreases
    c. alternately increases and decreases
    d. it has no effect

A[287]

296. Which of the following is measured by the volt?
    1. potential difference
    2. electromotive force
    3. resistance
       a. 1 & 2 only
       b. 1 & 3 only
       c. 2 & 3 only
       d. 1, 2, & 3

A[288]

297. What constant factor is used to determine heat units for a three-phase, twelve-pulse generator?
    a. 1.00
    b. 1.35
    c. 1.41
    d. 1.50

C[289]

298. What component of a cathode ray tube controls the location of the electron stream on the screen?
    1. anode
    2. electron gun
    3. deflecting coils
       a. 1 only
       b. 2 only
       c. 3 only
       d. 1, 2, & 3

B[290]

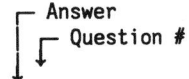

A³⁰⁹

C³¹⁰

D³¹¹

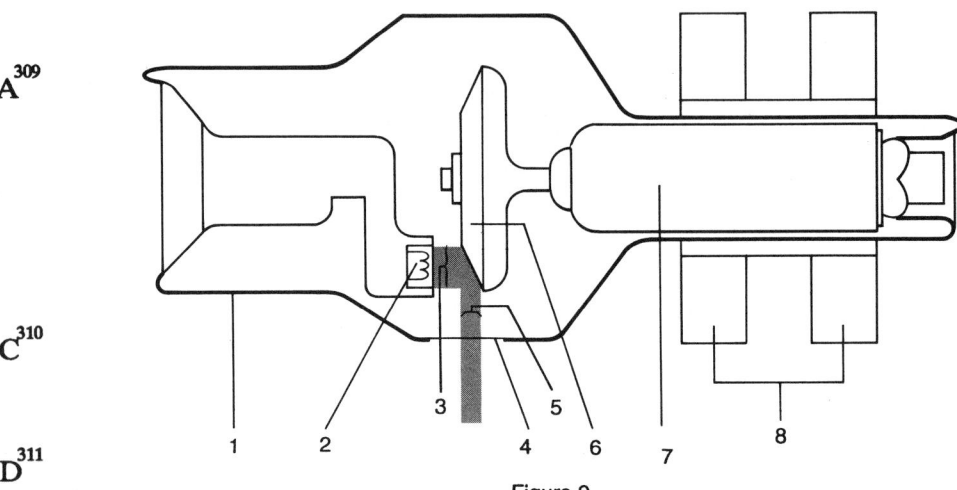

Figure 9

299. What is #4 in Figure 9?
   a. filament
   b. tube housing
   c. window
   d. stator

A³¹²

300. What is #2 in Figure 9?
   a. filament
   b. tube housing
   c. anode
   d. stator

301. What is #3 in Figure 9?
   a. effective focal spot
   b. actual focal spot
   c. filament diameter
   d. off-focus radiation

D³¹³

302. What is #8 in Figure 9?
   a. actual focal spot
   b. filament
   c. rotor
   d. stator

303. What is #7 in Figure 9?
    a. actual focal spot
    b. filament
    c. rotor
    d. stator

304. What is #5 in Figure 9?
    a. effective focal spot
    b. actual focal spot
    c. filament diameter B^{294}
    d. off-focus radiation

305. Where in the basic x-ray circuit is the timer circuit located?
    a. between incoming line and exposure switch
    b. in filament circuit between incoming line and step-down
       transformer A^{295}
    c. between exposure switch and step-up transformer
    d. separate circuit to stator of anode motor

306. Which of the following will prolong x-ray tube life?
    1. using lower mA stations
    2. pressing the exposure switch before the rotor when possible
    3. warming up the tube before first use
    a. 1 & 2 only A^{296}
    b. 1 & 3 only
    c. 2 & 3 only
    d. 1, 2, & 3

307. Which terms are used to describe the area of the anode that is struck by the high-speed electrons from the cathode filament?
    1. focal point C^{297}
    2. focal spot
    3. target
    a. 1 & 2 only
    b. 1 & 3 only
    c. 2 & 3 only
    d. 1, 2, & 3

308. At what temperature does an x-ray tube filament exhibit significant thermionic emission?
    a.   500°C
    b. 1,000°C
    c. 2,500°C C^{298}
    d. 10,000°C

309. What factor drops during a falling load exposure?
    a. mA
    b. time
    c. kVp
    d. filtration

C³²⁰

310. Which of the following are located in the filament circuit?
    1. exposure switch
    2. step-down transformer
    3. amperage control
    a. 1 & 2 only
    b. 1 & 3 only
    c. 2 & 3 only
    d. 1, 2, & 3

C³²¹

311. What is the approximate minimum exposure time range for modern electronic x-ray timers?
    a. 0.001 ms
    b. 0.01 ms
    c. 0.1 ms
    d. 1.0 ms

D³²²

312. Which are required as indicators on the x-ray exposure switch?
    1. audible
    2. visible
    3. tactile
    a. 1 & 2 only
    b. 1 & 3 only
    c. 2 & 3 only
    d. 1, 2, & 3

A³²³

313. What are the functions of the electrostatic lenses in a fluoroscopic image intensification tube?
    1. focus the electrons from the input screen and photocathode
    2. increase the speed with which electrons travel from input to output screen
    3. condense the image to increase its brightness
    a. 1 & 2 only
    b. 1 & 3 only
    c. 2 & 3 only
    d. 1, 2, & 3

C³²⁴

B³²⁵

314. Which of the following is another term for a generator?
    a. motor
    b. dynamo
    c. solenoid
    d. capacitor

C³⁰³

315. In which direction do electrons move through an x-ray tube?
    a. from negative to negative
    b. from positive to positive
    c. from negative to positive
    d. from positive to negative

A³⁰⁴

316. What term is used to describe the movement of an electrical charge in an object due to the repulsion of electrons from one another when a strongly charged object is brought close to it?
    a. valence
    b. repulsion
    c. attraction
    d. induction

C³⁰⁵

317. Why is a charge applied to the focusing cup?
    a. It increases the repulsion of electrons, thus producing higher-energy x-ray photons.
    b. It repels electrons from the focusing cup, focusing them into a narrow beam.
    c. It attracts electrons to the focusing cup, eliminating leakage radiation.
    d. It pulses electrons, reducing voltage ripple.

D³⁰⁶

318. Which of the following factors are included in Ohm's Law?
    1. heat
    2. voltage
    3. ohms
    a. 1 & 2 only
    b. 1 & 3 only
    c. 2 & 3 only
    d. 1, 2, & 3

D³⁰⁷

319. Which anode angles will produce effective focal spots that are smaller than the actual focal spot?
    a. 12° and 17°
    b. 35° and 45°
    c. 45° and 50°
    d. 50° and 55°

C³⁰⁸

320. What is the power rating of a three-phase x-ray generator capable of 140 kVp at 1,000 mA?
    a.   7.1 kVp/mA
    b.   140 watts
    c.   140 kilowatts
    d. 1,140 watts

B³³² 321. Which type of x-ray generator configuration permits the mA to decrease as the tube load increases?
    a. single-phase, two-pulse
    b. three-phase, six-pulse
    c. falling load
    d. capacitor discharge

322. Where in the basic x-ray circuit is the rotor switch located?
    a. between incoming line and exposure switch
    b. in filament circuit between incoming line and step-down transformer
    c. between exposure switch and step-up transformer
    d. separate circuit to stator of anode motor

323. Which of the following are step-up transformers?
    1. 1,000 turns in primary coil, 10,000 turns in secondary coil
    2. 200 turns in primary coil, 10,000 turns in secondary coil
    3. 1,000 turns in primary coil, 400 turns in secondary coil
    a. 1 & 2 only
    b. 1 & 3 only
    c. 2 & 3 only
    d. 1, 2, & 3

324. What device is designed to vary the x-ray tube circuit current prior to the high-voltage, step-up transformer?
    a. primary step-up transformer
    b. filament step-down transformer
A³³³ c. autotransformer
    d. rectification circuit

325. What conversion occurs in the image at the input phosphor of an image intensification tube?
    a. x-rays are converted to electrons
    b. x-rays are converted to light
A³³⁴ c. light is converted to electrons
    d. electrons are converted to light

326. Which of the following is capable of measuring both voltage and amperage in a DC circuit?
    a. voltmeter
    b. ammeter
    c. galvanometer
    d. densitometer

B³¹⁴

327. Which type of motor is most powerful?
    a. induction
    b. synchronous
    c. solenoid
    d. commutator

C³¹⁵

328. What symbol is used to represent power phase, as in a three-phase generator?
    a. τ
    b. φ
    c. Ω
    d. μ

D³¹⁶

329. What is the frequency of incoming line voltage in the U.S.?
    a. 20 rpm
    b. 20 Hz
    c. 60 Hz
    d. 120 Hz

330. What device is used to convert alternating current to direct current as it is transmitted from a generator?
    a. slip rings
    b. commutator ring
    c. rotor
    d. stator

B³¹⁷

331. What term is used to describe the tendency of an alternating current to oppose its own flow of current?
    a. mutual induction
    b. self induction
    c. primary induction
    d. secondary induction

C³¹⁸

A³¹⁹

Answer
Question #

332. What is the primary effect observed if the strength of magnetic lines of
force are varied through a stationary conductor?
1. magnetic field strength is increased
2. electricity is generated
3. x-rays are created
a. 1 only
b. 2 only
c. 3 only
d. 1, 2, & 3

A³⁴¹

D³⁴²

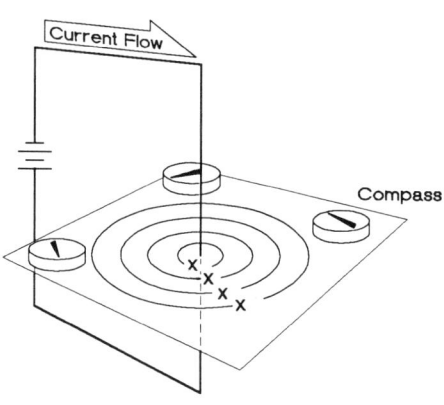

A³⁴³

Figure 10 (reproduced by permission; Principles of Radiographic Imaging by Richard R.
Carlton and Arlene McKenna Adler. Delmar Publishers Inc., Albany, NY; copyright 1992)

C³⁴⁴

333. In Figure 10, how should the magnetic flux line arrows appear where
the x's are indicated on the circular lines?
a. pointing right
b. pointing left
c. pointing up
d. pointing down

334. What effect does a long conductor have on resistance?
a. increases
b. decreases
c. alternately increases and decreases
d. it has no effect

335. Where does the greatest concentration of electrical charge accumulate?
    a. on the flattest surface
    b. at the area of highest atomic density
    c. at the point of greatest curvature
    d. at the point of generation

C^{326}

336. What is the normal rotational speed of the high speed anode in a diagnostic x-ray tube?
    a. 20,000 to 30,000 rpm
    b. 10,000 to 12,000 rpm
    c. 2,000 to 3,000 rpm
    d. 100 to 200 rpm

A^{327}

337. What is the charge on the electrostatic lenses in an image intensification tube?
    a. positive
    b. negative
    c. neutral
    d. positive or negative depending on the voltage

B^{328}

338. What is the function of a backup time when using an automatic exposure control?
    a. it reduces the mA
    b. it terminates the exposure in case of improper control settings
    c. it lengthens the exposure if the automatic exposure control fails to act quickly enough
    d. it protects the x-ray tube from overload

C^{329}

339. Which of the following would produce multiphase power?
    1. a generator with more than one armature
    2. a motor with more than one armature
    3. a motor with more than one rotor
    a. 1 only
    b. 2 only
    c. 3 only
    d. 1, 2, & 3

B^{330}

B^{331}

340. Which formula solves for electromotive force?
    a. V/I = R
    b. IR = V
    c. V/R = I
    d. R/V = I

341. What is the total resistance of a circuit including three parallel resistances of 0.4, 0.8, and 2.4 ohms?
  a. 0.24 ohm
  b. 0.75 ohm
  c. 3.6 ohms
  d. 4.15 ohms

B³⁵⁰

342. What charge does the x-ray tube glass envelope have during the production of x-rays?
  a. negative
  b. positive
  c. alternating current
  d. neutral

D³⁵¹

343. Which of the following suppress half the alternating current wave?
  1. half-wave rectification
  2. self rectification
  3. full-wave rectification
  a. 1 & 2 only
  b. 1 & 3 only
  c. 2 & 3 only
  d. 1, 2, & 3

D³⁵²

344. If a transformer receives 220 volts into 1,000 turns on the primary coil and the secondary coil has 12,000 turns, what is the voltage in the secondary coil?
  a. 16.7 volts
  b. 18.3 volts
  c. 2,640 volts
  d. 18.3 kilovolts

B³⁵³

D³⁵⁴

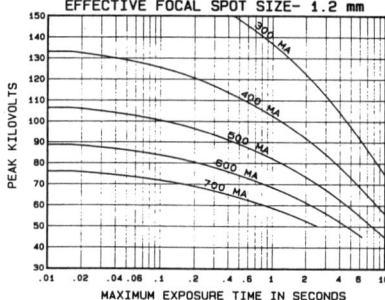

Figure 11 (courtesy of Varian Power Grid & X-ray Tube Products, Salt Lake City, Utah)

345. According to the tube rating chart in Figure 11, which of the
following technical factors would be safe?
     1. 70 kVp, 700 mA, 0.1 s
     2. 80 kVp, 600 mA, 0.3 s
     3. 80 kVp, 600 mA, 0.4 s
        a. 1 & 2 only
        b. 1 & 3 only
        c. 2 & 3 only
        d. 1, 2, & 3

C[335]

346. According to the tube rating chart in Figure 11, which of the
following technical factors would not be safe?
        a. 90 kVp, 500 mA, 0.3 s
        b. 80 kVp, 600 mA, 0.2 s
        c. 70 kVp, 600 mA, 0.6 s
        d. 70 kVp, 700 mA, 0.1 s

B[336]

347. According to the tube rating chart in Figure 11, which of the
following technical factors would be safe?
        a. 130 kVp, 400 mA, 0.05 s
        b. 120 kVp, 400 mA, 0.2 s
        c. 110 kVp, 400 mA, 0.4 s
        d.   80 kVp, 600 mA, 0.5 s

A[337]

348. Which of the following is used to describe current loss in the core
of a transformer due to lagging AC magnetization?
        a. hysteresis loss
        b. eddy current loss
        c. capacitance loss
        d. copper resistance (I^2R) loss

B[338]

349. Which of the following affect resistance?
     1. length of conductor
     2. diameter of conductor
     3. temperature of conductor
        a. 1 & 2 only
        b. 1 & 3 only
        c. 2 & 3 only
        d. 1, 2, & 3

A[339]

B[340]

350. What is the maximum number of electrons that can occupy the L shell of an atom?
    a. 2
    b. 8
    c. 18
    d. 32

A360

351. Which of the following factors are included in Ohm's Law?
    1. electromotive force
    2. resistance
    3. current
        a. 1 & 2 only
        b. 1 & 3 only
        c. 2 & 3 only
        d. 1, 2, & 3

A361

A362

352. When high-speed electrons are stopped at the anode of an x-ray tube, approximately what percentage of their energy is converted to heat?
    a. <1%
    b. 50%
    c. 75%
    d. >99%

A363

353. What component of a cathode ray tube creates the electron stream from the incoming pulsed signal?
    1. anode
    2. electron gun
    3. deflecting coils
        a. 1 only
        b. 2 only
        c. 3 only
        d. 1, 2, & 3

D364

354. Which of the following light converter tubes has been used in fluoroscopic imaging systems?
    1. plumbicon (TM)
    2. orthicon
    3. vidicon
        a. 1 only
        b. 2 only
        c. 3 only
        d. 1, 2, & 3

A365

355. Which of the following will affect the total brightness gain of an image intensification tube?
   1. flux gain
   2. minification gain
   3. incident primary beam intensity
     a. 1 & 2 only
     b. 1 & 3 only
     c. 2 & 3 only
     d. 1, 2, & 3

B [345]

356. Which of the following are correct differences between series and parallel circuits?
   1. given the same resistances, the total resistance of a parallel circuit will be less than a series
   2. given the same voltage, the total voltage of a series and parallel circuit will be the same
   3. amperage remains the same in all resistances of a series circuit
     a. 1 & 2 only
     b. 1 & 3 only
     c. 2 & 3 only
     d. 1, 2, & 3

A [346]

C [347]

357. Which of the following best describes the electrical properties of copper?
     a. conductor
     b. semiconductor
     c. superconductor
     d. insulator

A [348]

358. What constant factor is used to determine heat units for a single-phase, two-pulse generator?
     a. 1.00
     b. 1.35
     c. 1.41
     d. 1.50

359. Which of the following generators produces the smallest ripple in exposure output from a diagnostic x-ray tube?
     a. single-phase, two-pulse
     b. three-phase, six-pulse
     c. three-phase, twelve-pulse
     d. high frequency at 12 KHz

D [349]

┌ Answer
│ ┌ Question #
↓ ↓

360. What term describes the negatively charged electrode of a modern diagnostic x-ray tube?
   a. cathode
   b. anode
   c. input phosphor
   d. output phosphor

A^371

361. What unit is used to measure current?
   a. ampere
   b. volt
   c. ohm
   d. watt

A^372

362. Which of the following can be replaced by a charge-coupled device (CCD)?
   a. the fluoroscopic video camera light converter
   b. a cathode ray tube electron gun
   c. a spot filming device
   d. the image intensification tube

D^373

363. How many pulses per cycle are produced by a single-phase half-wave rectified circuit?
   a. 1
   b. 2
   c. 6
   d. 12

C^374

364. What is the unit of capacitance?
   a. watt
   b. volt
   c. ohm
   d. farad

A^375

365. Which of the following are step-down transformers?
   1. 800 turns in primary coil, 1,000 turns in secondary coil
   2. 10,200 turns in primary coil, 1,000 turns in secondary coil
   3. 500 turns in primary coil, 400 turns in secondary coil
   a. 1 & 2 only
   b. 1 & 3 only
   c. 2 & 3 only
   d. 1, 2, & 3

B^376

B^377

366. Which of the following is used to describe current loss in the core of a transformer due to swirling electromagnetic fields?
    a. hysteresis loss
    b. eddy current loss
    c. capacitance loss
    d. copper resistance (I^2R) loss

367. What term describes the left-hand to right-hand indexing of a video display terminal electron gun? D^{355}
    a. raster pattern
    b. half scan
    c. hypocycloidal
    d. multiphase

368. What conversion occurs in the image at the photocathode of an image intensification tube?
    a. x-rays are converted to electrons
    b. x-rays are converted to light
    c. light is converted to electrons B^{356}
    d. electrons are converted to light

369. Which of the following can be used to increase the voltage produced by an electrical generator?
    1. increasing the strength of the magnetic field
    2. increasing the number of turns in the conducting coil
    3. increase the angle between the magnetic field and the conductors A^{357}
    a. 1 & 2 only
    b. 1 & 3 only
    c. 2 & 3 only
    d. 1, 2, & 3

370. What is the primary effect observed if magnetic lines of force are caused to move through a stationary conductor? C^{358}
    1. magnetic field strength is increased
    2. electricity is generated
    3. x-rays are created
    a. 1 only
    b. 2 only D^{359}
    c. 3 only
    d. 1, 2, & 3

371. What is indicated by the direction of the thumb in the right-hand and left-hand generator and motor rules?
B[383]
    a. movement of conductor
    b. direction of magnetic lines of force
    c. direction of current or electron flow
    d. generator force velocity

372. Which magnetic classification includes rubber and plastic?
    a. nonmagnetic
    b. diamagnetic
    c. paramagnetic
    d. ferromagnetic

C[384]
373. What term describes materials that resist the flow of electrons?
    a. conductors
    b. semiconductors
    c. superconductors
    d. insulators

B[385]
374. What is the maximum number of electrons that can occupy the M shell of an atom?
    a. 2
    b. 8
    c. 18
    d. 32

D[386]
375. Which formula solves for resistance?
    a. $V/I = R$
    b. $IV = R$
    c. $V/R = I$
    d. $R/V = I$

D[387]
376. In the 80 to 100 kVp range, approximately what percentage of emitted x-ray photons are produced by characteristic interactions?
    a. 1
    b. 10
    c. 50
    d. 90

377. What is the effect of an increase in amperage?
A[388]
    a. more electrons flow with more force
    b. more electrons flow with the same force
    c. the same number of electrons flow with more force
    d. fewer electrons flow with more force

378. Which are located on the low voltage side of the x-ray circuit?
    1. exposure switch
    2. autotransformer
    3. primary side of high-voltage transformer
        a. 1 & 2 only
        b. 1 & 3 only
        c. 2 & 3 only
        d. 1, 2, & 3

B[366]

**Maintenance and Malfunctions of Radiographic Unit
and Accessories 4% (56) 379-434**

A[367]

379. Which device can be used to estimate x-ray tube focal spot size?
    1. pinhole camera
    2. star resolution test tool
    3. dosimeter
        a. 1 & 2 only
        b. 1 & 3 only
        c. 2 & 3 only
        d. 1, 2, & 3

C[368]

380. If a quality control test of a generator indicates that several milliamperage stations are inaccurate, which of the following terms can be used to describe the problem?
    a. timer accuracy
    b. milliamperage half value layer
    c. milliamperage linearity
    d. mR/mAs calculation

381. Within what percentage limits must the congruency of the collimator light beam to actual radiation field be maintained?
    a. 1 to 2%
    b. 10 to 15%
    c. 50 to 60%
    d. 85 to 90%

D[369]

382. Which of the following could seriously damage the anode disk of a high-speed rotor x-ray tube due to the gyroscopic effect?
    a. sequential high heat load exposures
    b. inadequate warm-up procedures
    c. rapid rotation of the tube housing from perpendicular to horizontal
    d. rapid movement of the tube housing to change FFD

B[370]

B³⁹⁴ 383. Which of the following would result from using a blue sensitive film with green emitting intensifying screens?
a. streak artifacts
b. insufficient density
c. excessive density
d. short scale contrast

B³⁹⁵ 384. What is the most likely cause of a mobile abdominal radiograph exhibiting satisfactory density and contrast in the center of the image, from the sternum to symphysis, but severely lacking density along the lateral margins of the image?
a. insufficient kVp
b. insufficient mAs
c. upside-down focused grid
d. failure to use a grid

A³⁹⁶ 385. Which of the following will increase intensifying screen efficiency?
a. higher temperature
b. higher kVp
c. lower mAs
d. greater filtration

B³⁹⁷ 386. What term is used to describe the process of monitoring technical equipment to maintain standards?
a. administrative review
b. continuing education
c. clinical previewing
d. quality control

387. Which of the following is radiographed in place over a cassette to evaluate film/screen contact?
a. an anatomical model or phantom
b. a plastic penetrometer (step wedge)
c. an aluminum penetrometer (step wedge)
d. a wire mesh

A³⁹⁸ 388. For what is a collimator test tool used?
a. to assure the congruence of collimator light field with primary beam field
b. to test the collimator for leakage radiation
c. to test the intensity of the primary beam as it exits the collimator
A³⁹⁹ d. to measure off-focus radiation

389. What is the primary cause of quantum mottle?
    a. low kVp
    b. high kVp
    c. low mA
    d. high mA

390. What is the function of a dosimeter?   B[378]
    a. it measures the density of radiographic film
    b. it measures radiation dose
    c. it measures radiation biological damage
    d. it calculates keV from kVp and mAs readings

391. What effect occurs due to the addition of a tint to intensifying screens?
    1. increased speed
    2. increased resolution
    3. higher conversion efficiency
    a. 1 only
    b. 2 only   A[379]
    c. 3 only
    d. 1, 2, & 3

392. Which of the following is the primary cause of decreased intensifying screen efficiency after several years of use?
    a. exposure to light
    b. exposure to x-rays
    c. abrasion of screen surface   C[380]
    d. exposure to heat

393. Which of the following will result from a more sensitive intensifying screen phosphor?
    1. lower resolution
    2. higher speed
    3. greater conversion efficiency   A[381]
    a. 1 & 2 only
    b. 1 & 3 only
    c. 2 & 3 only
    d. 1, 2, & 3

                                                            C[382]

A⁴⁰⁵

394. What term is used to describe the ability of an intensifying screen phosphor to emit the maximum amount of light for each incident x-ray photon?
   a. brightness gain
   b. conversion efficiency
   c. phosphor inversion
   d. screen lag

395. Which is a reasonable range of acceptable timer accuracy error?
   a. 0.1%
   b. 5%
   c. 30%
   d. 50%

C⁴⁰⁶

396. Which of the following are affected by half value layer?
   1. patient exposure dose
   2. image quality
   3. x-ray tube life
   a. 1 & 2 only
   b. 1 & 3 only
   c. 2 & 3 only
   d. 1, 2, & 3

A⁴⁰⁷

397. What is the purpose of a radiographic room log?
   a. to record the number and type of clinical procedures
   b. to record problems and service of equipment
   c. to maintain sufficient room supplies
   d. to document the number of rooms and their equipment for accreditation purposes

C⁴⁰⁸

398. Which are desirable qualities of intensifying screen base material?
   1. chemically inert
   2. flexible
   3. transparent
   a. 1 & 2 only
   b. 1 & 3 only
   c. 2 & 3 only
   d. 1, 2, & 3

B⁴⁰⁹

399. Which of the following is true regarding intensifying screens?
   a. they emit more light at low temperatures than at high
   b. thinner phosphor layers increase conversion efficiency
   c. resolution can be increased by the use of higher kVp settings
   d. smaller crystal sizes increase their speed

400. Which of the following will result from smaller intensifying screen phosphor crystals?
     1. higher resolution
     2. faster speed
     3. lower conversion efficiency
         a. 1 & 2 only
         b. 1 & 3 only
         c. 2 & 3 only
         d. 1, 2, & 3

C^{389}

401. Which is the best definition of an isotropical emission?
         a. it occurs in all directions
         b. it occurs in one predominant direction
         c. it occurs only under heavy bombardment by electrons
         d. it occurs only when phosphors are heated to a threshold temperature

B^{390}

402. Why are high atomic number phosphors desirable for intensifying screens?
         a. they promote more interactions with incident x-ray photons
         b. they are more durable
         c. they recapture more light photons for re-emission
         d. they reduce the amount of characteristic radiation emitted

B^{391}

403. Which of the following ancillary equipment items should be included in a total quality control program?
     1. viewbox reproducibility
     2. cassette cleaning
     3. cassette film/screen contact evaluation
         a. 1 & 2 only
         b. 1 & 3 only
         c. 2 & 3 only
         d. 1, 2, & 3

C^{392}

404. When a PBL mechanism is activated, which of the following is possible?
     1. increase primary beam field size larger than image receptor
     2. decrease primary beam field size smaller than image receptor
     3. eliminate off-focus radiation
         a. 1 only
         b. 2 only
         c. 3 only
         d. 1, 2, & 3

C^{393}

┌─ Answer
│ ┌─ Question #
↓ ↓

405. What is the normal cause of the grainy, speckled appearance of fluoroscopic images?
    a. quantum mottle
    b. screen lag
    c. proton failure
    d. mA saturation

B⁴¹⁵

406. Which of the following quality control tests requires loading four cassettes with film, placing all four with edges touching in a square, and then exposing one corner of all four at once by centering the x-ray tube to the point where all four cassettes meet?
    a. reproducibility
    b. mA linearity
    c. image receptor speed/linearity
    d. kVp accuracy

B⁴¹⁶

407. Which of the following will result from a more densely packed layer of intensifying screen phosphor crystals?
    1. higher resolution
    2. faster speed
    3. lower conversion efficiency
    a. 1 & 2 only
    b. 1 & 3 only
    c. 2 & 3 only
    d. 1, 2, & 3

A⁴¹⁷

408. Which of the following is the active layer of an intensifying screen?
    a. protective coating
    b. reflective layer
    c. phosphor layer
    d. base

B⁴¹⁸

409. Which of the following could result in differences in the amount of light transmitted by a viewbox?
    1. thickness of white plastic
    2. alignment of radiographs on viewbox
    3. brightness level of light bulb/s
    a. 1 & 2 only
    b. 1 & 3 only
    c. 2 & 3 only
    d. 1, 2, & 3

D⁴¹⁹

410. Which of the following is a reasonable range of acceptable kVp accuracy error?
     a. 0.1%
     b. 5%
     c. 30%
     d. 50%

411. Which of the following should be part of a total quality control program?
     1. angulator accuracy
     2. collimator congruence
     3. mA linearity
     a. 1 & 2 only
     b. 1 & 3 only
     c. 2 & 3 only
     d. 1, 2, & 3

B^{400}

A^{401}

412. What term is used to describe the amount of filtration necessary to reduce a beam to one half its original intensity?
     a. half-life
     b. half value layer
     c. attenuation coefficient
     d. filtration coefficient

A^{402}

413. Which of the following devices would most accurately estimate x-ray tube focal spot size?
     1. pinhole camera
     2. star resolution test tool
     3. dosimeter
     a. 1 only
     b. 2 only
     c. 3 only
     d. 1, 2, & 3

D^{403}

414. What is the primary reason intensifying screens must be cleaned on a regular basis?
     a. to remove dust and dirt particles
     b. to re-activate the phosphors
     c. to remove film emulsion residue
     d. to de-activate the phosphors

B^{404}

┌ Answer
│ ┌ Question #
↓ ↓

415. What is the approximate resolving capability of an average speed intensifying screen?
    a. 0.1 to 0.5 lp/mm
    b. 10 to 12 lp/mm
    c. 100 to 150 lp/mm
    d. 500 to 1,000 lp/mm

B[425]

416. visual effect would result from an intensifying screen that had been stained with brown spots from developer solution?
    a. a dark area because intensifying screen light photons would be attracted to the area
    b. a light area because intensifying screen light photons would be absorbed by the stain
    c. an area that would underdevelop because development would begin while the film was in the cassette in contact with the stains
    d. an area that would overdevelop because development would begin while the film was in the cassette in contact with the stains

B[426]

D[427]

417. Which is a desirable type of luminescence for intensifying screens?
    a. fluorescence
    b. phosphorescence
    c. incandescence
    d. isotropical

A[428]

418. Which of the following is the most critical quality control evaluation for an automatic exposure control?
    1. mA linearity
    2. exposure reproducibility
    3. timer accuracy
    a. 1 only
    b. 2 only
    c. 3 only
    d. 1, 2, & 3

D[429]

419. Which of the following are x-ray generator quality control tests?
    1. timer accuracy
    2. mA linearity
    3. kVp accuracy
    a. 1 & 2 only
    b. 1 & 3 only
    c. 2 & 3 only
    d. 1, 2, & 3

B[430]

420. Which of the following is the most appropriate action when there is doubt that an exposure occurred during a procedure?
    a. repeat the exposure immediately
    b. process and check the film before repeating the exposure B[410]
    c. eliminate the projection from the examination
    d. repeat the exposure at half the mAs

421. What is the function of a thin lead sheet in the back of a cassette?
    a. filter the primary beam
    b. reduce backscatter
    c. absorb the exit radiation
    d. strengthen the back

422. Which will result from a thicker intensifying screen phosphor D[411]
layer?
    1. higher resolution
    2. faster speed
    3. greater conversion efficiency
    a. 1 & 2 only
    b. 1 & 3 only
    c. 2 & 3 only   B[412]
    d. 1, 2, & 3

423. Which of the following can be evaluated by a collimator test tool?
    1. congruence of collimator light field with primary beam field
    2. central ray alignment
    3. leakage radiation from the collimator
    a. 1 & 2 only
    b. 1 & 3 only
    c. 2 & 3 only   A[413]
    d. 1, 2, & 3

424. What test can be used to assure the accuracy of a single-phase timer?
    a. kVp test cassette
    b. recycling test
    c. spinning top test
    d. gyroscope test

A[414]

425. If the half value layer of a diagnostic unit is too low, how should it be corrected?
    a. decrease primary beam filtration
    b. increase primary beam filtration
    c. increase minimum FFD
    d. decrease minimum FFD

426. If an exposure is made with a single-phase, half-wave, rectified x-ray unit on 60 Hz current at 0.2 s, how many dots should be imaged with a spinning top test?
    a. 18
    b. 12
    c. 6
    d. 3

427. What is the primary reason for using intensifying screens?
    a. increased anatomical detail
    b. decreased scatter dose to the radiographer
    c. their ability to record dynamic information
    d. reduced patient dose

B⁴³⁵

428. Which are desirable qualities of intensifying screen base material?
    1. uniformly radiolucent
    2. flexible
    3. high atomic number
    a. 1 & 2 only
    b. 1 & 3 only
    c. 2 & 3 only
    d. 1, 2, & 3

C⁴³⁶

429. Which are rare earths have been used in of intensifying screens?
    a. calcium tungstate, zinc sulfide, gadolinium
    b. calcium tungstate, lanthanum, barium lead sulfate
    c. gadolinium, lanthanum, barium lead sulfate
    d. gadolinium, lanthanum, yttrium

B⁴³⁷

430. What is the function of the reflective layer of an intensifying screen?
    a. reflect incident x-ray photons back into the intensifying screen phosphor layer
    b. reflect light emitted away from the film back toward the film
    c. it creates a second, fainter image on the back intensifying screen, thus avoiding light backscatter
    d. it prevents x-ray photons from scattering back toward the film after they have penetrated the cassette

A⁴³⁸

431. Which of the following focal spot size measuring standards have been adopted by the National Electrical Manufacturers Association (NEMA)?
    1. focal spots smaller than 0.8 mm may be 50% larger than stated
    2. focal spots between 0.8 and 1.5 mm may be 40% larger than stated
    3. focal spots larger than 1.5 mm may be 100% larger than stated
       a. 1 & 2 only
       b. 1 & 3 only
       c. 2 & 3 only
       d. 1, 2, & 3

B [420]

B [421]

432. What is the most common non-rare earth intensifying screen phosphor?
       a. zinc cadmium sulfide
       b. calcium tungstate
       c. iron oxide
       d. silver iodide

433. Which of the following artifacts indicates that intensifying screens need cleaning?
    1. half moon marks
    2. branching tree artifacts
    3. white specks
       a. 1 only
       b. 2 only
       c. 3 only
       d. 1, 2, & 3

C [422]

A [423]

434. Which of the following should be part of a quality control program for a diagnostic tomographic unit?
    1. section thickness accuracy
    2. uniformity and completeness of motion
    3. section depth indicator accuracy
       a. 1 & 2 only
       b. 1 & 3 only
       c. 2 & 3 only
       d. 1, 2, & 3

C [424]

Answer
Question #

Selection of Technical Factors 16% (224) 435-658

D⁴⁴⁴

For items 435 to 438 use the following information: A satisfactory radiograph of a lateral skull has been produced using the technical factors listed below. In each of the questions one factor has been changed. Indicate the result that will be seen on the radiograph as a result of each factor change.

B⁴⁴⁵

200 mA
0.25 s
65 kVp
40" FFD
2" OFD
8:1 grid ratio
100 relative speed film/screens
1.0 mm focal spot
10" x 12" field size

B⁴⁴⁶

435. Changing the OFD to 4" would result in:
    a. reduced magnification
    b. greater magnification
    c. higher recorded detail
    d. lower contrast

A⁴⁴⁷

436. The use of a 400 relative speed film/screen combination would result in:
    a. increased magnification
    b. decreased magnification
    c. increased density
    d. decreased density

C⁴⁴⁸

437. Collimating to a 4" x 4" primary beam field would result in:
    a. increased density
    b. decreased density
    c. grid cut-off
    d. focal spot blooming

438. Changing the grid ratio to 12:1 would result in:
    a. decreased density and higher contrast
    b. decreased density and lower contrast
    c. increased density and higher contrast
    d. increased density and lower contrast

C⁴⁴⁹

439. Which of the following technical factors would produce a radiograph with the shortest scale contrast?
   a. 50 mA, 1 s, 72 kVp
   b. 100 mA, 1/2 s, 75 kVp
   c. 150 mA, 1/5 s, 79 kVp
   d. 200 mA, 1/8 s, 78 kVp

440. Which of the following physical interactions between radiation and matter most assists in providing radiographic contrast?
   a. photoelectric
   b. Compton effect
   c. pair production
   d. photodisintegration

A[431]

441. Which of the following best illustrates magnification factor?
   a. MF = FOD/FFD
   b. MF = FFD/FOD
   c. MF = OFD/FOD
   d. MF = OFD/FFD

For items 442 to 445, choose the technical factors that would produce the greatest density on radiographic film if all other factors were to remain identical.

B[432]

442.

	mA	s	kVp	FFD	grid	film/screen
a.	300	1/4	74	40"	12:1	100
b.	200	3/8	76	40"	12:1	100
c.	150	1/2	74	40"	8:1	100
d.	100	3/4	76	40"	6:1	100

C[433]

443.

	mA	s	kVp	FFD	grid	film/screen
a.	50	1	78	36"	8:1	50
b.	200	1/4	76	40"	8:1	100
c.	100	3/4	74	36"	8:1	100
d.	150	1/10	78	40"	8:1	50

D[434]

Answer

Question #

444.

	mA	s		kVp	FFD	grid	film/screen
a.	150	1		65	36"	8:1	100
b.	100	3/4		65	40"	8:1	50
c.	200	6/10		65	36"	8:1	100
d.	100	1		65	40"	8:1	50

B⁴⁵⁵   445.

	mA	s		kVp	FFD	grid	film/screen
a.	200	1/8		76	40"	12:1	100
b.	150	1/6		76	40"	12:1	400
c.	100	1/4		68	40"	12:1	100
d.	50	1/2		68	40"	12:1	50

D⁴⁵⁶   446. What effect will be seen if the mA is decreased for an automatic exposure device exposure?
   a. time will decrease
   b. time will increase
   c. density will increase
   d. density will decrease

447. Which of the four primary radiographic exposure factors is controlled primarily by mAs?

C⁴⁵⁷   a. density
   b. contrast
   c. recorded detail
   d. distortion

448. Which of the four primary radiographic exposure factors is most effected by a change in focal spot size?

B⁴⁵⁸   a. density
   b. contrast
   c. recorded detail
   d. distortion

449. Which of the following will increase as a result of using a compressi on band on the abdomen of a large patient?
   1. subject density
   2. subject contrast

A⁴⁵⁹   3. radiographic density
      a. 1 & 2 only
      b. 1 & 3 only
      c. 2 & 3 only
      d. 1, 2, & 3

Question # ⌐
Answer ⌐│
        ↓│
         ↓

450. Which of the following will produce a change in contrast without changing density?
   a. increasing kVp and decreasing mAs
   b. increasing kVp and increasing mAs
   c. decreasing mAs with no change in kVp
   d. decreasing kVp with no change in mAs

A⁴³⁹

451. Which of the following will produce visible changes in radiographic density?
   1. kVp
   2. primary beam field size
   3. grid ratio
      a. 1 & 2 only
      b. 1 & 3 only
      c. 2 & 3 only
      d. 1, 2, & 3

A⁴⁴⁰

452. Which of the following has the ability to reduce image density by reducing x-ray tube output?
   1. a low vacuum inside the glass envelope
   2. a smooth anode focal track
   3. increased added filtration
      a. 1 only
      b. 2 only
      c. 3 only
      d. 1, 2, & 3

B⁴⁴¹

453. Which of the following will cause loss of recorded detail?
   a. kVp changes
   b. mAs changes
   c. subject motion
   d. subject density changes

D⁴²¹

454. What is the optimal kVp to produce the highest contrast with iodine based contrast media?
   a. 35
   b. 68
   c. 80
   d. 120

C⁴²²

Image Production and Evaluation

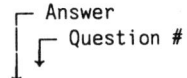
455. Which of the following time station changes would produce a visible change in radiographic density?
   1. from 0.03 s to 0.04 s
   2. from 0.75 s to 0.60 s
   3. from 0.80 s to 1.00 s
       a. 1 & 2 only
       b. 1 & 3 only
       c. 2 & 3 only
       d. 1, 2, & 3

A⁴⁶⁵

456. Which of the following mA stations would most reduce patient motion if the same mAs is used for two exposures?
       a. 100
       b. 200
       c. 400
       d. 1200

A⁴⁶⁶

457. In the production of x-ray film, potassium bromide and silver nitrate are added to the gelatin solution in total darkness. Why is total darkness necessary?
       a. a precipitate of the potassium bromide and silver nitrate cannot be produced when light photons are present
       b. light photons will initiate a destructive chemical reaction
       c. light photons will cause exposure of the silver bromide crystals
       d. light photons will cause exposure of the potassium nitrate crystals

A⁴⁶⁷

458. What term is used to describe the curve that illustrates the relationship between exposure and density?
       a. modulation curve
       b. characteristic curve
       c. resolution curve
       d. exposure curve

C⁴⁶⁸

459. What term describes the image that is produced by the interaction of electromagnetic radiation with the emulsion of a radiographic film prior to development?
       a. latent
       b. negative
       c. radiograph
       d. reflection

B⁴⁶⁹

128

Question #
Answer

460. Which of the following are reducing agents used in automatic film processing developer solutions?
    a. hydroquinone and metol
    b. hydroquinone and phenidone
    c. hydroquinone and potassium bromide
    d. metol and phenidone

A [450]

461. Which chemical assists in reducing swelling of the emulsion in the developer and aids in preventing film from sticking to automatic processor transport rollers?
    a. sodium sulfite
    b. potassium bromide
    c. glutaraldehyde
    d. acetic acid

D [451]

462. Why should the top of an automatic film processor be opened when it is shut down?
    a. condensation can cause cross-contamination of developer and fixer
    b. to reduce oxidation of the developer solution
    c. to prevent reduction of the developer solution strength
    d. to cool the processor down faster

463. Which automatic film processor replenishment rate is lowest?
    1. developer
    2. fixer
    3. wash
    a. 1 only
    b. 2 only
    c. 3 only
    d. 1, 2, & 3

B [452]

C [453]

464. What is the primary variable in a fixed kVp radiographic exposure technique system?
    a. distance
    b. filtration
    c. kVp
    d. mAs

B [454]

465. Which of the following silver recovery systems is most efficient under moderate radiology department use?
    1. electrolytic
    2. sludge
    3. metallic replacement
        a. 1 only
        b. 2 only
        c. 3 only
        d. 1, 2, & 3

D⁴⁷³

466. Which kVp ranges are appropriate for imaging a finger?
        a. 30 to 40
        b. 50 to 60
        c. 80 to 90
        d. 110 to 120

D⁴⁷⁴

467. Which of the following would increase radiographic density?
    1. increased developer temperature
    2. low temperature in film storage area
    3. decreased fixing time
        a. 1 only
        b. 2 only
        c. 3 only
        d. 1, 2, & 3

A⁴⁷⁵

468. Which of the following characteristics are common for radiographic films with wide latitude gradient?
    1. high contrast
    2. low-speed
    3. low average gradient
        a. 1 & 2 only
        b. 1 & 3 only
        c. 2 & 3 only
        d. 1, 2, & 3

469. Which pathologic conditions would require increased technical factors to maintain image density as compared to normal tissue?
    1. pleural effusion
    2. pneumothorax
    3. congestive heart failure
        a. 1 & 2 only
        b. 1 & 3 only
        c. 2 & 3 only
        d. 1, 2, & 3

470. Which of the following will change if the grid ratio is increased?
     1. recorded detail
     2. density
     3. contrast
        a. 1 & 2 only
        b. 1 & 3 only
        c. 2 & 3 only
        d. 1, 2, & 3

B⁴⁶⁰

For items 471 to 474 use the following information: A satisfactory lateral cervical spine radiograph has been produced using the technical factors listed below. In each of the questions one factor has been changed. Indicate the result that will be seen on the radiograph as a result of each factor change if all other factors remain the same.

C⁴⁶¹

200 mA
0.06 s
74 kVp
72" FFD
6" OFD
10:1 grid ratio
200 relative speed film/screens
2.5 mm focal spot
8" x 11" field size

A⁴⁶²

471. Changing the OFD to 7" would result in:
     1. increased magnification
     2. decreased recorded detail
     3. higher contrast
        a. 1 & 2 only
        b. 1 & 3 only
        c. 2 & 3 only
        d. 1, 2, & 3

A⁴⁶³

472. What mAs would be required to maintain the density if a 100 relative speed film/screen combination were used?
        a. 3
        b. 6
        c. 12
        d. 20

D⁴⁶⁴

┌─ Answer
│ ┌─ Question #
│ │
↓ ↓

473. Which of the following would result if collimation were changed to 1
    1" x 14"?
    1. lower contrast
    2. increased density
    3. increased patient exposure dose
        a. 1 & 2 only
        b. 1 & 3 only
        c. 2 & 3 only
        d. 1, 2, & 3

A⁴⁸⁰

474. Changing the distance to 40" would result in:
        a. decreased density and no change in recorded detail
        b. decreased density and decreased recorded detail
        c. increased density and decreased recorded detail
        d. increased density and no change in recorded detail

B⁴⁸¹

475. Which of the following technical factors would produce a radiograph
    with the highest contrast?
        a. 200 mA, 0.10 s, 102 kVp
        b. 200 mA, 0.05 s, 120 kVp
        c. 400 mA, 0.05 s, 120 kVp
        d. 400 mA, 0.10 s, 120 kVp

D⁴⁸²

D⁴⁸³

C⁴⁸⁴

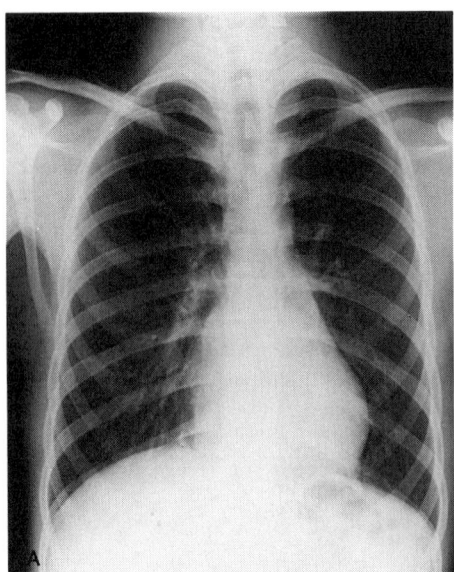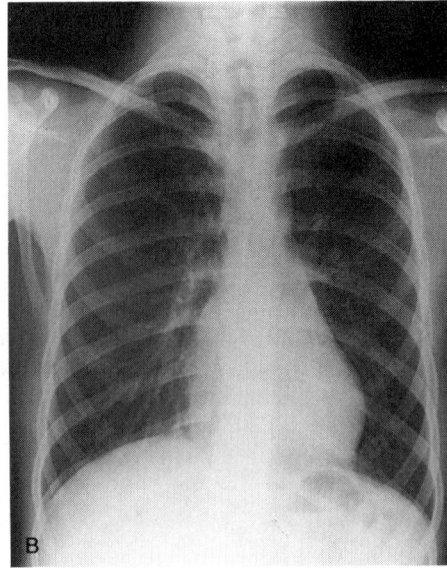

Figure 12 (courtesy of Bruce Long, Indiana University Medical Center, Indianapolis, Indiana)

476. If Figure 12A was produced with technical factors of 80 kVp and 15 mAs, which of the following technical factors were most likely used to produce Figure 12B?
   1. 68 kVp, 30 mAs
   2. 80 kVp, 30 mAs
   3. 92 kVp, 15 mAs
      a. 1 only
      b. 2 only
      c. 3 only
      d. 1, 2, & 3

C⁴⁷⁰ C^{470}

477. Which of the following is true about Figure 12B?
   1. longer scale contrast is exhibited
   2. the same mAs was used
   3. greater FFD was used
      a. 1 & 2 only
      b. 1 & 3 only
      c. 2 & 3 only
      d. 1, 2, & 3

For items 478 to 481, choose the technical factors that would produce the greatest density on radiographic film if all other factors were to remain identical.

478.

	mA	s	kVp	FFD	grid	film/screen
a.	400	0.02	102	40"	10:1	100
b.	200	0.04	120	40"	10:1	100
c.	400	0.02	102	40"	12:1	100
d.	800	0.01	120	40"	12:1	100

479.

A^{471}

	mA	s	kVp	FFD	grid	film/screen
a.	500	0.03	64	40"	12:1	50
b.	300	1/20	62	36"	12:1	100
c.	200	0.08	62	36"	12:1	200
d.	100	0.15	65	40"	12:1	400

B^{472}

480.

	mA	s	kVp	FFD	grid	film/screen
a.	200	0.18	80	40"	10:1	250
b.	300	0.12	82	40"	10:1	200
c.	400	0.12	82	40"	10:1	100
d.	400	0.09	78	40"	10:1	400

A[490]

481.

	mA	s	kVp	FFD	grid	film/screen
a.	200	1/6	90	40"	12:1	100
b.	200	0.08	77	40"	10:1	400
c.	400	1/12	90	40"	10:1	100
d.	400	0.08	77	40"	12:1	200

D[491]

482. What result is expected if a single automatic exposure control ion chamber is activated for an AP abdomen and bowel gas is positioned directly over it?
   a. increased density over the entire abdomen including bowel gas
   b. increased density over the entire abdomen except bowel gas areas

C[492]
   c. decreased density over the entire abdomen including bowel g as areas
   d. decreased density over the entire abdomen except bowel gas areas

B[493]
483. Which of the following are affected by film/screen combination?
   1. density
   2. contrast
   3. recorded detail
      a. 1 & 2 only
      b. 1 & 3 only
      c. 2 & 3 only
      d. 1, 2, & 3

B[494]
484. Which of the following does not affect density?
   1. distance
   2. kVp
   3. focal spot size
      a. 1 only
B[495]
      b. 2 only
      c. 3 only
      d. 1, 2, & 3

485. Which of the following directly affect shape distortion?
    1. alignment of tube to part
    2. alignment of tube to image receptor
    3. alignment of part to image receptor
        a. 1 & 2 only
        b. 1 & 3 only
        c. 2 & 3 only
        d. 1, 2, & 3

C^{476}

486. Which of the following technical exposure factor changes would compensate for tissue with a disease process that has increased the attenuation of the primary beam?
    1. increased mAs
    2. decreased distance
    3. increased kVp
        a. 1 & 2 only
        b. 1 & 3 only
        c. 2 & 3 only
        d. 1, 2, & 3

A^{477}

487. Which of the following changes will occur with an increase in abdominal compression?
    1. increased density
    2. higher contrast
    3. decreased recorded detail
        a. 1 & 2 only
        b. 1 & 3 only
        c. 2 & 3 only
        d. 1, 2, & 3

B^{478}

488. What is the magnification factor for a lung mass that casts a shadow 0.4 cm wide on a PA chest radiograph produced at 100cm when the mass is located 6.2 cm from the film?
        a. 0.94
        b. 1.01
        c. 1.07
        d. 1.12

D^{479}

489. Which describes the number of grid lines per inch or centimeter?
        a. grid ratio
        b. grid type
        c. grid frequency
        d. grid interspace material

490. Which of the following technical factors would produce a radiograph with the longest scale contrast?
      a. 100 mA, 0.12 s, 69 kVp
      b. 100 mA, 0.24 s, 60 kVp
      c. 100 mA, 0.24 s, 60 kVp
      d. 200 mA, 0.24 s, 51 kVp

D^{501}

491. Which of the following terms correctly describes a gross distortion of an object in which the image, usually one end, appears to be smaller than the original object while the other end is an accurate representation or even enlarged?
      a. spatial distortion
      b. geometric unsharpness
      c. elongation
      d. foreshortening

A^{502}

492. Which radiographic quality factor can be described as the overall blackening of the image?
      a. recorded detail
      b. distortion
      c. density
      d. contrast

A^{503}

493. What is the primary function of a radiographic grid?
      a. reduce patient exposure dose
      b. increase image contrast
      c. increase image density
      d. decrease image magnification

494. What effect does increased primary beam attenuation have on the radiographic image?
      a. density increases
      b. density decreases
      c. recorded detail increases
      d. recorded detail decreases

D^{504}

495. Which radiographic quality factor can be described as misrepresentation of the size or shape of a structure?
      a. recorded detail
      b. distortion
      c. density
      d. contrast

C^{505}

496. Which of the following will result in distortion of the knee joint?
 1. centering central ray 2" superior to the joint
 2. positioning joint 2" superior to central ray
 3. centering film 2" superior to joint
 a. 1 & 2 only
 b. 1 & 3 only
 c. 2 & 3 only
 d. 1, 2, & 3

D[485]

497. Which is the proper formula for calculating magnification?
 a. FFD/FOD
 b. FFD/OFD
 c. FOD/FFD
 d. OFD/FOD

498. Which of the following will decrease the effects of patient motion
 if the time is compensated to maintain the same density?
 1. increased mA
 2. increased kVp
 3. increased film/screen speed
 a. 1 & 2 only
 b. 1 & 3 only
 c. 2 & 3 only
 d. 1, 2, & 3

D[486]

499. Which of the following will increase recorded detail?
 1. decreased FFD
 2. decreased film/screen speed
 3. decreased OFD
 a. 1 & 2 only
 b. 1 & 3 only
 c. 2 & 3 only
 d. 1, 2, & 3

A[487]

500. Which film/screen characteristic/s best meet/s the needs where the
 primary consideration is high-speed?
 1. wide latitude
 2. increased patient exposure dose requirements
 3. high contrast
 a. 1 only
 b. 2 only
 c. 3 only
 d. 1, 2, & 3

C[488]

C[489]

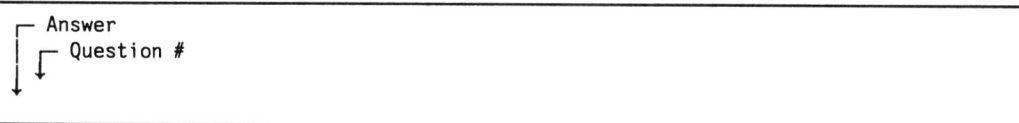

Answer
Question #

501. What is the grid ratio of a grid with lead strips 3.2 mm high, 0.3 mm wide, and with a distance between strips of 0.20 mm?
    a. 6:1
    b. 9:1
    c. 10:1
    d. 16:1

A⁵¹¹

502. Which of the following pathologic conditions would require increased technical factors to maintain image density as compared to normal tissue?
    1. tumor
    2. edema
    3. atrophy
    a. 1 & 2 only
    b. 1 & 3 only
    c. 2 & 3 only
    d. 1, 2, & 3

D⁵¹²

503. Which of the following time station changes would produce a visible change in radiographic density?
    1. from 0.03 s to 0.04 s
    2. from 0.75 s to 0.50 s
    3. from 0.80 s to 1.00 s
    a. 1 & 2 only
    b. 1 & 3 only
    c. 2 & 3 only
    d. 1, 2, & 3

B⁵¹³

C⁵¹⁴

504. Which of the following factors affect radiographic image density?
    1. distance
    2. filtration
    3. anatomic part size
    a. 1 & 2 only
    b. 1 & 3 only
    c. 2 & 3 only
    d. 1, 2, & 3

A⁵¹⁵

505. If a satisfactory radiograph is produced with 20 mAs at 40", what m As change should be made to produce an identical radiograph at 72"?
    a. 0.007 mAs
    b. 6.2 mAs
    c. 65 mAs
    d. 165 mAs

A⁵¹⁶

506. Which of the following will occur if exposure time is increased?
    1. mA will increase
    2. density will increase
    3. OFD will increase
        a. 1 only
        b. 2 only
        c. 3 only
        d. 1, 2, & 3

A^{496}

507. Which of the following factors are most often changed to correct the quality of the radiographic image?
    1. mAs
    2. kVp
    3. distance
        a. 1 & 2 only
        b. 1 & 3 only
        c. 2 & 3 only
        d. 1, 2, & 3

A^{497}

508. Which of the following is most effected by central ray alignment?
        a. density
        b. contrast
        c. distortion
        d. recorded detail

D^{498}

509. Which of the following are typical of high resolution film?
    1. slow-speed
    2. high contrast
    3. low patient dose requirements
        a. 1 & 2 only
        b. 1 & 3 only
        c. 2 & 3 only
        d. 1, 2, & 3

C^{499}

510. Which of the following affect radiographic density?
    1. average atomic number of tissue
    2. thickness of anatomic part
    3. disease processes that decrease tissue density
        a. 1 & 2 only
        b. 1 & 3 only
        c. 2 & 3 only
        d. 1, 2, & 3

C^{500}

511. What effect will be seen if the mA is increased for an automatic exposure device exposure?
    a. time will decrease
    b. time will increase
    c. density will increase
    d. density will decrease

512. Which radiographic quality factor can be described as the difference between adjacent densities?
    a. recorded detail
    b. distortion
    c. density
    d. contrast

513. What is the actual size of a lung mass that casts a shadow 1.5 cm wide on a PA chest radiograph produced at 180 cm when the mass is located 10.4 cm from the film?
    a. 1.06 cm
    b. 1.4 cm
    c. 1.5 cm
    d. 1.6 cm

A^{521}

514. Which of the following kVp ranges are appropriate for imaging the lumbar spine?
    a. 30 to 40
    b. 50 to 60
    c. 80 to 90
    d. 110 to 120

D^{522}

515. Which of the following chemicals are used in both the developer and fixer for automatic film processing solutions?
    a. sodium sulfite
    b. glutaraldehyde
    c. potassium bromide
    d. sodium carbonate

B^{523}

516. Which of the following will decrease recorded detail?
    a. decreased FFD
    b. decreased film/screen speed
    c. decreased OFD
    d. decreased focal spot size

D^{524}

Question # ⌐
Answer ⌐ |
↓ |
↓

517. Which of the following substances is most dense?
    a. fat
    b. muscle
    c. water
    d. bone

518. Which of the following are not affected by the use of radiographic   B⁵⁰⁶
    contrast media?
    1. recorded detail
    2. distortion
    3. density
        a. 1 & 2 only
        b. 1 & 3 only
        c. 2 & 3 only
        d. 1, 2, & 3

519. A 16:1 ratio grid has a non-grid conversion factor of 6.5, and a   A⁵⁰⁷
    12:1 grid has a non-grid conversion factor of 5.5. What mAs
    should be used to produce a radiograph of similar density with the
    12:1 grid when a satisfactory radiograph is produced using 120
    kVp and 3 mAs with the 16:1 ratio grid?
        a.   2.5 mAs   C⁵⁰⁸
        b.   3.5 mAs
        c. 10 mAs
        d. 19 mAs

520. Which of the four primary radiographic exposure factors is
    controlled primarily by kVp?
        a. density
        b. contrast
        c. recorded detail   A⁵⁰⁹
        d. distortion

                                                              D⁵¹⁰

141

B⁵³⁰

For items 521 to 525 use the following information: A satisfactory radiograph of an AP abdomen has been produced using the technical factors listed below. In each of the questions one factor has been changed. Indicate the result that will be seen on the radiograph as a result of each factor change.

C⁵³¹

400 mA
0.08 s
75 kVp
40" FFD
1" OFD
12:1 grid ratio
400 relative speed film/screens
2.5 mm focal spot
12" x 16" field size

C⁵³²

521. Changing the OFD to 0.5" would result in:
    a. decreased magnification
    b. increased magnification
    c. increased recorded detail
    d. lower contrast

C⁵³³

522. Which of the following sets of technical factors would maintain the same radiographic density if the 400 relative speed film/screen combination is changed to 200?
    a. 75 kVp, 400 mA, 0.04 s
    b. 75 kVp, 800 mA, 0.04 s
    c. 75 kVp, 800 mA, 0.16 s
    d. 86 kVp, 400 mA, 0.08 s

523. Collimating to a 4" x 4" primary beam field would result in:
    a. increased density
    b. decreased density
    c. grid cut-off
    d. focal spot blooming

D⁵³⁴

524. Changing the grid ratio to 10:1 would result in:
    a. decreased density and higher contrast
    b. decreased density and lower contrast
    c. increased density and higher contrast
    d. increased density and lower contrast

525. Which of the following sets of technical factors would achieve the same radiographic density?
    a. 64 kVp, 400 mA, 0.08 s
    b. 64 kVp, 200 mA, 0.32 s
    c. 75 kVp, 400 mA, 0.16 s
    d. 86 kVp, 400 mA, 0.08 s

D^{517}

526. What is the magnification factor for a foreign object that casts a shadow 5.4 cm wide on a PA abdomen radiograph produced at 100 cm when the mass is located 4.4 cm from the film?
    a. 0.96
    b. 1.01
    c. 1.04
    d. 1.05

A^{518}

527. Which technical factor exposure system has the advantage of being easier to remember?
    a. fixed kVp
    b. variable kVp
    c. high kVp
    d. anatomic proportion

528. Which of the following are not affected by the use of a grid?
    1. recorded detail
    2. distortion
    3. density
    a. 1 & 2 only
    b. 1 & 3 only
    c. 2 & 3 only
    d. 1, 2, & 3

A^{519}

529. Which of the following characteristics are common for radiographic films with a high average gradient?
    1. high contrast
    2. low-speed
    3. narrow latitude
    a. 1 & 2 only
    b. 1 & 3 only
    c. 2 & 3 only
    d. 1, 2, & 3

B^{520}

530. Which of the following best describes a grid cassette?
    a. a cassette without a lead back
    b. a cassette with a grid built into the front
    c. a cassette with a grid built into the back
    d. a cassette with a slight curvature toward the front

A^{538}

531. Which of the following is an older name for an automatic exposure control device?
    a. automatic brightness control
    b. orthocon tube
    c. phototimer
    d. valve tube

D^{539}

532. Which of the following generator types will produce the greatest radiographic density if all other factors remain the same?
    1. single-phase, 2-pulse
    2. three-phase, 6-pulse
    3. three-phase, 12-pulse
    a. 1 only
    b. 2 only
    c. 3 only
    d. 1, 2, & 3

A^{540}

533. Which of the following describes the relationship between mAs, x-ray exposure, and radiographic density?
    a. inverse square law
    b. density maintenance formula (direct square law)
    c. reciprocity law
    d. reciprocity law failure

B^{541}

534. Which of the following factors affect radiographic image density?
    1. grids
    2. film processing
    3. anatomic part size
    a. 1 & 2 only
    b. 1 & 3 only
    c. 2 & 3 only
    d. 1, 2, & 3

A^{542}

B^{543}

For items 535 to 538 use the following information: A
satisfactory oblique abdomen radiograph has been produced using
the technical factors listed below. In each of the questions one
factor has been changed. Indicate the result that will be seen on   B^{525}
the radiograph as a result of each factor change if all other factors
remain the same.

800 mA
0.04 s
76 kVp
40" FFD
2" OFD
10:1 grid ratio
200 relative speed film/screens
2.5 mm focal spot
13" x 17" field size

D^{526}

535. Changing the FFD to 36" would result in:
  1. increased magnification
  2. decreased recorded detail
  3. increased density
      a. 1 & 2 only
      b. 1 & 3 only
      c. 2 & 3 only
      d. 1, 2, & 3

A^{527}

536. If the kVp were raised by 10, what mAs would be required to
maintain the density if a 100 speed film/screen combination were
used?
      a. 8
      b. 16
      c. 32
      d. 64

A^{528}

537. Which of the following would result if collimation were changed
to 11" x 14"?
  1. higher contrast
  2. increased density
  3. decreased patient exposure dose
      a. 1 & 2 only
      b. 1 & 3 only
      c. 2 & 3 only
      d. 1, 2, & 3

B^{529}

538. Changing the distance to 55" would result in:
    a. decreased density and increased recorded detail
    b. decreased density and decreased recorded detail
    c. increased density and decreased recorded detail

B^{549}

539. A film/screen combination is rated with an arbitrary number of 400. If another film/screen combination is rated at 200, what adjustment must be made to correctly compensate radiographic density?
    a. decrease kVp by 7%
    b. decrease kVp by 15%
    c. decrease mAs to 1/2
    d. increase mAs by a factor of 2

B^{550}

540. Which technical factor exposure system has the advantage of providing maximum overall reductions in patient exposure dose?
    a. fixed kVp
    b. variable kVp
    c. high kVp
    d. anatomic proportion

541. What is the actual size of a lung mass that casts a shadow 3.4 cm wide on a PA chest radiograph produced at 100 cm when the mass is located 10.8 cm from the film?
    a. 1.16 cm
    b. 3.0 cm
    c. 3.4 cm
    d. 3.8 cm

A^{551}

542. Which of the following kVp ranges are appropriate for imaging the hand?
    a. 40 to 60
    b. 70 to 80
    c. 80 to 90
    d. 110 to 120

C^{552}

543. Which automatic film processing chemical rapidly produces fine recorded detail shades of gray on the film?
    a. hydroquinone
    b. phenidone
    c. potassium bromide
    d. sodium carbonate

C^{553}

Question # ⌐
Answer ⌐ │
          ↓ │
            │
            ↓

544. Which of the following will minimize size distortion?
     1. increased FFD
     2. increased film/screen speed
     3. decreased OFD
        a. 1 & 2 only
        b. 1 & 3 only
        c. 2 & 3 only
        d. 1, 2, & 3

545. Which demonstrates proper use of the anode heel theory?
     1. AP femur with anode toward hip
     2. AP thoracic spine with cathode toward neck
     3. lateral lumbar spine with cathode toward pelvis
        a. 1 only
        b. 2 only
        c. 3 only
        d. 1, 2, & 3

546. Which of the following is/are size distortion?
        a. elongation and foreshortening
        b. elongation and magnification
        c. foreshortening and magnification
        d. magnification

547. Which of the following material/s is/are commonly used for
     interspace material in radiographic grids?
     1. iodine
     2. barium
     3. aluminum
        a. 1 only
        b. 2 only
        c. 3 only
        d. 1, 2, & 3

D^{535}

548. Which pathological conditions would require decreased technical
     factors to maintain image density as compared to normal tissue?
     1. degenerative arthritis
     2. fibrosarcoma
     3. osteoporosis
        a. 1 & 2 only
        b. 1 & 3 only
        c. 2 & 3 only
        d. 1, 2, & 3

C^{536}

B^{537}

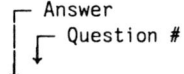

Answer
Question #

549. Which of the following mAs values would produce a visible density difference from a radiograph of the same part at 12 mAs?
   1. 8
   2. 14
   3. 16
      a. 1 & 2 only
      b. 1 & 3 only
      c. 2 & 3 only
      d. 1, 2, & 3

550. Which of the following physical interactions between radiation and matter most inhibits the production of high radiographic contrast?
      a. photoelectric
      b. Compton effect
      c. pair production
      d. photodisintegration

551. Which of the following would require approximately twice the mAs to maintain the same radiographic density as a film produced at 80 kVp with a 6:1 ratio grid?
   1. 80 kVp with an 8:1 grid
   2. 92 kVp with a 10:1 grid
   3. 92 kVp with a 16:1 grid
      a. 1 & 2 only
      b. 1 & 3 only
      c. 2 & 3 only
      d. 1, 2, & 3

C^{558}

552. What happens to the optical density value (OD) as measured by a densitometer from a sensitometric step wedge after a sensitometric film curve passes D$_{max}$?
      a. remains the same
      b. increases
      c. decreases
      d. varies inversely with the square of the OD value

B^{559}

553. What effects does increased collimation of the primary beam have on radiographic image contrast and density?
      a. contrast and density increase
      b. contrast and density decrease
      c. contrast increases and density decreases
      d. contrast decreases and density increases

D^{560}

554. What effect will be seen if the mA is decreased for an automatic exposure device exposure?
    a. time will decrease
    b. time will increase
    c. density will increase
    d. density will decrease

B[544]

555. Which of the following will increase size distortion?
    1. increased OFD
    2. decreased film/screen speed
    3. decreased FFD
    a. 1 & 2 only
    b. 1 & 3 only
    c. 2 & 3 only
    d. 1, 2, & 3

C[545]

556. Which of the following would require approximately a 15% decrease in kVp to maintain the same radiographic density as a film produced at 90 kVp with a 12:1 ratio grid?
    1. 90 kVp with an 8:1 grid
    2. 90 kVp with a 10:1 grid
    3. 120 kVp with a 16:1 grid
    a. 1 & 2 only
    b. 1 & 3 only
    c. 2 & 3 only
    d. 1, 2, & 3

D[546]

557. What is the primary rule for determining kVp changes in a variable kVp radiographic exposure technique system?
    a. 2 kVp per cm
    b. 5 kVp per cm
    c. kVp x 15% cm
    d. kVp x cm x 3.

D[547]

D[548]

149

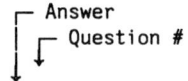

D⁵⁶⁶

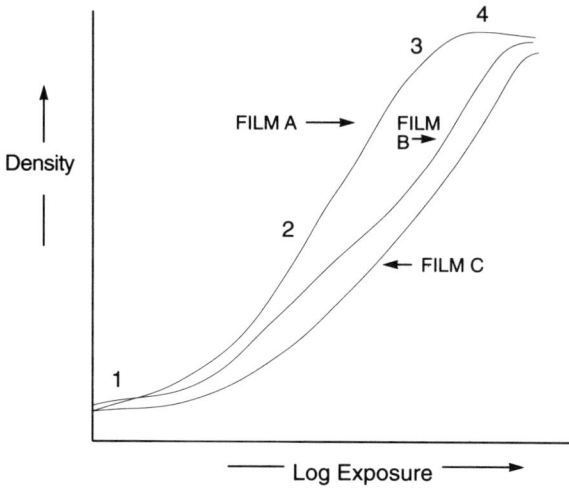

Figure 13

B⁵⁶⁷

D⁵⁶⁸

558. What term is used to describe the portion of the curve in Figure 13 that is labeled 1?
   a. D_{max}
   b. straight line portion
   c. toe
   d. shoulder

559. What term is used to describe the portion of the curve in Figure 13 that is labeled 2?
   a. D_{max}
   b. straight line portion
   c. toe
   d. shoulder

C⁵⁶⁹

560. What term is used to describe the portion of the curve in Figure 13 that is labeled 3?
   a. D_{max}
   b. straight line portion
   c. toe
   d. shoulder

561. What term is used to describe the portion of the curve in Figure 13 that is labeled 4?
    a. D_{max}
    b. straight line portion
    c. toe
    d. shoulder

B^{554}

562. Which of the curves in Figure 13 has the greatest speed?
    1. film A
    2. film B
    3. film C
       a. 1 only
       b. 2 only
       c. 3 only
       d. 1, 2, & 3

B^{555}

563. Which of the curves in Figure 13 has the greatest contrast?
    1. A
    2. B
    3. C
       a. 1 only
       b. 2 only
       c. 3 only
       d. 1, 2, & 3

C^{556}

564. Which of the curves in Figure 13 has the widest latitude?
    1. A
    2. B
    3. C
       a. 1 only
       b. 2 only
       c. 3 only
       d. 1, 2, & 32

A^{557}

565. Which of the following time station changes would produce a visible change in radiographic density?
    1. from 0.12 s to 0.16 s
    2. from 0.35 s to 0.30 s
    3. from 0.02 s to 0.03 s
       a. 1 & 2 only
       b. 1 & 3 only
       c. 2 & 3 only
       d. 1, 2, & 3

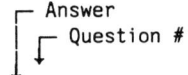

566. Which of the following factors affect radiographic image density?
    1. beam restriction
    2. film/screen combination
    3. filtration
       a. 1 & 2 only
       b. 1 & 3 only
       c. 2 & 3 only
       d. 1, 2, & 3

B⁵⁷⁵ 567. Which of the following are primarily controlled by the characteristics of the radiographic film?
    1. latitude
    2. resolution
    3. contrast
D⁵⁷⁶   a. 1 & 2 only
       b. 1 & 3 only
       c. 2 & 3 only
       d. 1, 2, & 3

568. If a focused grid is used off-level so that it is not parallel to the image receptor or perpendicular to the central ray, how will the resulting image appear?
B⁵⁷⁷   a. decreased density from edge to edge
       b. increased density from edge to edge
       c. increased density at both edges
       d. decreased density at one edge

569. Which of the following pathologic conditions would require decreased technical factors to maintain image density as compared to normal
D⁵⁷⁸   tissue?
    1. pneumonia
    2. pneumothorax
    3. emphysema
       a. 1 & 2 only
B⁵⁷⁹   b. 1 & 3 only
       c. 2 & 3 only
       d. 1, 2, & 3

570. Which of the following will change as a result of using a compression band on the abdomen of a large patient?
1. subject density
2. subject contrast
3. radiographic density
   a. 1 & 2 only
   b. 1 & 3 only
   c. 2 & 3 only
   d. 1, 2, & 3

A⁵⁶¹

571. Which of the following technical factors would produce a radiograph with the highest scale contrast?
   a. 800 mA, 0.02 s, 72 kVp
   b. 600 mA, 0.03 s, 82 kVp
   c. 400 mA, 0.04 s, 82 kVp
   d. 200 mA, 0.04 s, 94 kVp

A⁵⁶²

572. Which of the following will produce a decrease in contrast without changing density?
   a. increasing kVp and decreasing mAs
   b. increasing kVp and increasing mAs
   c. decreasing mAs with no change in kVp
   d. decreasing kVp with no change in mAs

A⁵⁶³

573. Which of the primary radiographic exposure factor/s is/are controlled by geometric factors such as distance?
1. density
2. contrast
3. recorded detail
   a. 1 only
   b. 2 only
   c. 3 only
   d. 1, 2, & 3

C⁵⁶⁴

574. Which of the following conditions contribute to increased recorded detail?
1. small effective focal spot size
2. long FFD
3. short OFD
   a. 1 & 2 only
   b. 1 & 3 only
   c. 2 & 3 only
   d. 1, 2, & 3

B⁵⁶⁵

Image Production and Evaluation

For items 575 to 578, choose the technical factors that would produce the greatest density on radiographic film if all other factors were to remain unknown?

A⁵⁸⁵ 575.

	mA	s	kVp	FFD	grid	film/screen
a.	400	0.01	98	40"	10:1	100
b.	200	0.04	85	40"	8:1	100
c.	400	0.02	85	40"	12:1	100
d.	800	0.01	85	40"	12:1	100

576.

C⁵⁸⁶

	mA	s	kVp	FFD	grid	film/screen
a.	100	8/10	50	40"	12:1	100
b.	200	2/10	58	40"	12:1	100
c.	200	1/10	67	40"	12:1	100
d.	400	1/20	77	40"	12:1	100

577.

	mA	s	kVp	FFD	grid	film/screen
a.	200	0.08	60	40"	10:1	200
b.	400	0.02	79	40"	10:1	400
c.	400	0.01	79	40"	10:1	400
d.	800	0.01	91	40"	10:1	100

B⁵⁸⁷ 578.

	mA	s	kVp	FFD	grid	film/screen
a.	100	0.6	90	40"	2:1	100
b.	200	0.3	77	40"	12:1	200
c.	200	0.2	90	40"	12:1	100
d.	400	0.15	77	40"	12:1	100

579. Which exposure system permits minute density adjustments?
   a. fixed kVp
   b. variable kVp
   c. high kVp
   d. anatomic proportion

B⁵⁸⁸

580. Which radiographic quality factor can be described as the amount of geometric sharpness or accuracy of the image?
   a. recorded detail
   b. distortion
   c. density
   d. contrast

A⁵⁸⁹

581. Which film/screen characteristics meet the needs in a clinical situation such as mobile radiography where the primary consideration is wide latitude?
  1. slow-speed
  2. increased patient exposure dose requirements
  3. high contrast
     a. 1 & 2 only
     b. 1 & 3 only
     c. 2 & 3 only
     d. 1, 2, & 3

D^{570}

582. Which of the following are typical of low resolution film?
  1. high-speed
  2. narrow latitude
  3. low patient dose requirements
     a. 1 & 2 only
     b. 1 & 3 only
     c. 2 & 3 only
     d. 1, 2, & 3

D^{571}

583. A 5:1 ratio grid has a non-grid conversion factor of 3, and a 12:1 grid has a non-grid conversion factor of 5. What mAs should be used to produce a radiograph of similar density with the 5:1 grid when a satisfactory radiograph is produced using 65 kVp and 12 mAs with the 12:1 ratio grid?
     a. 7 mAs
     b. 10 mAs
     c. 20 mAs
     d. 36 mAs

A^{572}

584. What is the grid ratio of a grid with lead strips 1.5 mm high, 0.25mm wide, and with a distance between strips of 0.19 mm?
     a. 6:1
     b. 8:1
     c. 10:1
     d. 16:1

C^{573}

D^{574}

155

585. Which technical factor exposure system has the advantage of maintaining nearly equal contrast from one projection to another within a single procedure?
    a. fixed kVp
    b. variable kVp
    c. high kVp
    d. anatomic proportion

A⁵⁹⁵

586. Which of the following projections takes advantage of the divergence of the primary beam to reduce distortion?
    1. AP lumbar spine
    2. PA thoracic spine
    3. lateral L5-S1 lumbar spot
    a. 1 only
    b. 2 only
    c. 3 only
    d. 1, 2, & 3

C⁵⁹⁶

587. Which of the following are affected by intensifying screen phosphor size and layer thickness?
    1. density
    2. distortion
    3. recorded detail
    a. 1 & 2 only
    b. 1 & 3 only
    c. 2 & 3 only
    d. 1, 2, & 3

B⁵⁹⁷

588. Which of the following characteristics are common for radiographic films with high contrast?
    1. high average gradient
    2. low-speed
    3. narrow latitude
    a. 1 & 2 only
    b. 1 & 3 only
    c. 2 & 3 only
    d. 1, 2, & 3

B⁵⁹⁸

589. Which end of the x-ray tube produces less intensity due to the anode heel effect?
    a. anode
    b. cathode
    c. window side
    d. opposite of window side

D⁵⁹⁹

590. What effects will be seen if the density control is increased for an automatic exposure device exposure?
    1. time will decrease
    2. time will increase
    3. density will increase
        a. 1 & 2 only
        b. 1 & 3 only
        c. 2 & 3 only
        d. 1, 2, & 3

A^{581}

591. What is the optimal kVp to produce the highest contrast with barium contrast media?
        a. 35
        b. 68
        c. 80
        d. 120

592. What is the minimum change necessary to produce a visible radiographic density difference?
        a. 5%
        b. 15%
        c. 30%
        d. 75%

B^{582}

593. Which of the following have the ability to increase image density by increasing x-ray tube output?
    1. a high vacuum inside the glass envelope
    2. a smooth anode focal track
    3. decreased added filtration
        a. 1 & 2 only
        b. 1 & 3 only
        c. 2 & 3 only
        d. 1, 2, & 3

A^{583}

594. Which of the following will produce visible changes in radiographic contrast?
    1. mAs
    2. primary beam field size
    3. grid ratio
        a. 1 & 2 only
        b. 1 & 3 only
        c. 2 & 3 only
        d. 1, 2, & 3

B^{584}

595. If a satisfactory radiograph is produced with 18 mAs at 72", what mAs change should be made to produce an identical radiograph at 40"?
    a. 6 mAs
    b. 10 mAs
    c. 16 mAs
    d. 58 mAs

A^{605} 596. Which of the following factors is considered to be the prime factor that regulates radiographic contrast?
    1. mA
    2. time
    3. kVp
        a. 1 only
        b. 2 only
        c. 3 only
        d. 1, 2, & 3

B^{606} 597. Which of the following physical interactions between radiation and matter most assists in producing long scale radiographic contrast?
    a. photoelectric
    b. Compton effect
    c. pair production
    d. photodisintegration

B^{607} 598. Which of the following kVp ranges is appropriate for imaging the knee?
    a. 40 to 50
    b. 60 to 70
    c. 80 to 90
    d. 110 to 120

599. Which of the following can be used to compensate for a faster film/screen combination?
    1. decrease mAs
    2. decrease kVp
    3. increase FFD
        a. 1 only
        b. 2 only
        c. 3 only
        d. 1, 2, & 3

D^{608}

C^{609}

Question # ┐
Answer ┐ │
↓ │
↓

600. Which automatic film processing chemical slowly produces heavy densities on the film?
    a. hydroquinone
    b. phenidone
    c. potassium bromide
    d. sodium carbonate

601. Which of the following will increase recorded detail?   C^{590}
    1. decreased focal spot size
    2. decreased OFD
    3. decreased FFD
      a. 1 & 2 only
      b. 1 & 3 only   D^{591}
      c. 2 & 3 only
      d. 1, 2, & 3

602. Which of the following demonstrates proper use of the anode heel theory?
    1. AP femur with anode toward knee
    2. lateral humerus with anode toward elbow   C^{592}
    3. lateral thoracic spine with cathode toward neck
      a. 1 only
      b. 2 only
      c. 3 only
      d. 1, 2, & 3

603. Which of the following substances is least dense?
      a. fat
      b. muscle
      c. water   D^{593}
      d. bone

604. Which of the following are advantages of rare earth intensifying screens?
    1. reduced patient exposure dose
    2. use of lower power generators
    3. increased tube life
      a. 1 & 2 only
      b. 1 & 3 only
      c. 2 & 3 only
      d. 1, 2, & 3   C^{594}

┌ Answer
│ ┌ Question #
↓ ↓

D^{615}

605. Which of the following conditions best uses a parallel grid?
1. long FFD
2. small angle anode
3. small focal spot
   a. 1 only
   b. 2 only
   c. 3 only
   d. 1, 2, & 3

C^{616}

606. Which pathologic conditions would require increased technical factors to maintain image density as compared to normal tissue?
1. ascites
2. bowel obstruction
3. cirrhosis
   a. 1 & 2 only
   b. 1 & 3 only
   c. 2 & 3 only
   d. 1, 2, & 3

B^{617}

607. In which kVp range does the 15% rule function best?
1. 30 to 50
2. 50 to 80
3. 80 to 120
   a. 1 only
   b. 2 only
   c. 3 only
   d. 1, 2, & 3

A^{618}

608. Which will produce visible changes in radiographic contrast?
1. kVp
2. primary beam field size
3. grid ratio
   a. 1 & 2 only
   b. 1 & 3 only
   c. 2 & 3 only
   d. 1, 2, & 3

B^{619}

609. A film/screen combination is rated with an arbitrary number of 400. If another film/screen combination is rated at 200, what adjustment must be made to correctly compensate radiographic density?
   a. decrease kVp by 7%
   b. decrease kVp by 15%
   c. increase kVp by 15%
   d. decrease mAs by 1/2

Question # ⌐
Answer ⌐ |
↓ |
↓

610. Which of the following technical factors would produce a radiograph with the shortest scale contrast?
    a. 100 mA, 0.02 s, 58 kVp
    b. 100 mA, 0.04 s, 50 kVp
    c. 400 mA, 0.01 s, 50 kVp
    d. 400 mA, 0.02 s, 43 kVp
          A[600]

611. Which of the following will decrease patient motion?
    1. increased mA
    2. decreased kVp
    3. decreased FFD
    a. 1 & 2 only
    b. 1 & 3 only
    c. 2 & 3 only
    d. 1, 2, & 3
          A[601]

612. Which of the following will decrease if film-screen contact is poor?
    1. resolution
    2. density
    3. magnification
    a. 1 only
    b. 2 only
    c. 3 only
    d. 1, 2, & 3
          D[602]

613. Which of the following is increased by decreasing part thickness?
    a. recorded detail
    b. distortion
    c. contrast
    d. density
          A[603]

614. Which of the following will change as a result of increasing the x-ray tube angle in relationship to the film?
    1. density
    2. contrast
    3. distortion
    a. 1 only
    b. 2 only
    c. 3 only
    d. 1, 2, & 3
          D[604]

615. Which automatic film processing chemical maintains the pH of the fixer and controls oxidation of the developer?
    a. hydroquinone
    b. phenidone
    c. potassium bromide
    d. sodium sulfite

C[624]

616. Which of the following will minimize size distortion?
    a. decreased FFD
    b. increased film/screen speed
    c. decreased OFD
    d. increased focal spot size

617. Which of the following demonstrates improper use of the anode heel theory?
    1. AP lower leg with anode toward hip
A[625]
    2. AP thoracic spine with cathode toward neck
    3. AP lumbar spine with cathode toward pelvis
    a. 1 only
    b. 2 only
    c. 3 only
    d. 1, 2, & 3

618. Which of the following is/are shape distortion?
    a. elongation and foreshortening
D[626]
    b. elongation and magnification
    c. foreshortening and magnification
    d. magnification

619. Which of the following is controlled primarily by the characteristics of the intensifying screen?
    1. latitude
A[627]
    2. resolution
    3. contrast
    a. 1 only
    b. 2 only
    c. 3 only
    d. 1, 2, & 3

620. Which of the following characteristics are common for radiographic films with a high speed?
    1. low average gradient
    2. high contrast
    3. narrow latitude
        a. 1 & 2 only
        b. 1 & 3 only
        c. 2 & 3 only
        d. 1, 2, & 3

D^{610}

621. A focused grid has an imaginary line, often called the convergence line, that exists in space at an established distance over the grid. What object must be placed along the convergence line to avoid grid cut-off?
        a. the patient entrance skin surface
        b. the structures of interest within the patient
        c. the tabletop
        d. the x-ray tube focal spot

B^{611}

622. Which of the following technical exposure factor changes would compensate for tissue with a disease process that has decreased the attenuation of the primary beam?
    1. decreased mAs
    2. increased distance
    3. increased kVp
        a. 1 & 2 only
        b. 1 & 3 only
        c. 2 & 3 only
        d. 1, 2, & 3

A^{612}

623. What function is served by calipers in a radiographic room?
        a. verification of tabletop to bucky tray distance
        b. measurement of size of primary beam field
        c. measurement of patient part size for establishing technical factors
        d. absorbing scattered radiation during skull radiography

D^{613}

D^{614}

624. Which of the following time station changes would not produce a visible change in radiographic density?
    1. from 0.15 s to 0.20 s
    2. from 0.50 s to 0.40 s
    3. from 2.00 s to 1.50 s
        a. 1 & 2 only
        b. 1 & 3 only
        c. 2 & 3 only
        d. 1, 2, & 3

C⁶³²

625. Which of the following mAs values would not produce a visible density difference from a radiograph of the same part at 35 mAs?
    1. 30
    2. 40
    3. 47
        a. 1 & 2 only
        b. 1 & 3 only
        c. 2 & 3 only
        d. 1, 2, & 3

A⁶³³

D⁶³⁴

626. Which of the following factors affect radiographic image density?
    1. distance
    2. grids
    3. anatomic part size
        a. 1 & 2 only
        b. 1 & 3 only
        c. 2 & 3 only
        d. 1, 2, & 3

B⁶³⁵

627. Which of the following has the greatest effect on recorded detail?
        a. focal spot size
        b. mAs
        c. kVp
        d. anode target angle

D⁶³⁶

For items 628 to 631 use the following information: A satisfactory axial shoulder radiograph has been produced using the technical factors listed below. In each of the questions one factor has been changed. Indicate the result that will be seen on the radiograph as a result of each factor change if all other factors remain the same.

100 mA
0.06 s
65 kVp
40" FFD
3" OFD
no grid
200 relative speed film/screens   C[620]
1.2 mm focal spot
6" x 9" field size

628. Changing to a 0.8 focal spot would result in:
    1. increased magnification
    2. increased recorded detail
    3. increased density
        a. 1 only
        b. 2 only
        c. 3 only   D[621]
        d. 1, 2, & 3

629. If the kVp were changed to 55, what mAs would be required to
    maintain the density if a 100 speed film/screen combination were
    used?
        a. 3
        b. 6
        c. 12
        d. 24

630. Which of the following would result if collimation were changed A[622]
    to 11" x 14"?
    1. higher contrast
    2. increased density
    3. increased patient exposure dose
        a. 1 & 2 only
        b. 1 & 3 only
        c. 2 & 3 only   C[623]
        d. 1, 2, & 3

631. Changing the distance to 55" would result in:
        a. decreased density and no change in recorded detail
        b. decreased density and decreased recorded detail
        c. increased density and decreased recorded detail
        d. increased density and no change in recorded detail

Image Production and Evaluation

A⁶⁴²

632. Which of the following terms correctly describes a gross distortion of an object in which the image, usually one end, appears to be larger than the original object while the other end is an accurate, although slightly enlarged, representation?
    a. spatial distortion
    b. geometric unsharpness
    c. elongation
    d. foreshortening

D⁶⁴³

633. Which of the following physical interactions between x-rays and matter most assists in producing high radiographic contrast?
    a. photoelectric
    b. Compton effect
    c. pair production
    d. photodisintegration

C⁶⁴⁴

634. Which of the following technical factors would produce a radiograph with the longest contrast?
    a. 100 mA, 0.60 s, 72 kVp
    b. 100 mA, 0.30 s, 82 kVp
    c. 200 mA, 0.15 s, 82 kVp
    d. 200 mA, 0.08 s, 94 kVp

635. Which automatic film processor replenishment rate is highest?
    1. developer
    2. fixer
    3. wash
    a. 1 only
    b. 2 only
    c. 3 only
    d. 1, 2, & 3

636. Which of the following will not cause loss of recorded detail?
    1. kVp changes
    2. mAs changes
    3. subject density changes
    a. 1 only
    b. 2 only
    c. 3 only
    d. 1, 2, & 3

C⁶⁴⁵

637. Which of the following will produce an increase in contrast without changing density?
    a. increasing kVp and decreasing mAs
    b. increasing kVp and increasing mAs
    c. decreasing kVp and decreasing mAs
    d. decreasing kVp and increasing mAs

For items 638 to 641, choose the technical factors that would produce the greatest density on radiographic film if all other factors were to remain identical.

638.

	mA	s	kVp	FFD	grid	film/screen
a.	400	0.02	85	72"	10:1	100
b.	200	0.04	85	72"	10:1	100
c.	400	0.02	85	40"	10:1	100
d.	800	0.01	85	72"	10:1	100

C [628]

639.

	mA	s	kVp	FFD	grid	film/screen
a.	200	8/10	80	40"	12:1	100
b.	400	2/10	80	40"	12:1	100
c.	400	1/10	92	40"	12:1	100
d.	800	1/20	106	40"	12:1	100

B [629]

640.

	mA	s	kVp	FFD	grid	film/screen
a.	100	0.16	60	40"	10:1	400
b.	400	0.04	79	40"	10:1	400
c.	800	0.01	79	40"	10:1	400
d.	800	0.02	91	40"	10:1	400

641.

	mA	s	kVp	FFD	grid	film/screen
a.	100	0.3	90	40"	12:1	100
b.	100	0.3	77	40"	12:1	200
c.	100	0.2	90	40"	12:1	100
d.	400	0.3	77	40"	12:1	100

B [630]

A [631]

642. If a satisfactory radiograph is produced with 2.4 mAs at 40", what m As change should be made to produce an identical radiograph at 32"?
   a. 1.5 mAs
   b. 1.9 mAs
   c. 3.0 mAs
   d. 3.8 mAs

D⁶⁵¹

643. A film/screen combination is rated with an arbitrary number of 200. If another film/screen combination is rated at 400, what adjustment must be made to correctly compensate radiographic density?
   a. increase kVp by 7%
   b. increase kVp by 15%
   c. increase mAs by a factor of 2
   d. decrease mAs to 1/2

B⁶⁵²

644. If there is a choice of right, left, and center ion chambers with an automatic exposure device, which should be activated when radiographing an AP lumbar spine?
   a. right, left, and center
   b. right and left
   c. center only
   d. right only

B⁶⁵³

For items 645 to 650 use the following information: A satisfactory radiograph of an AP knee has been produced using the technical factors listed below. In each of the questions one factor has been changed. Indicate the result that will be seen on the radiograph as a result of each factor change.

100 mA
0.08 s
60 kVp
40" FFD
0.5" OFD
12:1 grid ratio
100 relative speed film/screens
2.5 mm focal spot
10" x 12" field size

A⁶⁵⁴

645. Changing the focal spot to 1.0 mm would result in:
   a. decreased magnification
   b. increased magnification
   c. increased recorded detail
   d. lower contrast

646. Which of the following sets of technical factors would maintain the same radiographic density if the mA station was changed to 50?
    a. 51 kVp and 0.08 s
    b. 51 kVp and 0.16 s
    c. 60 kVp and 0.16 s
    d. 69 kVp and 0.16 s

D^{637}

647. Which of the following would compensate for removing the grid?
    1. decreasing mAs
    2. increasing kVp
    3. increasing FFD
    a. 1 & 2 only
    b. 1 & 3 only
    c. 2 & 3 only
    d. 1, 2, & 3

C^{638}

648. If the field size is changed to 14" x 17", which of the following would occur?
    1. contrast would decrease
    2. density would increase
    3. recorded detail would decrease
    a. 1 & 2 only
    b. 1 & 3 only
    c. 2 & 3 only
    d. 1, 2, & 3

A^{639}

649. Changing the film/screen combination relative speed to 80 would result in:
    a. increased density
    b. decreased density
    c. increased recorded detail
    d. decreased recorded detail

B^{640}

650. Which of the following sets of technical factors would achieve the same radiographic density?
    a. 51 kVp, 100 mA, 0.08 s
    b. 51 kVp, 200 mA, 0.08 s
    c. 60 kVp, 200 mA, 0.04 s
    d. 69 kVp, 200 mA, 0.04 s

D^{641}

651. Which of the following are used to determine the resolving ability of a film/screen combination?
    1. modulation transfer function
    2. line spread function
    3. line pairs per millimeter
        a. 1 & 2 only
        b. 1 & 3 only
        c. 2 & 3 only
        d. 1, 2, & 3

A⁶⁵⁹

652. Which of the following is typical of high resolution film?
    1. high-speed
    2. high contrast
    3. low patient dose requirements
        a. 1 only
        b. 2 only
        c. 3 only
        d. 1, 2, & 3

C⁶⁶⁰

653. Which of the following would increase radiographic density?
    1. decreased developer temperature
    2. high temperature in film storage area
    3. decreased fixing time
        a. 1 only
        b. 2 only
        c. 3 only
        d. 1, 2, & 3

A⁶⁶¹

654. An 8:1 ratio grid has a non-grid conversion factor of 4, and a 16:1 grid has a non-grid conversion factor of 7. What mAs should be used to produce a radiograph of similar density with the 16:1 grid when a satisfactory radiograph is produced using 90 kVp and 4 mAs with the 8:1 ratio grid?
        a.   7 mAs
        b. 10 mAs
        c. 20 mAs
        d. 36 mAs

A⁶⁶²

A⁶⁶³

655. Which of the following pathologic conditions would require increased technical factors to maintain image density as compared to normal tissue?
    1. chronic osteomyelitis
    2. acromegaly C^{646}
    3. aseptic necrosis
      a. 1 & 2 only
      b. 1 & 3 only
      c. 2 & 3 only
      d. 1, 2, & 3

656. Which of the following films would most likely have the highest speed?
    1. low contrast B^{647}
    2. narrow latitude
    3. low base-plus-fog
      a. 1 only
      b. 2 only
      c. 3 only
      d. 1, 2, & 3

657. Which of the following describes the effect that occurs when extremely long exposure times (in excess of 10 s) may cause the proportional relationship between mAs and density to change?
      a. inverse square law A^{648}
      b. density maintenance formula (direct square law)
      c. reciprocity law
      d. reciprocity law failure

658. Which of the primary radiographic exposure factors are controlled by geometric factors such as distance?
    1. contrast B^{649}
    2. distortion
    3. recorded detail
      a. 1 & 2 only
      b. 1 & 3 only
      c. 2 & 3 only
      d. 1, 2, & 3 C^{650}

┌─ Answer
│ ┌─ Question #
↓ ↓

Film Processing and Quality Assurance 5% (70) 659-728

659. Which sensitometric measures of processor quality control would be expected as a result of developer contamination by fixer?
    1. increased base-plus-fog
    2. decreased speed
    3. higher contrast index
        a. 1 & 2 only
        b. 1 & 3 only
        c. 2 & 3 only
        d. 1, 2, & 3

A⁶⁶⁹

660. What causes a black, crescent, half moon artifact on a radiograph?
        a. static discharge
        b. handling with dry hands
        c. bending the film
        d. improperly aligned guide shoe deflectors

C⁶⁷⁰

661. What is a typical fixer replenishment rate for an automatic film processor?
        a. 6 to 8 ml/in
        b. 25 to 50 ml/in
        c. 100 to 200 ml/in
        d. 500 to 600 ml/in

D⁶⁷¹

662. Which of the following are functions of an automatic processor transport system?
    1. control of film immersion time
    2. agitation of solutions
    3. seal emulsions
        a. 1 & 2 only
        b. 1 & 3 only
        c. 2 & 3 only
        d. 1, 2, & 3

B⁶⁷²

663. Which of the following information are appropriate for the identification blocker area of the film?
    1. patient name
    2. procedure performed
    3. physician age
        a. 1 & 2 only
        b. 1 & 3 only
        c. 2 & 3 only
        d. 1, 2, & 3

A⁶⁷³

664. What conditions will cause static discharge artifacts on film?
    a. high humidity
    b. high temperature
    c. low humidity
    d. low temperature

665. Which metric size is equivalent to a 14" x 17" cassette?
    a. 18 cm x 24 cm
    b. 24 cm x 30 cm
    c. 30 cm x 35 cm
    d. 35 cm x 43 cm

A^{655}

666. Which type of intensifying screen cassette would produce the lowest patient exposure dose?
    a. detail calcium tungstate
    b. medium-speed calcium tungstate
    c. high-speed calcium tungstate
    d. high-speed rare earth

667. Which of the following is the most likely result of an improperly seated crossover network in an automatic film processor?
    a. black lines the length of the radiograph
    b. white lines the length of the radiograph
    c. regularly repeated black marks the length of the radiograph
    d. black, crescent, half moon marks

B^{656}

668. What is the approximate fixer immersion time for a film in a 90-second processor?
    a. 1 to 5 seconds
    b. 20 to 25 seconds
    c. 45 to 60 seconds
    d. 90 seconds

D^{657}

C^{658}

┌ Answer
│ ┌ Question #
↓ ↓

669. Which of the following are potential causes of films exiting an automatic processor with an overall light gray appearance, lacking cl ear white or completely black densities?
1. weak developer solution
2. developer solution contamination
3. insufficient washing
   a. 1 & 2 only
   b. 1 & 3 only
   c. 2 & 3 only
   d. 1, 2, & 3

D^{679}

670. Which of the following best describes an artifact?
   a. an object embedded within the film emulsion
   b. a device used to extract films from cassettes
   c. a mark or other foreign image on a radiograph
   d. a bubbling of the emulsion due to failure of the base adhesive

C^{680}

671. Which of the following color safelights would produce safe conditions for working with blue-violet sensitive film?
   a. blue-violet
   b. yellow-green
   c. dark red
   d. orange-brown

B^{681}

672. What is the proper method of mixing concentrated film processing solutions?
   a. add water to concentrated chemicals
   b. add concentrated chemicals to water
   c. add water and concentrated chemicals simultaneously
   d. concentrated chemicals must be diluted before adding to water

B^{682}

673. Which of the following are subsystems of an automatic processor transport system?
1. crossover network
2. transport rack drive system
3. replenishment system
   a. 1 & 2 only
   b. 1 & 3 only
   c. 2 & 3 only
   d. 1, 2, & 3

C^{683}

674. Which of the following are true about the radiograph?
1. it is a legal medical record
2. it can be subpoenaed by a court of law
3. it is the property of the patient
   a. 1 & 2 only
   b. 1 & 3 only
   c. 2 & 3 only
   d. 1, 2, & 3

C^{664}

675. A test is performed where an unexposed film is placed on the darkroom work bench and covered with a light-proof piece of cardboard while 2" portions are uncovered at 10-second intervals until the entire film is uncovered. The film is then processed. Which of the following describes this procedure?
   a. static discharge test
   b. safelight test
   c. base-plus-fog test
   d. film-screen contact test

D^{665}

D^{666}

676. Which of the following would cause white artifacts on a radiograph?
   a. dirt in the cassette
   b. handling film with damp hands
   c. abrasion of the film surface during handling
   d. sharp bending of the film during handling

B^{667}

677. Which of the following contribute to the regulation of solution temperatures in an automatic film processor?
1. recirculation system
2. developer heater
3. dryer blower
   a. 1 & 2 only
   b. 1 & 3 only
   c. 2 & 3 only
   d. 1, 2, & 3

B^{668}

678. What is a penetrometer?
   a. a step wedge, usually of aluminum or plastic
   b. a device that produces a uniform optical scale of densities on a film
   c. a device to measure film density
   d. a device to measure radiation exposure dose

679. Which of the following are sensitometric measurements that should be taken daily on all radiographic film processors?
    1. base-plus-fog
    2. contrast index
    3. speed
        a. 1 & 2 only
        b. 1 & 3 only
        c. 2 & 3 only
        d. 1, 2, & 3

C⁶⁸⁹

680. Which of the following types of silver recovery methods is dangerous because of the fumes produced by the silver recovery process?
        a. metallic replacement
        b. electrolytic
        c. chemical precipitation
        d. resin

C⁶⁹⁰

681. What is an appropriate power light bulb for a safelight approximately 4 feet from a film working surface?
        a. 1 to 2 watts
        b. 7 to 15 watts
        c. 60 to 100 watts
        d. 200 to 250 watts

B⁶⁹¹

682. Which of the following could produce increased base-plus-fog levels during sensitometric evaluation of radiographic film?
    1. fixer fumes
    2. rough handling of film
    3. increased developer temperature
        a. 1 & 2 only
        b. 1 & 3 only
        c. 2 & 3 only
        d. 1, 2, & 3

A⁶⁹²

C⁶⁹³

683. Which of the following color light emissions will expose orthochromatic film?
    1. red
    2. blue
    3. yellow
        a. 1 & 2 only
        b. 1 & 3 only
        c. 2 & 3 only
        d. 1, 2, & 3

A⁶⁹⁴

Question # ┐
Answer   ┐ │
         ↓ │
           ↓

684. Which type of intensifying screen cassette would produce the highest patient exposure dose?
     a. detail calcium tungstate
     b. medium-speed calcium tungstate
     c. high-speed calcium tungstate
     d. high-speed rare earth

685. Which of the following sensitometric measures of processor quality control would be expected as a result of a clogged developer replenishment filter?   C⁶⁷⁴
     1. increased base-plus-fog
     2. decreased speed
     3. lower contrast index
        a. 1 & 2 only
        b. 1 & 3 only
        c. 2 & 3 only
        d. 1, 2, & 3

686. What causes a white scratch artifact that runs the length of a radiograph?   B⁶⁷⁵
     a. static discharge
     b. handling with dry hands
     c. bending the film
     d. improperly aligned guide shoe deflectors

687. Which of the following types of silver recovery methods is considered most cost efficient for an average hospital diagnostic radiology department?   A⁶⁷⁶
     a. metallic replacement
     b. electrolytic
     c. chemical precipitation
     d. resin

688. What is a typical developer replenishment rate for an automatic film processor?   A⁶⁷⁷
     a. 0.1 to 0.5 ml/in
     b. 4 to 5 ml/in
     c. 20 to 30 ml/in
     d. 100 to 200 ml/in

A⁶⁷⁸

C^{700}

689. Which of the following are components of an automatic processor transport rack?
    1. recirculation pump
    2. guide shoe deflectors
    3. planetary roller
      a. 1 & 2 only
      b. 1 & 3 only
      c. 2 & 3 only
      d. 1, 2, & 3

A^{701}

690. Who is responsible for recording identification information on the radiograph correctly?
      a. radiologist
      b. attending physician
      c. radiographer
      d. administrative technologist

A^{702}

691. What is the appropriate humidity for proper film storage?
      a. 0 to 10%
      b. 30 to 60%
      c. 70 to 80%
      d. 90 to 100%

692. Which U.S. Customary size is equivalent to a 20 cm x 25 cm cassette?
      a. 8" x 10"
      b. 10" x 12"
      c. 11" x 14"
      d. 14" x 17"

B^{703}

693. What is a typical automatic processor dryer air temperature?
      a. 40 to 50°F
      b. 90 to 100°F
      c. 120 to 150°F
      d. 200 to 250°F

B^{704}

694. Which automatic film processor system controls the replenishment system pumps?
      a. entrance roller
      b. transport
      c. replenishment
      d. dryer

695. What is the cause of reticulation marks over the surface of a radiograph?
    a. rapid temperature changes during processing
    b. abrasive trauma to the emulsion during processing   A[684]
    c. failure of the emulsion to base adhesive
    d. over saturation of the emulsion by fixer

696. Which of the following colors is acceptable for darkroom walls and working benches?
    1. white
    2. black
    3. orange-red
    a. 1 only
    b. 2 only
    c. 3 only   C[685]
    d. 1, 2, & 3

697. Why do crossover networks require cleaning more often than transport rollers?
    a. they are porous and absorb chemicals, which may then precipitate and form deposits
    b. they are positioned partly in solution and partly in air   D[686] which permits chemical deposits to readily accumulate
    c. they turn at half the speed of the transport rollers
    d. they turn at twice the speed of the transport rollers

698. Which automatic processor system replaces depleted chemicals in both the developer and fixer?
    1. recirculation system
    2. replenishment system   B[687]
    3. dryer system
    a. 1 only
    b. 2 only
    c. 3 only
    d. 1, 2, & 3

699. Why is a lead blocker placed in one corner of most radiographic   B[688] cassettes?
    a. to provide a base-plus-fog measurement area
    b. to reserve a space for the identification marker
    c. to reduce backscatter
    d. to indicate the tube side of the cassette

Image Production and Evaluation

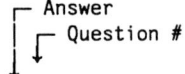

700. At what temperature should radiographic film be stored?
    a. >94 to 96°F
    b. >68°F
    c. <68°F
    d. <32°F

B⁷¹¹

701. Which of the following is an acceptable storage method for unexposed radiographic film?
    1. on end
    2. flat
    3. at an angle
    a. 1 only
    b. 2 only
    c. 3 only
    d. 1, 2, & 3

C⁷¹²

702. Which type of intensifying screen cassette would produce the best resolution?
    a. detail calcium tungstate
    b. medium-speed calcium tungstate
    c. high-speed calcium tungstate
    d. high-speed rare earth

A⁷¹³

703. Which of the following sensitometric measures of processor quality control would be expected as a result of an increase in developer temperature?
    1. increased base-plus-fog
    2. decreased speed
    3. lower contrast index
    a. 1 & 2 only
    b. 1 & 3 only
    c. 2 & 3 only
    d. 1, 2, & 3

C⁷¹⁴

704. What causes an artifact that is repeated at regular intervals for the length of the radiograph?
    a. static discharge
    b. dirt on a processor transport roller
    c. bending the film
    d. improperly aligned guide shoe deflectors

705. Which of the following types of silver recovery methods filters used fixer through steel wool permitting the silver to precipitate onto it?
    a. metallic replacement
    b. electrolytic
    c. chemical precipitation
    d. resin

A[695]

706. Why are guide shoe deflectors ribbed?
    a. to prevent wet films from sticking to their surface
    b. to begin the drying process
    c. to avoid scratching the wet film
    d. to increase solution agitation

707. Which of the following are the most desirable conditions for storing processed film?
    a. <20% humidity, >80°F
    b. 40% humidity, 32°F
    c. 60% humidity, 70°F
    d. 100% humidity, 100°F

D[696]

708. Which metric size is equivalent to an 11" x 14" cassette?
    a. 18 cm x 24 cm
    b. 24 cm x 30 cm
    c. 28 cm x 35 cm
    d. 35 cm x 43 cm

B[697]

709. Which automatic film processor system uses tubes with a slit for air to exit?
    a. entrance roller
    b. transport
    c. replenishment
    d. dryer

710. Which of the following would cause jamming of films in an automatic processor?
    1. improperly seated crossover networks
    2. improperly seated transport racks
    3. improperly aligned films on feed tray
    a. 1 & 2 only
    b. 1 & 3 only
    c. 2 & 3 only
    d. 1, 2, & 3

B[698]

B[699]

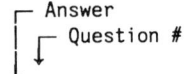

711. Which of the following are most likely to be the cause of white lines occurring over the length of a radiograph processed in an automatic film processor?
    1. improperly seated crossover network
    2. dirt on transport rollers
    3. maladjusted guide shoe deflectors
        a. 1 & 2 only
        b. 1 & 3 only
        c. 2 & 3 only
        d. 1, 2, & 3

D^{719}

712. Which of the following are potential causes of films exiting an automatic processor with a slimy, wet feel?
    1. developer solution contamination
    2. insufficient washing
    3. insufficient drying
        a. 1 & 2 only
        b. 1 & 3 only
        c. 2 & 3 only
        d. 1, 2, & 3

A^{720}

713. Which of the following describes an artifact produced when chemistry is not properly removed from a film, and it runs up or down the film leaving a stain?
        a. curtain effect
        b. alabaster effect
        c. crescent half moon
        d. pi line

B^{721}

714. What devices are used in an automatic film processor to turn the film at the bottom and top of each solution tank?
        a. transport rollers
        b. squeegee rollers and hot air
        c. crossover networks and guide shoes
        d. master and planetary rollers

D^{722}

B^{723}

715. Which of the following pieces of information are appropriate for the identification blocker area of the radiograph?
    1. patient age
    2. physician name
    3. hospital name
        a. 1 & 2 only
        b. 1 & 3 only
        c. 2 & 3 only
        d. 1, 2, & 3

A^{705}

716. What types of artifact occur as a result of static discharge in the darkroom?
    1. black tree branching
    2. black smudges
    3. white abrasion lines
        a. 1 & 2 only
        b. 1 & 3 only
        c. 2 & 3 only
        d. 1, 2, & 3

A^{706}

717. What conditions will cause water-spot artifacts on film?
        a. high humidity
        b. high temperature
        c. low humidity
        d. low temperature

C^{707}

718. Which of the following should be avoided when loading radiographic cassettes?
    1. fully opening cassette on darkroom loading bench
    2. using lotion on hands
    3. wearing a ring with a large stone
        a. 1 & 2 only
        b. 1 & 3 only
        c. 2 & 3 only
        d. 1, 2, & 3

C^{708}

D^{709}

D^{710}

719. Which of the following color light emissions will expose panchromatic film?
    1. red
    2. blue
    3. yellow
        a. 1 & 2 only
        b. 1 & 3 only
        c. 2 & 3 only
        d. 1, 2, & 3

A⁷²⁸

720. Which of the following are acceptable base-plus-fog optical density (OD) levels?
    1. 0.12
    2. 0.16
    3. 0.26
        a. 1 & 2 only
        b. 1 & 3 only
        c. 2 & 3 only
        d. 1, 2, & 3

D⁷²⁹

721. Why is it critical that immediate notification be given if a film bin is accidently left open in full light?
        a. so that responsibility for the wasted expense can be properly noted
        b. to avoid repeated exposures to patients due to fogged films
        c. to avoid the loss of silver when the fogged films are processed
        d. to notify the film supplier for free replacement of the fogged films

C⁷³⁰

722. Which of the following can be used to place identification information on a radiograph?
    1. lead markers
    2. light exposure through paper
    3. permanent felt tip markers
        a. 1 & 2 only
        b. 1 & 3 only
        c. 2 & 3 only
        d. 1, 2, & 3

A⁷³¹

723. What is the cause of a pi line artifact on a radiograph?
        a. static discharge
        b. dirt on a processor transport roller
        c. bending the film
        d. improperly aligned guide shoe deflectors

A⁷³²

724. Which of the following types of silver recovery methods passes a current from a cathode to an anode through the fixer, permitting the ionized silver in the used fixer to be attracted to the negatively charge cathode where it plates for removal?
    a. metallic replacement
    b. electrolytic
    c. chemical precipitation
    d. resin

D^{715}

725. Which automatic processor system removes excess water and shrinks and seals the emulsion?
    1. temperature control system
    2. recirculation system
    3. dryer system
    a. 1 only
    b. 2 only
    c. 3 only
    d. 1, 2, & 3

A^{716}

726. Which of the following types of cases should be retained in storage longer than routine films?
    1. poor quality films
    2. films involved in litigation
    3. pediatric cases
    a. 1 & 2 only
    b. 1 & 3 only
    c. 2 & 3 only
    d. 1, 2, & 3

A^{717}

727. What type of artifact occurs when a cardboard or paper sheet is quickly removed from inside a box of film?
    a. black tree branching
    b. black smudges
    c. black abrasion lines
    d. white abrasion lines

D^{718}

┌ Answer
│ ┌ Question #
↓ ↓

C⁷³⁸

728. Which of the following will arrest film aging?
1. freezing
2. storage <68°F
3. low humidity
   a. 1 only
   b. 2 only
   c. 3 only
   d. 1, 2, & 3

A⁷³⁹

Evaluation of Radiographs 6% (84) 729-812

729. If a satisfactory radiograph is produced at 100 mA and 2 s, but the time needs to be changed to 0.5 s, what mA produces a similar density?
   a. 150
   b. 200
   c. 300
   d. 400

D⁷⁴⁰

730. What term describes an image lacking a great difference between adjacent shades of gray?
   a. light
   b. dark
   c. low contrast
   d. high contrast

C⁷⁴¹

731. Which of the following will decrease image distortion?
1. increased FOD
2. decreased OFD
3. decreased grid ratio
   a. 1 & 2 only
   b. 1 & 3 only
   c. 2 & 3 only
   d. 1, 2, & 3

A⁷⁴²

732. Which of the following exposure factors is most closely related to the quality of photons in the x-ray beam?
1. kVp
2. mAs
3. distance
   a. 1 only
   b. 2 only
   c. 3 only
   d. 1, 2, & 3

D⁷⁴³

733. What is the relationship between film latitude and contrast?
    a. equal
    b. directly proportional
    c. inversely proportional
    d. linearly related

For items 734 and 735, choose the technical factors that would produce the highest contrast on radiographic film if all other factors were to remain identical.   B[724]

734.

	mA	s	kVp	FFD	grid	film/screen
a.	200	0.12	85	40"	10:1	100
b.	400	0.12	72	40"	10:1	100
c.	400	0.06	85	40"	10:1	100
d.	500	0.05	98	40"	10:1	100

C[725]

735.

	mA	s	kVp	FFD	grid	film/screen
a.	200	0.08	85	40"	8:1	100
b.	400	0.04	85	40"	8:1	100
c.	400	0.06	85	40"	10:1	100
d.	800	0.04	85	40"	12:1	100

736. Which of the following will produce a visible change in contrast?   C[726]
    1. 50% increase in mA
    2. 30% increase in kVp
    3. 30% decrease in kVp
    a. 1 & 2 only
    b. 1 & 3 only
    c. 2 & 3 only
    d. 1, 2, & 3

737. If a satisfactory image is achieved using 68 kVp and 2.5 mAs, which of the following sets of technical factors would maintain the same image density while raising contrast?   C[727]
    a. 79 kVp at 1.3 mAs
    b. 68 kVp at 1.3 mAs
    c. 57 kVp at 2.5 mAs
    d. 57 kVp at 5 mAs

738. Which of the following does not directly affect subject contrast?
     a. subject thickness
     b. subject density
     c. atomic valence
     d. atomic number

D ^{750}

739. What is the relationship between exposure latitude and kilovoltage?
     a. directly proportional
     b. inversely proportional
     c. linearly related
     d. equal

B ^{751}

740. Which radiographic quality factors require satisfactory density prior to being properly evaluated?
     1. contrast
     2. recorded detail
     3. distortion
     a. 1 & 2 only
     b. 1 & 3 only
     c. 2 & 3 only
     d. 1, 2, & 3

A ^{752}

741. Which of the following would be nearly impossible to visualize if it were swallowed by a small child?
     a. a coin
     b. a battery
     c. a small plastic ball
     d. a screw

C ^{753}

742. Which body habitus would produce an image with the least density if no technical factors compensation were made?
     a. hypersthenic
     b. hyposthenic
     c. sthenic
     d. asthenic

B ^{754}

743. Which of the following have an effect on radiographic density?
     1. film speed
     2. developer activity
     3. collimation
     a. 1 & 2 only
     b. 1 & 3 only
     c. 2 & 3 only
     d. 1, 2, & 3

A ^{755}

Question # ⌐
Answer ⌐ |
↓ |
↓

744. Which of the following could produce an overexposed image?
     a. increased developer time
     b. decreased developer temperature
     c. increased fixer temperature
     d. increased grid ratio

C⁷³³

745. What type of image would be produced by using a focused grid at an angle so that the central ray was angled into the grid lines?
     a. equal but light density across the image
     b. normal image on one side, light on the other
     c. light image on the edges, dark image at center
     d. dark image on the edges, light image at center

746. Which of the following affects recorded detail?
     a. kVp
     b. mA
     c. time
     d. distance

D⁷³⁴

747. What term describes the area of distinct and sharp edges around an image?
     a. blur
     b. mottle
     c. penumbra
     d. umbra

D⁷³⁵

748. Which of the following are controlled by changing time?
     1. average photon wavelength
     2. photon quantity
     3. number of photons
     a. 1 & 2 only
     b. 1 & 3 only
     c. 2 & 3 only
     d. 1, 2, & 3

C⁷³⁶

749. Which of the following will produce greater image density?
     1. decreased FOD
     2. increased kVp
     3. decreased OFD
     a. 1 & 2 only
     b. 1 & 3 only
     c. 2 & 3 only
     d. 1, 2, & 3

D⁷³⁷

750. Approximately what change in mAs will reduce image density by half the diagnostic range of kVp and within average part sizes?
    a. 5%
    b. 15%
    c. 25%
    d. 50%

A^{761}

751. Which of the following will improve recorded detail of an extremity?
    a. using a larger focal spot
    b. using a slower film/screen combination
    c. decreasing FFD
    d. increasing developer temperature

B^{762}

752. Which abdominal region would produce an image with the least density if the right kidney were the location of a large staghorn calculus and no technical factors compensation were made?
    a. right lumbar
    b. left iliac
    c. right hypochondriac
    d. left hypochondriac

D^{763}

753. What change in kVp would maintain image density if the mA must stay the same and time must be decreased by 50%?
    a. decrease 15%
    b. decrease 50%
    c. increase 15%
    d. increase 100%

B^{764}

754. Which of the following will produce a poor recorded detail image?
    1. decreased FFD
    2. high kVp
    3. increased OFD
    a. 1 & 2 only
    b. 1 & 3 only
    c. 2 & 3 only
    d. 1, 2, & 3

A^{765}

755. Which of the following would result in a 50% increase in density from an image that was produced at 70 kVp and 22 mAs?

mA	s	kVp	FFD	grid	film/screen	
a.	200	0.11	76	40"	10:1	100
b.	200	0.11	70	40"	10:1	100
c.	400	0.03	81	40"	10:1	100
d.	400	0.06	70	40"	10:1	100

756. Approximately what percentage change in kVp will reduce image density by half within the diagnostic range of kVp and within average patient part sizes?
    a. 5%
    b. 15%
    c. 25%
    d. 50%

A [744]

757. Which body habitus would produce an image with the greatest density if no technical factors compensation were made?
    a. hypersthenic
    b. hyposthenic
    c. sthenic
    d. asthenic

B [745]

758. Which of the following have an effect on radiographic contrast?
    1. film latitude
    2. developer activity
    3. collimation
    a. 1 & 2 only
    b. 1 & 3 only
    c. 2 & 3 only
    d. 1, 2, & 3

D [746]

759. Approximately how many 30% density values below optimal density can be considered within the acceptance range for most diagnostic radiography?
    a. 0
    b. 2
    c. 4
    d. 8

D [747]

760. Which factors has an effect on image contrast?
    1. grid ratio
    2. kVp
    3. film/screen combination speed
    a. 1 only
    b. 2 only
    c. 3 only
    d. 1, 2, & 3

C [748]

D [749]

Answer
Question #

761. Which of the following are controlled by changing kVp?
1. average photon wavelength
2. photon quality
3. number of photons
    a. 1 & 2 only
    b. 1 & 3 only
    c. 2 & 3 only
    d. 1, 2, & 3

B⁷⁷¹

762. Which of the following will increase image distortion?
1. decreased FOD
2. increased kVp
3. increased OFD
    a. 1 & 2 only
    b. 1 & 3 only
    c. 2 & 3 only
    d. 1, 2, & 3

763. Which of the following projections is most likely to decrease recorded detail?
    a. supine AP cervical spine
    b. erect sitting AP cervical spine
    c. erect standing AP cervical spine
    d. erect standing PA cervical spine

764. Which of the following would result in halving density from an image that was produced at 85 kVp and 48 mAs?

	mA	s	kVp	FFD	grid	film/screen
a.	100	0.24	98	40"	10:1	100
b.	200	0.06	98	40"	10:1	100
c.	200	0.48	85	40"	10:1	100
d.	400	0.24	72	40"	10:1	100

A⁷⁷²

765. Which of the following sets of technique factors will produce an image with the highest contrast?
    a. 60 kVp, 100 mA, 0.5 s, 40"
    b. 70 kVp, 100 mA, 0.5 s, 40"
    c. 80 kVp, 200 mA, 0.12 s, 40"
    d. 92 kVp, 200 mA, 0.06 s, 40"

B⁷⁷³

Question # ⌐
Answer ⌐ |
↓ |
↓

766. If a satisfactory radiograph is produced at 100 mA and 0.12 s but the image exhibits patient motion, requiring the time to be changed to 0.04 s, what mA is required to produce a similar density?
    a. 150
    b. 200
    c. 300
    d. 400

B[756]

767. Which of the following includes changes in the shape of an image of an object?
    a. density
    b. contrast
    c. recorded detail
    d. distortion

D[757]

768. Which body habitus would produce an image with the lowest contrast if no technical factors compensation were made?
    a. hypersthenic
    b. hyposthenic
    c. sthenic
    d. asthenic

D[758]

769. What effect does a relatively long wavelength beam have on image quality?
    1. decreases contrast
    2. decreases density
    3. increases recorded detail
    a. 1 only
    b. 2 only
    c. 3 only
    d. 1, 2, & 3

B[759]

770. What are the effects of lower grid frequency on image quality?
    1. contrast decreases
    2. density increases
    3. recorded detail increases
    a. 1 & 2 only
    b. 1 & 3 only
    c. 2 & 3 only
    d. 1, 2, & 3

D[760]

┌ Answer
│ ┌ Question #
↓ ↓

771. Which of the following factors is used to describe image density?
    a. average gradient
    b. speed
    c. base-plus-fog
    d. modulation transfer function

A⁷⁷⁹

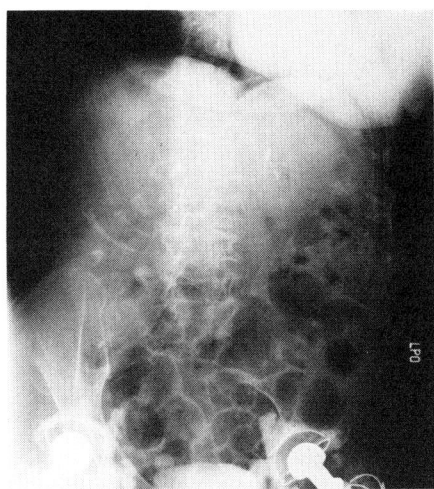

Figure 14

B⁷⁸⁰

D⁷⁸¹

772. What is the best solution to produce a better oblique intravenous pyelogram of the older patient shown in Figure 14?
    a. increase mAs
    b. decrease time
    c. increase kVp
    d. decrease kVp

B⁷⁸²

773. Which of the following kVp levels was most likely used to produce the image in Figure 14?
    a. 40 to 50
    b. 60 to 70
    c. 80 to 90
    d. 100 to 110

A⁷⁸³

774. Which of the following will not decrease recorded detail?
    1. increased OFD
    2. increased grid ratio
    3. decreased film/screen speed
        a. 1 & 2 only
        b. 1 & 3 only   C⁷⁶⁶
        c. 2 & 3 only
        d. 1, 2, & 3

775. What term describes an image with a great difference between adjacent shades of gray?
        a. light
        b. dark   D⁷⁶⁷
        c. low contrast
        d. high contrast

776. Which of the following will produce decreased image density?
    1. decreased FOD
    2. increased grid ratio   A⁷⁶⁸
    3. increased OFD
        a. 1 & 2 only
        b. 1 & 3 only
        c. 2 & 3 only
        d. 1, 2, & 3

777. Which of the following projections would produce the best detail of the posterior lumbar facets?
        a. AP
        b. PA   A⁷⁶⁹
        c. RAO and LAO
        d. RPO and LPO

778. Which of the following have an effect on radiographic density?
    1. film latitude
    2. OFD
    3. collimation
        a. 1 & 2 only
        b. 1 & 3 only   A⁷⁷⁰
        c. 2 & 3 only
        d. 1, 2, & 3

Image Production and Evaluation

779. Which of the following are part of subject contrast?
    1. tissue thickness
    2. tissue composition
    3. tissue metabolic rate
        a. 1 & 2 only
        b. 1 & 3 only
A^{789} c. 2 & 3 only
        d. 1, 2, & 3

780. What effect would be expected on the image if a blue sensitive film is used with a green-emitting intensifying screen?
    1. higher contrast
    2. decreased density
D^{790} 3. increased recorded detail
        a. 1 only
        b. 2 only
        c. 3 only
        d. 1, 2, & 3

781. What are the two primary types of distortion?
A^{791} a. long and short
        b. density and contrast
        c. size and contrast
        d. size and shape

782. Which factor has an effect on image contrast?
    1. anode heel effect
    2. film speed
C^{792} 3. central ray alignment
        a. 1 only
        b. 2 only
        c. 3 only
        d. 1, 2, & 3

A^{793} 783. What term describes an image with few silver atoms deposited in the silver halides of the film?
        a. light
        b. dark
        c. low contrast
        d. high contrast

A^{794}

784. Which of the following is controlled by changing milliamperage?
    1. average photon wavelength
    2. photon quantity
    3. number of photons
        a. 1 & 2 only
        b. 1 & 3 only   C[774]
        c. 2 & 3 only
        d. 1, 2, & 3

785. Which of the following will produce a low contrast image?
    1. use of a grid
    2. high kVp
    3. reduced OFD   D[775]
        a. 1 & 2 only
        b. 1 & 3 only
        c. 2 & 3 only
        d. 1, 2, & 3

786. Which of the following would result in a 33% increase (adding approximately one density level) in density from an image that was produced at 50 kVp and 3 mAs?   C[776]

mA	s	kVp	FFD	grid	film/screen
a. 100	0.06	50	40"	none	100
b. 100	0.12	50	40"	none	100
c. 100	0.03	58	40"	none	100
d. 100	0.02	58	40"	none	100

787. Which of the following is within the resolving ability of a diagnostic film/screen combination?   D[777]
        a.   0.5 to 1.0 lp/mm
        b.   1 to 10 lp/mm
        c.   50 to 100 lp/mm
        d.   200 to 400 lp/mm

788. Approximately what percentage change in mAs will double image density within the diagnostic range of kVp and within average patient part sizes?
        a.   15%   D[778]
        b.   25%
        c.   50%
        d.   100%

┌─ Answer
│ ┌─ Question #
│ │
↓ ↓

789. Which effects occurs when a radiographic image is magnified?
    1. recorded detail is decreased
    2. density is increased
    3. contrast is increased
        a. 1 only
        b. 2 only
        c. 3 only
        d. 1, 2, & 3

B^{800}

790. Which body habitus would produce an image with the highest contrast if no technical factors compensation were made?
        a. hypersthenic
        b. hyposthenic
        c. sthenic
        d. asthenic

B^{801}

791. What change in kVp would maintain image density if the mA is increased by 100% and all other factors remain the same?
        a. decrease 15%
        b. decrease 50%
        c. increase 15%
        d. increase 100%

B^{802}

792. What type of image would be produced by using a focused grid upside down?
        a. equal but light density across the image
        b. dark image on one side, light on the other
        c. light image on the edges, dark image at center
        d. dark image on the edges, light image at center

C^{803}

793. Which projections is most likely to increase recorded detail?
        a. supine AP cervical spine
        b. erect standing AP cervical spine
        c. erect sitting AP cervical spine
        d. erect sitting PA cervical spine

794. Which of the following will decrease recorded detail?
    1. increased OFD
    2. decreased FFD
    3. lower contrast
        a. 1 & 2 only
        b. 1 & 3 only
        c. 2 & 3 only
        d. 1, 2, & 3

B^{804}

795. What term describes the unsharp edges around an image?
   a. blur
   b. mottle
   c. penumbra
   d. umbra

796. Which of the following will produce a high-resolution image?   C[784]
   1. increased FOD
   2. high kVp
   3. reduced OFD
      a. 1 & 2 only
      b. 1 & 3 only
      c. 2 & 3 only
      d. 1, 2, & 3

797. Which of the following would result in halving density from an   C[785]
   image that was produced at 120 kVp and 8 mAs?

	mA	s	kVp	FFD	grid	film/screen
a.	100	0.08	120	40"	12:1	200
b.	200	0.04	120	40"	12:1	200
c.	200	0.02	120	40"	12:1	200
d.	400	0.02	120	40"	12:1	200

798. Which of the following projections would produce the poorest   D[786]
   recorded detail of the right sacroiliac joint?
      a. AP
      b. PA
      c. RAO and LAO
      d. RPO and LPO

799. Which of the following types of technical factors would produce   B[787]
   less contrast while maintaining image density?
      a. increasing kVp and increasing mAs
      b. increasing kVp and decreasing mAs
      c. decreasing kVp and increasing mAs
      d. decreasing kVp and decreasing mAs

D[788]

Image Production and Evaluation

800. If a satisfactory radiograph is produced at 100 mA and 0.3 s but the image exhibits patient motion, requiring the time to be changed to 0. 15 s, what mA is required to produce a similar density?
    a. 150
    b. 200
    c. 300
    d. 400

A⁸¹⁰

801. Which of the following have an effect on radiographic contrast?
    1. film speed
    2. FFD
    3. base-plus-fog
        a. 1 & 2 only
        b. 1 & 3 only
        c. 2 & 3 only
        d. 1, 2, & 3

C⁸¹¹

802. Approximately how many 30% density values above optimal density can be considered within the acceptance range for most diagnostic radiography?
        a. 1
        b. 3
        c. 5
        d. 9

D⁸¹²

803. What type of film is capable of recording a wide range of exposures?
    1. high contrast, high speed
    2. high contrast, slow speed
    3. low contrast, slow speed
        a. 1 only
        b. 2 only
        c. 3 only
        d. 1, 2, & 3

D⁸¹³

804. Which of the following will reduce scattered radiation?
    1. decreased kVp
    2. decreased FFD
    3. increased grid frequency
        a. 1 & 2 only
        b. 1 & 3 only
        c. 2 & 3 only
        d. 1, 2, & 3

C⁸¹⁴

Question # ⌐
Answer ⌐ |
↓ |
↓

805. What is the primary reason FFD is not used to control image density?
    a. contrast also changes
    b. kVp settings do not permit appropriate compensation on most units
    c. recorded detail also changes
    d. mA stations do not go high enough to permit appropriate compensation

C^{795}

806. What will the magnification factor be for an object placed 20" from the x-ray tube source and 20" from the image receptor?
    a. 1X
    b. 1.5X
    c. 2X
    d. 4X

B^{796}

807. Which of the following has little effect on image density?
    1. anode heel effect
    2. intensifying screen speed
    3. central ray alignment
    a. 1 only
    b. 2 only
    c. 3 only
    d. 1, 2, & 3

C^{797}

808. What term describes an image which has experienced a great amount of reduction during development?
    a. light
    b. dark
    c. low contrast
    d. high contrast

C^{798}

809. Which of the following are controlled by changing kVp?
    1. average photon wavelength
    2. number of photons
    3. photon penetrating ability
    a. 1 & 2 only
    b. 1 & 3 only
    c. 2 & 3 only
    d. 1, 2, & 3

B^{799}

Answer
Question #

810. Which of the following will produce a high contrast image?
    1. use of a grid
    2. low kVp
    3. reduced OFD
        a. 1 & 2 only
        b. 1 & 3 only
        c. 2 & 3 only
        d. 1, 2, & 3

B 821

811. Which of the following would result in halving density from an image that was produced at 60 kVp and 14 mAs?

	mA	s	kVp	FFD	grid	film/screen
a.	100	0.28	60	40"	6:1	100
b.	100	0.07	69	40"	6:1	100
c.	200	0.04	60	40"	6:1	100
d.	200	0.07	60	40"	6:1	100

C 822

812. Which of the following sets of technique factors will produce an image with the longest scale of contrast?
        a. 60 kVp, 200 mA, 0.5 s, 40"
        b. 70 kVp, 200 mA, 0.5 s, 40"
        c. 80 kVp, 400 mA, 0.24 s, 56"
        d. 92 kVp, 400 mA, 0.06 s, 40"

D 823

General Procedural Considerations 2% (28) 813-840

813. What are the proper breathing instructions for an AP projection of the upper ribs?
        a. inspiration
        b. expiration
        c. suspension of breathing
        d. continued breathing

A 824

814. What radiographic procedure will permit measurements of the inlet and outlet of the female pelvis?
        a. aortography
        b. sialography
        c. pelvimetry
        d. hysterosalpingography

A 825

B 826

Question #
Answer

815. What term best describes the position of the body when standing
upright with the palms of the hand facing forward?
   a. anatomic position
   b. erect position
   c. coronal position
   d. trendelenburg position

816. Which term describes the direction away from the body?   C[805]
   a. proximal
   b. distal
   c. cephalad
   d. caudal

817. Which part of the patient's body is closest to the image receptor if   C[806]
the patient is in a left decubitus position?
   a. anterior
   b. posterior
   c. right side
   d. left side

818. What are the proper breathing instructions for a lateral projection   C[807]
of the cervicothoracic region?
   a. inspiration
   b. expiration
   c. suspension of breathing
   d. continued breathing

819. Which term describes rotation of the hand to place the palm
down?   B[808]
   a. abduct
   b. adduct
   c. supinate
   d. pronate

820. Which term describes a position in which neither the coronal or
sagittal plane is perpendicular to the plane of the image receptor?   B[809]
   a. axial
   b. PA
   c. AP
   d. oblique

B⁸³⁴

821. Which of the following projections would reduce the probability of motion by a pediatric patient?
    1. PA projection
    2. AP projection
    3. AP half axial (Waters) projection
        a. 1 only
        b. 2 only
        c. 3 only
        d. 1, 2, & 3

B⁸³⁵

822. Which of the following should be removed prior to an examination of the stomach?
    1. dentures
    2. underwear with wide elastic banding
    3. pants with metallic or plastic fasteners

C⁸³⁶

        a. 1 & 2 only
        b. 1 & 3 only
        c. 2 & 3 only
        d. 1, 2, & 3

823. Which term describes an increase in the angle of a joint?
        a. adduction

B⁸³⁷

        b. pronation
        c. flexion
        d. extension

824. Into what divisions is the body divided by a transverse plane?
        a. superior and inferior

A⁸³⁸

        b. anterior and posterior
        c. medial and lateral
        d. right and left

825. What term describes the direction of x-ray beam travel?
        a. projection
        b. position

C⁸³⁹

        c. view
        d. body habitus

826. What are the proper breathing instructions for an AP projection of the lower ribs?
        a. inspiration

A⁸⁴⁰

        b. expiration
        c. suspension of breathing
        d. continued breathing

Question # ⌐
Answer ⌐ |
↓ |
↓

827. Which term describes a projection taken from one side?
    a. AP
    b. PA
    c. oblique   A[815]
    d. lateral

828. What term describes a movement toward the midline of the body?
    a. abduct
    b. adduct
    c. flex   B[816]
    d. circumduct

829. Which plane divides the body into front and rear halves?
    a. sagittal
    b. coronal
    c. transverse   D[817]
    d. medial

830. What are the proper breathing instructions for a lateral projection
of the thoracic spine?
    a. inspiration
    b. expiration
    c. suspension of breathing   C[818]
    d. continued breathing

831. Which term describes the direction of the feet?
    a. dorsal
    b. ventral
    c. cephalad   D[819]
    d. caudal

832. Which term describes the back of the body?
    a. dorsal
    b. ventral
    c. cephalad
    d. caudal

833. Into what divisions is the body divided by the sagittal plane?   D[820]
    a. superior and inferior
    b. anterior and posterior
    c. medial and lateral
    d. right and left

Answer
Question #

834. What are the proper breathing instructions for an AP projection of the abdomen?
    a. inspiration
    b. expiration
    c. suspension of breathing
    d. continued breathing

C[846]

835. Which term describes the direction toward the body?
    a. caudad
    b. cephalad
    c. distal
    d. proximal

B[847]

836. Which term describes a decrease in the angle of a joint?
    a. adduction
    b. pronation
    c. flexion
    d. extension

C[848]

837. Which term describes a movement away from the midline of the body?
    a. adduct
    b. abduct
    c. flex
    d. circumduct

C[849]

838. What are the proper breathing instructions for a PA projection of the chest?
    a. inspiration
    b. expiration
    c. suspension of breathing
    d. continued breathing

A[850]

839. If an object is located immediately inferior to the right lumbar region of the abdomen, in which region is it located?
    a. left lumbar
    b. epigastric
    c. right iliac
    d. hypogastric

B[851]

840. Which plane divides the body into right and left halves?
    a. sagittal
    b. coronal
    c. transverse
    d. medial

A[852]

Specific Imaging Procedures 26% (364) 841-1204

841. Which of the following demonstrates the humerus in the true lateral position?
    1. AP neutral rotation shoulder
    2. AP external rotation shoulder
    3. AP internal rotation shoulder
        a. 1 only
        b. 2 only
        c. 3 only
        d. 1, 2, & 3

D^{827}

B^{828}

842. Which of the following structures is located immediately distal to the head of the ulna?
        a. distal epicondyle
        b. lesser tuberosity
        c. bicipital groove
        d. styloid process

B^{829}

843. Which of the following is a small detached bone which frames the upper anterior portion of the larynx?
        a. hyoid
        b. thyroid cartilage
        c. C5
        d. C4

D^{830}

844. Which of the following is not a structure found in the mediastinum?
        a. esophagus
        b. trachea
        c. thyroid gland
        d. thymus gland

D^{831}

845. What term describes biologic catalysts which speed up the process of digestion?
        a. enzymes
        b. hormones
        c. hemolytic agents
        d. secretions

A^{832}

D^{833}

846. What term describes the semifluid mass that is produced when the stomach contents are churned with saliva and other stomach fluids?
    a. bolus
    b. fecal material
    c. chyme
    d. cachexia

847. What is the centering point for an average size RAO stomach?
    a. cardiac antrum
    b. duodenal bulb
    c. greater curvature
    d. iliac crest

848. Which term describes a surgical opening into a renal collecting system?
    a. hydronephrosis
    b. nephroptosis
    c. nephrotomy
    d. nephrectomy

849. Which of the following is not a normal function of the renal system?
    a. removal of nitrogenous wastes
    b. regulation of water levels
    c. discharge of red blood cells into the urine
    d. regulation of acid-base balance and electrolyte levels

C^{859} 850. Which term describes the expanded superior, most lateral portion of the scapular spine?
    a. acromion process
    b. coracoid process
    c. lateral border
    d. supraspinatus process

C^{860} 851. What is the other name for the os magnum?
    a. hamate
    b. capitate
    c. unciform
    d. trapezoid

C^{861} 852. In which direction is the finger rotated from the PA projection to properly position the 2nd digit for a lateral projection?
    a. medially
    b. laterally
    c. externally
    d. distally

853. What position of the elbow best demonstrates the olecranon process?
    a. lateromedial
    b. AP
    c. internal oblique
    d. external oblique

854. What is the correct central ray location for an AP foot?
    a. 3rd proximal interphalangeal joint
    b. head of the 3rd metatarsal   C^{841}
    c. base of the 3rd metatarsal
    d. 3rd metatarsophalangeal joint

855. What is the name of the depression on the lateral side of the coronoid process with which the head of the radius articulates?
    a. radial notch
    b. coronoid fossa   D^{842}
    c. capitellum
    d. trochlea

856. How many degrees of cephalic angulation are required for an axial plantodorsal projection of the os calcis?
    a. 20
    b. 30   A^{843}
    c. 35
    d. 40

857. In the lateral projection, which carpals are located most anteriorly?
    a. capitate and hamate
    b. capitate and os magnum   C^{844}
    c. navicular and lunate
    d. pisiform and greater multangular

858. Which of the following structures are best demonstrated with a lateral (external) oblique projection of the elbow?
    a. coronoid process
    b. trochlea
    c. radial head
    d. capitellum

Image Production and Evaluation

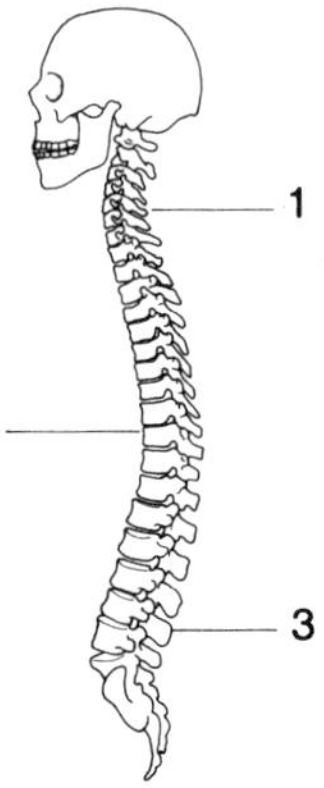

Figure 15 (from Akesson EJ, Loeb JA, Wilson-Pauwels L: Thompson's Core Textbook of Anatomy, 2nd ed. Philadelphia, JB Lippincott, 1990)

B^868

B^869

C^870   859. Which of the following describes the curve labeled 1 in Figure 15?
              1. kyphotic
              2. scoliotic
              3. lordotic
                 a. 1 only
B^871   b. 2 only
                 c. 3 only
                 d. 1, 2, & 3

          860. Which of the following describes the curve labeled 3 in Figure 15?
              1. kyphotic
              2. scoliotic
              3. lordotic
                 a. 1 only
A^872   b. 2 only
                 c. 3 only
                 d. 1, 2, & 3

          861. Which term describes an opacification study of the peripheral or central veins?
                 a. angiography
                 b. lymphangiography
                 c. venography
                 d. arteriography

Question # ⌐
Answer ⌐ |
↓ |
↓

862. Which of the following best demonstrate the hepatic flexure of the colon?
    a. RPO and LAO
    b. LPO and RAO
    c. RPO and LPO
    d. RAO and LAO

A[853]

863. Which term describes the accumulation of abnormal amounts of fluid in the intercellular spaces?
    a. abscess
    b. edema
    c. infarct
    d. hemorrhage

C[854]

864. What structure is not seen due to superimposition on an anteroposterior projection of the pelvis if the feet are not inverted?
    a. greater trochanter
    b. lesser trochanter
    c. bicipital groove
    d. ischial tuberosity

A[855]

865. Which intervertebral disc space is normally at the level of the umbilicus?
    a. T12-L1
    b. L2-L3
    c. L3-L4
    d. L4-L5

D[856]

866. Which surface of the foot should be closest to the image receptor for the best recorded detail when performing a lateral projection?
    a. plantar
    b. dorsal
    c. lateral
    d. medial

D[857]

867. Which temporal portion will be demonstrated in an anterior profile projection, or Arcelin method, if the head is turned to the left?
    a. right petrous portion
    b. left petrous portion
    c. foramen magnum
    d. palatine plate

C[858]

┌ Answer
│ ┌ Question #
↓ ↓

868. Which of the following is a localized dilation of the wall of an artery?
    a. edema
    b. aneurysm
    c. pneumothorax
    d. dissection

C⁸⁷⁶

869. When viewing a submentovertical projection of the skull, which sinus appears between the foramen magnum and the maxillary sinuses?
    1. sphenoidal
    2. frontal
    3. ethmoid
    a. 1 only
    b. 2 only
    c. 3 only
    d. 1, 2, & 3

870. Which of the carpal bones does not have a second or third name?
    a. navicular
    b. lunate
    c. pisiform
    d. unciform

871. Which of the following is more desirable when positioning the breast?
    a. compressing to profile the nipple
    b. compressing to demonstrate as much of the posterior breast as possible
    c. maintaining the medial side of the breast as far from the image receptor as possible
    d. avoiding compression to make the patient more comfortable

872. What term is used to describe the baseline between the external auditory meatus and the outer canthus of the eye?
    a. orbitomeatal line
    b. acanthiomeatal line
    c. mentomeatal line
    d. sagittal plane

C⁸⁷⁷

D⁸⁷⁸

Question # ⌐
Answer ⌐ |
↓ |
↓

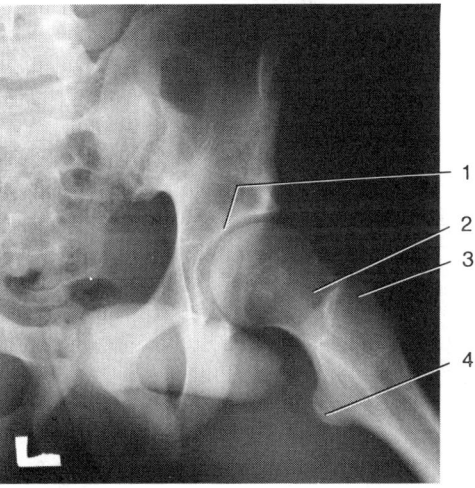

Figure 16

B⁸⁶²

B⁸⁶³

B⁸⁶⁴

873. Which number in Figure 16 illustrates the surgical neck?
    a. 1
    b. 2
    c. 3
    d. 4

C⁸⁶⁵

874. Which number in figure 16 illustrates the lesser trochanter?
    a. 1
    b. 2
    c. 3
    d. 4

D⁸⁶⁶

875. Which number in Figure 16 illustrates the acetabulum?
    a. 1
    b. 2
    c. 3
    d. 4

B⁸⁶⁷

┌─ Answer
│ ┌─ Question #
↓ ↓

876. What is the proper centering point for a routine posterioranterior chest projection?
  a. T2-T3
  b. T4-T5
  c. T6-T7
  d. T8-T9

D⁸⁸⁵

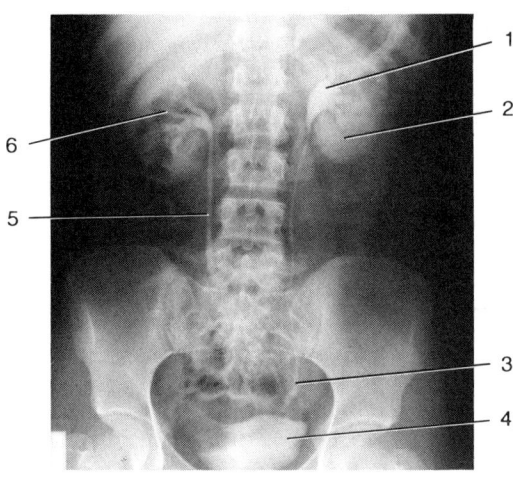

Figure 17

A⁸⁸⁶

D⁸⁸⁷

877. Which numbers in Figure 17 illustrate the ureter?
  1. 1
  2. 3
  3. 5
    a. 1 & 2 only
    b. 1 & 3 only
    c. 2 & 3 only
    d. 1, 2, & 3

B⁸⁸⁸

878. Which number in Figure 17 illustrates the renal pelvis?
  a. 1
  b. 2
  c. 4
  d. 6

D⁸⁸⁹

879. Which number in Figure 17 illustrates the lower pole of a kidney?
    a. 1
    b. 2
    c. 4
    d. 6

880. What is the proper central ray angulation to achieve a correct anteroposterior projection of the sacrum?
    a. 10° caudad
    b. 10° cephalad
    c. 15° caudad
    d. 15° cephalad

881. What is the proper term for the radiographic examination of the parotid glands?
    a. lymphangiography
    b. venography
    c. glandography
    d. sialography

882. Which projection best demonstrates the articular facets of the lumbar spine?
    a. anteroposterior
    b. posteroanterior
    c. lateral
    d. oblique

B⁸⁷³

883. What position should be assumed by the hand for a proper AP projection of the forearm?
    1. supinated
    2. pronated
    3. with the volar surface in contact with the image receptor
    a. 1 only
    b. 2 only
    c. 3 only
    d. 1, 2, & 3

C⁸⁷⁴

884. What degree of obliquity from lateral is required to visualize the apophyseal articulations of the thoracic spine?
    a. 10°
    b. 20°
    c. 30°
    d. 70°

A⁸⁷⁵

885. What term describes a guide wire in which the position of the inside portion can be varied?
     a. J guide wire
     b. straight guide wire
     c. fixed core
     d. moveable core

A^{893}

886. Which of the following correctly position the skull for a PA projecti on by the Caldwell method for a general survey of the cranium?
     1. orbitomeatal line perpendicular to the image receptor
     2. midsagittal plane is parallel to the central ray
     3. central ray is angled 15° cephalad
     a. 1 & 2 only
     b. 1 & 3 only
     c. 2 & 3 only
     d. 1, 2, & 3

A^{894}

887. Which of the following are considered part of the urinary system?
     1. ureters
     2. urethra
     3. kidneys
     a. 1 & 2 only
     b. 1 & 3 only
     c. 2 & 3 only
     d. 1, 2, & 3

C^{895}

888. Which of the following unite to form the common bile duct?
     1. common hepatic duct
     2. pancreatic duct
     3. cystic duct
     a. 1 & 2 only
     b. 1 & 3 only
     c. 2 & 3 only
     d. 1, 2, & 3

A^{896}

889. Which of the following structures should be visualized on a lateral chest radiograph?
     1. heart and diaphragm
     2. costophrenic angles and apices of lungs
     3. superimposition of the ribs posterior to the vertebral column
     a. 1 & 2 only
     b. 1 & 3 only
     c. 2 & 3 only
     d. 1, 2, & 3

A^{897}

Question # ⌐
Answer ⌐

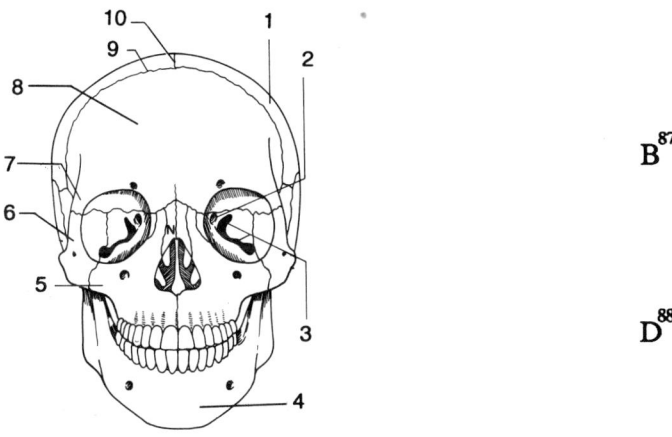

B⁸⁷⁹

D⁸⁸⁰

Figure 18 (from Akesson EJ, Loeb JA, Wilson-Pauwels L: Thompson's Core Textbook of Anatomy, 2nd ed. Philadelphia, JB Lippincott, 1990)

D⁸⁸¹

890. Which numbers in Figure 18 illustrate the frontal bone?
    1. 2 and 9
    2. 7 and 8
    3. 8 and 9
       a. 1 only
       b. 2 only
       c. 3 only
       d. 1, 2, & 3

D⁸⁸²

891. Which number in Figure 18 illustrates the sagittal suture?
       a. 2
       b. 5
       c. 9
       d. 10

A⁸⁸³

892. Which number in Figure 18 illustrates the maxillary bone?
       a. 1
       b. 3
       c. 5
       d. 8

B⁸⁸⁴

A⁹⁰³

893. What position outlines the lesser tuberosity between the humeral he ad and the greater tuberosity?
 a. AP humerus
 b. lateral humerus
 c. transthoracic lateral humerus
 d. axillary shoulder

D⁹⁰⁴

894. What projection is achieved if the patient is positioned so the midsagittal plane and orbitomeatal line are perpendicular to the image receptor and the central ray is perpendicular, exiting at the nasion?
 a. PA
 b. lateral
 c. parietoacanthial (Waters method)
 d. PA axial (Caldwell method)

895. What is the proper centering point for a lateral position of the sella turcica?
 a. 3/4" anterior and 3/4" inferior to the external auditory meatus
 b. 3/4" posterior and 3/4" inferior to the external auditory meatus
 c. 3/4" anterior and 3/4" superior to the external auditory meatus
 d. 1/2" posterior and 1/2" inferior to the external auditory meatus

B⁹⁰⁵

896. Which of the following correctly position the skull for a lateral projection?
 1. interpupillary line perpendicular to the image receptor
 2. midsagittal plane is parallel to the image receptor
 3. infraorbitomeatal line is parallel to the central ray

A⁹⁰⁶

 a. 1 & 2 only
 b. 1 & 3 only
 c. 2 & 3 only
 d. 1, 2, & 3

897. Where should supporting positioning sponges, pillows, or sandbags be placed to correct the angulation of the sagittal plane when positioning a hypersthenic patient for a lateral skull?
 a. under the parietal bone

D⁹⁰⁷

 b. under the mandible
 c. under the superior chest
 d. under the abdomen below the diaphragm

Question # ⌐
Answer ⌐ |
↓ |
↓

898. Which bones make up the zygomatic arch?
1. temporal
2. zygoma
3. maxillary
a. 1 & 2 only
b. 1 & 3 only
c. 2 & 3 only
d. 1, 2, & 3

899. What term is used to describe the opening between the duodenum and the stomach?
a. pyloric orifice
b. cardiac orifice
c. sphincter of Oddi
d. pylorus

900. Which of the following are names for the same salivary gland?
1. sublingual
2. submandibular
3. submaxillary
a. 1 & 2 only
b. 1 & 3 only
c. 2 & 3 only
d. 1, 2, & 3

901. What is the relationship of the esophagus to other thoracic structures?   C^{890}
1. anterior to the trachea
2. anterior to the vertebral column
3. medial to the heart
a. 1 & 2 only   C^{891}
b. 1 & 3 only
c. 2 & 3 only
d. 1, 2, & 3

902. What is another term for the body of the sternum?
a. gladiolus
b. xiphoid   C^{892}
c. manubrium
d. coracoid

Answer
Question #

903. What structure forms the eye of the apophyseal joint "scotty dog" th
at can be demonstrated on oblique projections of the lumbar spine?
   a. pedicle
   b. lamina
   c. superior articular process
   d. inferior articular process

C^{914}

904. What is the proper position of the patient for a lateral projection of
the proximal left femur?
   a. RAO
   b. LAO
   c. RPO
   d. LPO

905. Which of the following characterizes a brachycephalic skull?
   1. broad from side to side
   2. long from front to back
   3. has an angle of 54° between internal structures and the midsagittal
   plane
   a. 1 & 2 only
   b. 1 & 3 only
   c. 2 & 3 only
   d. 1, 2, & 3

906. What is the average normal transit time for the stomach to empty?
   a. 2 to 3 hours
   b. 10 to 12 hours
   c. 24 hours
   d. 48 hours

C^{915}

907. Which of the following can be detected with postoperative
cholangiography?
   1. the status of the sphincter of the hepatopancreatic ampulla
   2. the presence of previously undetected stones
   3. the patency of the ducts
   a. 1 & 2 only
   b. 1 & 3 only
   c. 2 & 3 only
   d. 1, 2, & 3

C^{916}

908. What are the proper breathing instructions for an AP abdomen?
    a. shallow breathing
    b. rapid breathing
    c. full inhalation
    d. full exhalation

909. Which of the following are part of the intervertebral disks?   A^{898}
    1. nucleus pulposus
    2. annulus fibrosus
    3. pedicles
        a. 1 & 2 only
        b. 1 & 3 only
        c. 2 & 3 only
        d. 1, 2, & 3

910. What structure is at the level of the iliac crest?   A^{899}
    a. T6
    b. T12
    c. L2
    d. L4

911. How many tarsals are there?
    a. 5   C^{900}
    b. 7
    c. 14
    d. 26

912. Which of the following indicates a presence of air in the pleural cavity resulting in a partial or complete collapse of the lung?
    a. pneumonia
    b. emphysema
    c. pneumothorax   C^{901}
    d. empyema

913. Which of the following is the normal, non-dislocated position of the humeral head in a scapular Y position of the shoulder joint?
    1. superimposed over the junction of the Y
    2. beneath the coracoid process   A^{902}
    3. beneath the acromion process
        a. 1 only
        b. 2 only
        c. 3 only
        d. 1, 2, & 3

914. Which bone appears immediately proximal to the carpometacarpal joint of the thumb?
     a. first metacarpal
     b. proximal phalanx of the thumb
     c. trapezium
     d. navicular

C⁹²²

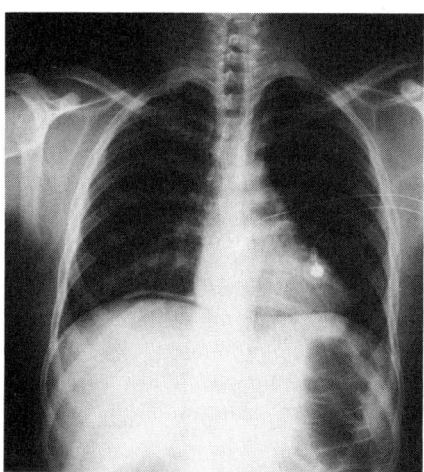

Figure 19

A⁹²³

C⁹²⁴

915. What are the two wires visible over the chest in Figure 19?
     a. arterial cardiac monitor
     b. Swan-Ganz catheter
     c. electrocardiographic leads
     d. ventilator O_2 hose

916. In what position was the patient when the exposure in Figure 19 was made?
     a. supine
     b. prone
     c. erect
     d. decubitus

917. Which position of the elbow projects the ulnar coronoid process from superimposition?
    a. lateral oblique
    b. medial oblique
    c. AP
    d. lateral

D^{908}

918. How many degrees of angulation are there between the orbitomeatal and infraorbitomeatal skull base lines?
    a. 5
    b. 6
    c. 7
    d. 8

A^{909}

919. Which of the following describes a retrograde pyelogram?
    1. cystography
    2. nephrotomography
    3. urography
    a. 1 only
    b. 2 only
    c. 3 only
    d. 1, 2, & 3

D^{910}

920. Which of the following signal completion of a small bowel study?
    1. 60 minutes after ingestion of barium
    2. barium in the cecum
    3. barium in the rectum
    a. 1 only
    b. 2 only
    c. 3 only
    d. 1, 2, & 3

B^{911}

921. Which position best demonstrates the ribs that overshadow the heart?
    a. AP
    b. PA
    c. LAO or RPO
    d. RAO or LPO

C^{912}

A^{913}

922. What is accomplished by instructing a patient to phonate "ah" during exposure of the atlas and axis in the AP open mouth position?
    a. occlusal surface is aligned with the base of the skull
    b. lips are opened
    c. tongue is affixed to the floor of the mouth
    d. patient concentrates on the phonation thereby holding the position better than without phonation

D ^{931}

923. At what structure does the femoral head articulate with the hip bone?
    a. acetabulum
    b. glenoid fossa
    c. apophyseal joint
    d. inferior pelvis facet

D ^{932}

924. Which of the following is a fatty tumor?
    a. adenoma
    b. sarcoma
    c. lipoma
    d. angioma

D ^{933}

A ^{934}

B ^{935}

D ^{936}

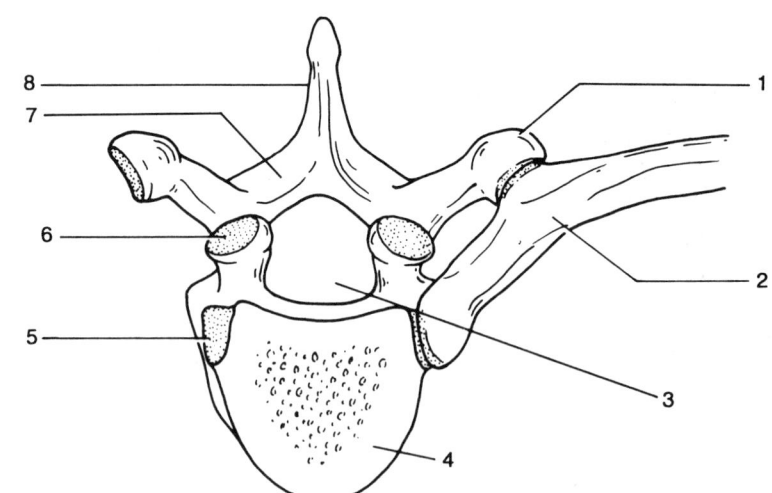

Figure 20 (from Akesson EJ, Loeb JA, Wilson-Pauwels L: Thompson's Core Textbook of Anatomy, 2nd ed. Philadelphia, JB Lippincott, 1990)

Question #
Answer

925. Which of the following is illustrated by #7 in Figure 20?
   a. pedicle
   b. lamina
   c. spinous process
   d. transverse process

B^917

926. Which number in Figure 20 illustrates the vertebral foramen?
   a. 1
   b. 3
   c. 6
   d. 7

927. Which number in Figure 20 illustrates the superior facet of an apophyseal joint?
   a. 1
   b. 5
   c. 6
   d. 8

C^918

928. Which of the following is illustrated by #2 in Figure 20?
   a. spinous process
   b. transverse process
   c. lamina
   d. rib

C^919

929. Which of the following should be perpendicular to the image receptor for a PA axial position (Caldwell method) of the sinuses?
   1. coronal plane
   2. midsagittal plane
   3. orbitomeatal line
   a. 1 & 2 only
   b. 1 & 3 only
   c. 2 & 3 only
   d. 1, 2, & 3

B^920

930. Which of the following bones are part of the orbit?
   1. zygoma
   2. sphenoid
   3. ethmoid
   a. 1 & 2 only
   b. 1 & 3 only
   c. 2 & 3 only
   d. 1, 2, & 3

C^921

┌ Answer
│ ┌ Question #
↓ ↓

931. Which of the following intersects the glabella, nasion, acanthion, and mental point of the skull?
    a. infraorbitomeatal line
    b. interpupillary line
    c. acanthiomeatal line
    d. midsagittal plane

B⁹⁴³

932. Which position best demonstrates the splenic flexure of the colon?
    a. PA
    b. lateral
    c. RAO
    d. LAO

B⁹⁴⁴

933. Which ribs lack anterior cartilage?
    a. 7th to 9th
    b. 7th to 12th
    c. 9th to 12th
    d. 11th to 12th

934. Which type of joint is formed between two vertebral bodies?
    a. amphidiarthrodial
    b. synarthrotic
    c. diarthrotic
    d. ball and socket

935. Which bone articulates with the proximal end of all three cuneiforms?
    a. cuboid
    b. navicular
    c. fifth metatarsal
    d. os calcis

936. What is the primary structure of interest if a patient is positioned supine with the body rotated approximately 35° to 45° toward the affected side, and the central ray is directed at the shoulder joint?
    a. greater tubercle of the humerus
    b. bicipital groove of the humerus
    c. acromioclavicular joint
    d. glenoid fossa

B⁹⁴⁵

Question #
Answer

937. Which bones form the acetabulum?
    1. ilium
    2. ischium
    3. pubis
      a. 1 & 2 only
      b. 1 & 3 only
      c. 2 & 3 only
      d. 1, 2, & 3

B^{925}

938. Which of the following temporal bone methods are complementary positions that produce similar projections by reversing central ray entrance and exit points?
      a. Henschen and Schuller
      b. Schuller and Laws
      c. Laws and Stenvers
      d. Stenvers and Arcelin

B^{926}

939. Which bone includes the inion?
      a. occipital
      b. frontal
      c. right and left parietal
      d. sphenoid

C^{927}

940. To which body system do the suprarenal glands belong?
      a. gastrointestinal
      b. urinary
      c. endocrine
      d. nervous

D^{928}

941. Which of the following secretes bile?
      a. gallbladder
      b. liver
      c. pancreas
      d. stomach

C^{929}

942. What term describes the bifurcation of the trachea?
      a. bronchus
      b. epiglottis
      c. carina
      d. coronoid

D^{930}

943. At which vertebral level does the trachea form a junction with the larynx?
    a. 4th cervical
    b. 6th cervical
    c. 2nd thoracic
    d. 4th thoracic

D⁹⁵²

944. Although the superior angle of the neck of the femur varies with age, sex, and body type, what is the approximate range?
    a. 5 to 10°
    b. 15 to 20°
    c. 45 to 50°
    d. 120 to 130°

D⁹⁵³

C⁹⁵⁴

A⁹⁵⁵

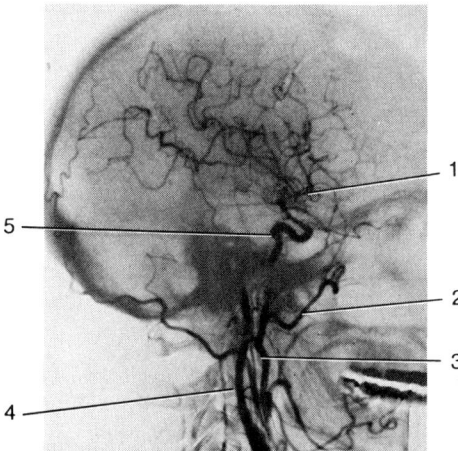

Figure 21

C⁹⁵⁶

945. What type of technique was used to produce the image in Figure 21?
    1. magnification
    2. subtraction
    3. minification
    a. 1 only
B⁹⁵⁷
    b. 2 only
    c. 3 only
    d. 1, 2, & 3

946. Which of the following is illustrated by #5 in Figure 21?
    a. middle cerebral artery
    b. carotid siphon
    c. internal carotid artery
    d. external carotid artery

947. Which number in Figure 21 illustrates the internal carotid artery? D^{937}
    a. 1
    b. 2
    c. 3
    d. 4

948. What term describes the angle of the mandible?
    a. glenoid D^{938}
    b. glabella
    c. mental point
    d. gonion

949. Which of the following describes the areas of incomplete ossification present in the newborn infant calvarium? A^{939}
    a. bregmatic fossae
    b. ossificans
    c. fontanels
    d. depressions

950. What is the primary direction in which the stomach will move C^{940} when a patient changes from an upright to recumbent position?
    a. posterior
    b. anterior
    c. superior
    d. lateral

951. Which of the following procedures uses a fiberoptic endoscope? B^{941}
    a. percutaneous transhepatic cholangiography
    b. endoscopic retrograde cholangiopancreatography
    c. postoperative cholangiography
    d. operative cholangiography

C^{942}

952. Which of the following soft tissues should be demonstrated on an AP abdomen projection?
    1. psoas muscles
    2. liver
    3. kidneys
        a. 1 only
        b. 2 only
        c. 3 only
        d. 1, 2, & 3

953. Which bones form the sternal angle?
        a. manubrium and xiphoid process
        b. manubrium and gladiolus
        c. manubrium and 2nd rib
        d. gladiolus and xiphoid process

954. What central ray angle should be used to demonstrate the coccyx when the patient is prone?
        a. 15° cephalad
        b. 15° caudad
        c. 10° cephalad
        d. 10° caudad

C⁹⁶³

955. Which of the following are contained within the pelvic cavity?
    1. urinary bladder
    2. rectum
    3. kidneys
        a. 1 & 2 only
        b. 1 & 3 only
        c. 2 & 3 only
        d. 1, 2, & 3

B⁹⁶⁴

956. What structure is at the level of the xiphoid tip?
        a. T4
        b. T8
        c. T10
        d. L1

A⁹⁶⁵

957. What is the largest foramina in the body?
        a. foramen magnum
        b. obturator foramen
        c. foramen ovale
        d. jugular foramen

B⁹⁶⁶

958. Which of the following includes the medial malleolus?
    a. tibia
    b. fibula   B[946]
    c. talus
    d. os calcis

959. What is the difference between a thrombosis and an embolism?
    a. a thrombosis is a fibrinogen clot while an embolism is a platelet clot   C[947]
    b. an embolism occurs when several thrombosis combine
    c. an embolism is a clot that has detached from a thrombosis and is moving free in the circulatory system
    d. an embolism is an infected thrombosis

960. What is the proper position of the arm for an inferosuperior axial D[948] shoulder joint projection?
    a. neutral
    b. internal rotation
    c. external rotation
    d. pulled across the chest to grip the opposite shoulder

961. What is the proper position of the hand for an AP elbow?   C[949]
    a. pronated
    b. supinated
    c. lateral
    d. lateral (external) oblique

962. How many lobes are normal in the left lung?
    1. 2
    2. 3   C[950]
    3. 4
    a. 1 only
    b. 2 only
    c. 3 only   B[951]
    d. 1, 2, & 3

A⁹⁷²

C⁹⁷³

C⁹⁷⁴

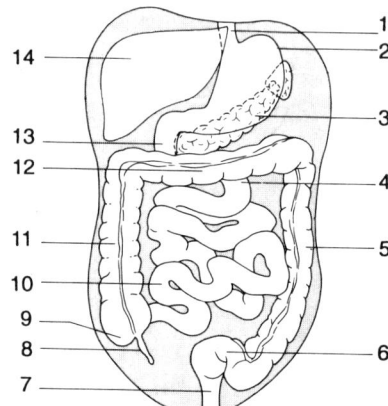

Figure 22 (from Akesson EJ, Loeb JA, Wilson-Pauwels L: Thompson's Core Textbook of Anatomy, 2nd ed. Philadelphia, JB Lippincott, 1990)

963. Which of the following is illustrated by #13 in Figure 22?
    a. ileum
    b. jejunum
    c. duodenum
    d. colon

964. Which number in Figure 22 illustrates the pancreas?
    a. 1
    b. 3
    c. 13
    d. 14

965. Which number in Figure 22 illustrates the descending colon?
    a. 5
    b. 6
    c. 9
    d. 11

966. Which of the following is illustrated by #9 in Figure 22?
    a. vermiform appendix
    b. cecum
    c. ileum
    d. ascending colon

Question # ┐
Answer ┐ │
↓ │
↓

967. What are rugae?
    a. regions of the duodenum prone to ulcers because of their
       thin walls
    b. out-pouchings of the wall of the colon   A⁹⁵⁸
    c. stones that may form in the gallbladder
    d. gastric mucosal folds

968. What structures are examined during sialography?
    1. salivary glands
    2. salivary ducts
    3. esophagus
    a. 1 & 2 only   C⁹⁵⁹
    b. 1 & 3 only
    c. 2 & 3 only
    d. 1, 2, & 3

969. What is the relationship of the thymus gland to other thoracic
structures?
    1. anterior to the trachea   C⁹⁶⁰
    2. superior to the heart
    3. medial to the sternoclavicular joints
    a. 1 & 2 only
    b. 1 & 3 only
    c. 2 & 3 only
    d. 1, 2, & 3

970. What is the primary reason for considering the use of a PA B⁹⁶¹
projection of the abdomen in place of an AP?
    a. magnification of the kidneys to increase recorded detail
    b. reduction of gonadal dose
    c. patient motion is reduced
    d. fecal material drops into the cecum or rectum

971. Which of the following would best demonstrate fluid in the right A⁹⁶²
pleural cavity?
    a. left lateral decubitus chest
    b. right lateral decubitus chest
    c. ventral decubitus chest
    d. dorsal decubitus chest

972. Which projection opens the intervertebral disk spaces of the cervical spine?
    a. AP with 15° to 20° cephalad angulation
    b. PA with 15° to 20° cephalad angulation
    c. RPO with 15° to 20° caudad angulation
    d. lateral

973. What is the proper position of the patient to produce an AP project ion of the left ilium?
    a. 25° LPO
    b. 25° RPO
    c. 40° LPO
    d. 40° RPO

974. Which of the following involves a cystic dilation of the distal ureter near the entrance to the bladder?
    a. polycystic renal disease
    b. cystitis
    c. ureterocele
    d. pyelonephritis

A 982

A 983

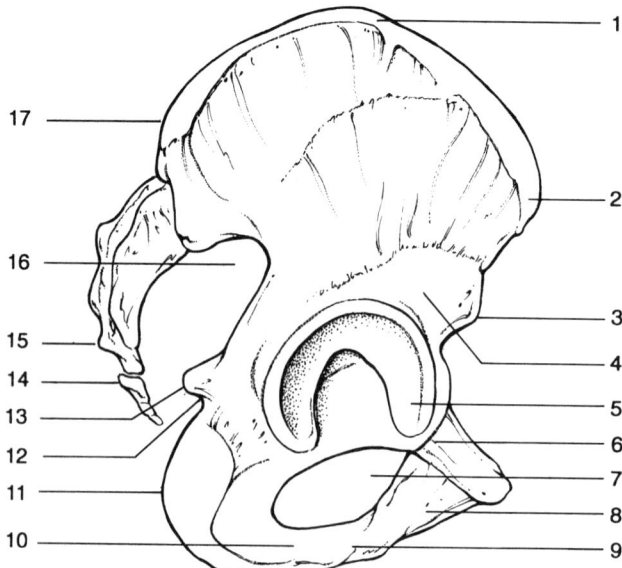

Figure 23 (from Akesson EJ, Loeb JA, Wilson-Pauwels L: Thompson's Core Textbook of Anatomy, 2nd ed. Philadelphia, JB Lippincott, 1990)

975. Which of the following is illustrated by #7 in Figure 23?
    a. superior ramus of pubis
    b. body of pubis
    c. inferior ramus of pubis   D^{967}
    d. ramus of ischium

976. Which number in Figure 23 illustrates the anterior superior spine of the ilium?
    a. 1
    b. 2
    c. 3
    d. 17

977. Which number in Figure 23 illustrates the sacrum?   A^{968}
    a. 13
    b. 14
    c. 15
    d. 17

978. Which of the following is illustrated by #3 in Figure 23?
    a. anterior superior iliac spine
    b. anterior inferior iliac spine
    c. posterior superior iliac spine   D^{969}
    d. greater sciatic notch

979. Which of the following is illustrated by #12 in Figure 23?
    a. ischial tuberosity
    b. ischial spine
    c. lesser sciatic notch
    d. greater sciatic notch

980. Which cuneiform is most lateral?   B^{970}
    a. first
    b. second
    c. third
    d. fourth

981. Which term describes a localized area of necrotic tissue?   B^{971}
    a. abscess
    b. edema
    c. infarct
    d. hemorrhage

┌─ Answer
│ ┌─ Question #
│ │
↓ ↓

B⁹⁹⁰

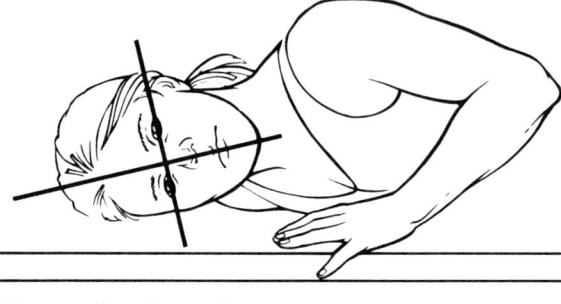

C⁹⁹¹

Hypersthenic patient

Figure 24 (reprinted with permission from Eisenberg RL, Dennis CA, May CR: Radiographic Positioning, Little, Brown and Company, copyright 1989)

B⁹⁹²

982. Which positioning baselines are not properly aligned for a lateral skull radiograph of the hypersthenic patient shown in Figure 24?
1. interpupillary
2. midsagittal
3. midcoronal
    a. 1 & 2 only
    b. 1 & 3 only
    c. 2 & 3 only
    d. 1, 2, & 3

983. Which of the following are complimentary methods that demonstrate the same anatomic structures in essentially the same relationships?
1. Arcelin
2. Stenvers
3. Waters
    a. 1 & 2 only
    b. 1 & 3 only
    c. 2 & 3 only
    d. 1, 2, & 3

Question # ⌐
Answer ⌐ |
↓ |
↓

984. Which bone serves as an attachment for the muscles of the throat
and tongue but does not articulate with any other bones?   B^{975}
    a. mandible
    b. clavicle
    c. hyoid
    d. 7th cervical vertebra

985. Which of the following are part of the sphenoid bone?
    1. anterior clinoid processes
    2. posterior clinoid processes   B^{976}
    3. crista galli
    a. 1 & 2 only
    b. 1 & 3 only
    c. 2 & 3 only
    d. 1, 2, & 3

986. What is the approximate respiratory excursion of the kidneys?   C^{977}
    a. 1 mm
    b. 1 cm
    c. 2.5 cm
    d. 5 cm

987. Which organ includes the duct of Wirsung?   B^{978}
    a. spleen
    b. liver
    c. pancreas
    d. kidney

988. What is the normal number of parathyroid glands?   C^{979}
    a. 2
    b. 3
    c. 4
    d. 5

989. Which is the longest rib?   C^{980}
    a. 1st
    b. 5th
    c. 7th
    d. 12th   C^{981}

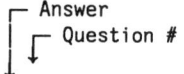

┌ Answer
│ ┌ Question #
│ │
↓ ↓

990. Which of the following is a malignant tumor arising from connective tissue?
   a. adenoma
   b. sarcoma
   c. lipoma
   d. angioma

C^{999}

991. Which body part is being examined if the patient is supine and the central ray is directed to a point approximately 2" inferior to the coracoid process?
   a. acromioclavicular joints
   b. shoulder
   c. scapula
   d. clavicle

D^{1000}

992. Which body part is examined with a carpal bridge tangential position?
   a. elbow
   b. wrist
   c. mandible
   d. maxilla

D^{1001}

C^{1002}

C^{1003}

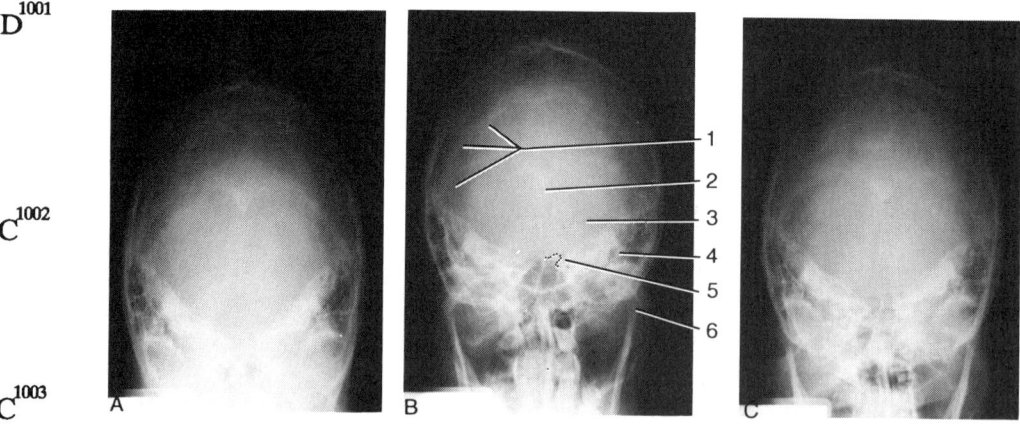

Figure 25

C^{1004}

Question # ⌐
Answer ⌐ |
↓ |
↓

993. Which of the following positions was used to produce the radiographs in Figure 25?
    a. PA axial Haas method
    b. AP axial Towne method
    c. PA Caldwell method
    d. submentovertical full basilar projection
C^{984}

994. What was the angle between the central ray and the orbitomeatal line for the radiograph in Figure 25a?
    a. 25°
    b. 30°
    c. 35°
    d. 40°

995. Which of the following is illustrated by #1 in Figure 25b?
    a. coronal suture
    b. sagittal suture
    c. lambdoidal suture
    d. petrous portion of the temporal bone
A^{985}

996. Which number in Figure 25b illustrates the inion?
    a. 1
    b. 2
    c. 3
    d. 5
C^{986}

997. Which of the following is illustrated by #5 in Figure 25b?
    a. dorsum sellae
    b. condyle of mandible
    c. posterior clinoid process
    d. petrous portion (pyramid)
C^{987}

998. What was the angle between the central ray and the orbitomeatal line for the radiograph in Figure 25b?
    a. 30°
    b. 35°
    c. 40°
    d. 45°
C^{988}

C^{989}

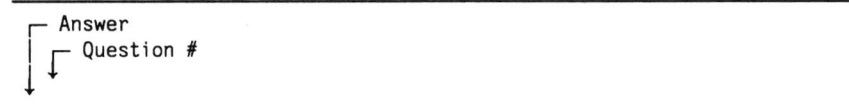

Answer
Question #

999. What is the proper angulation of the orbitomeatal line to the image receptor for a parietoacanthial projection (Waters method) of the paranasal sinuses?
    a. 15°
    b. 25°
D¹⁰¹¹   c. 37°
    d. 53°

1000. What is the proper angulation of the midsagittal plane for a parieto-orbital oblique position (Rhese method) of the optic foramen?
    a. 15°
    b. 25°
    c. 37°
    d. 53°

C¹⁰¹²   1001. Which of the following correctly position the skull for a general survey AP axial position by the Towne method?
    1. orbitomeatal line perpendicular to the image receptor
    2. midsagittal plane is parallel to the image receptor
    3. the central ray is directed 30° caudally
    a. 1 & 2 only
    b. 1 & 3 only
    c. 2 & 3 only
    d. 1, 2, & 3

A¹⁰¹³   1002. How many bones make up the facial bones?
    a. 4
    b. 8
    c. 14
    d. 22

B¹⁰¹⁴   1003. Where should a Colcher-Sussman ruler be placed for an AP?
    a. 10 cm above the tabletop
    b. 15 cm above the tabletop
    c. 10 cm below the symphysis pubis
    d. at the level of the symphysis pubis

1004. What is the normal time period from intravenous injection to the greatest concentration of urographic contrast media in the renal collecting system?
C¹⁰¹⁵
    a. 30 to 60 seconds
    b. 2 to 8 minutes
    c. 15 to 20 minutes
    d. 45 to 60 minutes

1005. What is the anatomic relationship of the prostate gland to the rectum?
    1. anterior
    2. posterior
    3. to the right
        a. 1 only
        b. 2 only
        c. 3 only
        d. 1, 2, & 3

B [993]

1006. Which position best demonstrates the rectum?
        a. PA
        b. lateral
        c. RAO
        d. LAO

D [994]

1007. What is the proper central ray angulation for a PA axial position of the colon?
        a. 10° to 20° caudad
        b. 10° to 20° cephalad
        c. 30° to 40° caudad
        d. 30° to 40° cephalad

C [995]

1008. What is the average normal transit time for food to travel from the mouth through the rectum?
        a. 2 to 3 hours
        b. 10 to 12 hours
        c. 24 hours
        d. 48 hours

B [996]

1009. What term describes the region in which all thoracic organs except the lungs are located?
        a. sternal cavity
        b. mediastinum
        c. diaphragm
        d. bronchial tree

C [997]

1010. Which of the following structures is most medial?
        a. greater trochanter
        b. lesser trochanter
        c. femoral neck
        d. femoral head

A [998]

1011. Which of the following will demonstrate the intercondyloid fossa?
 1. Beclere method
 2. Camp-Coventry method
 3. Holmblad method
  a. 1 & 2 only
  b. 1 & 3 only
  c. 2 & 3 only
  d. 1, 2, & 3

1012. Which of the following will demonstrate the lesser tubercle of the humerus medially and in profile?
 1. AP neutral rotation shoulder
 2. AP external rotation shoulder
 3. AP internal rotation shoulder
  a. 1 only
  b. 2 only
  c. 3 only
  d. 1, 2, & 3

1013. Which of the following is achieved by ulnar flexion of the wrist?
 1. navicular foreshortening is corrected
 2. spaces between adjacent carpals are closed
 3. the radius is superimposed over the navicular

B¹⁰²¹
  a. 1 only
  b. 2 only
  c. 3 only
  d. 1, 2, & 3

A¹⁰²² 1014. At what level is the duodenal bulb located?
  a. T10
  b. L2
  c. L4
  d. L5

1015. Which of the following provide evaluation of renal function?
 1. cystourethrogram
C¹⁰²³ 2. retrograde pyelogram
 3. intravenous urogram (IVP)
  a. 1 only
  b. 2 only
  c. 3 only
  d. 1, 2, & 3

Question #
Answer

1016. Which term describes the thin flap that covers the laryngeal entrance during swallowing?
    a. pharynx
    b. cricoid
    c. epiglottis
    d. hyoid

1017. Which of the following are reasons why foreign bodies entering   A^{1005}
the trachea are more likely to enter the right bronchus than the left?
    1. the right bronchus lies in a more vertical position
    2. the right bronchus is larger   B^{1006}
    3. the left bronchus is capped by a valve
    a. 1 & 2 only
    b. 1 & 3 only
    c. 2 & 3 only
    d. 1, 2, & 3

1018. What term describes the joint where the two pubic bones articulate?   C^{1007}
    a. interpubic articulation
    b. symphysis pubis
    c. sacroiliac joint
    d. acetabulum

1019. Which of the following are rationale for using a 72" FFD with the patient erect for a routine PA projection of the chest?
    1. avoid engorgement of the pulmonary vessels   C^{1008}
    2. decrease heart size magnification from 40" FFD
    3. increase image contrast
    a. 1 & 2 only
    b. 1 & 3 only
    c. 2 & 3 only
    d. 1, 2, & 3

1020. What is the proper central ray angulation for an AP projection of   B^{1009}
the cervical vertebrae?
    a. 10 to 15° cephalad
    b. 15 to 20° cephalad
    c. 10 to 15° caudad
    d. 15 to 20° caudad   D^{1010}

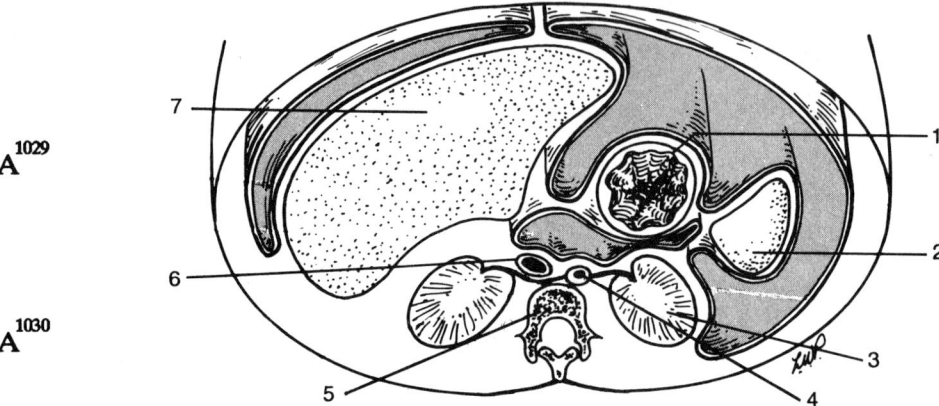

A¹⁰²⁹

A¹⁰³⁰

Figure 26 (from Akesson EJ, Loeb JA, Wilson-Pauwels L: Thompson's Core Textbook of Anatomy, 2nd ed. Philadelphia, JB Lippincott, 1990)

A¹⁰³¹   1021. Which of the following is illustrated by #7 in Figure 26?
a. stomach
b. liver
c. kidney
d. spleen

C¹⁰³²   1022. Which number in Figure 26 illustrates the stomach?
a. 1
b. 2
c. 3
d. 7

C¹⁰³³   1023. Which of the following is illustrated by #4 in Figure 26?
a. kidney
b. vena cava
c. aorta
d. vertebra

A¹⁰³⁴

1024. Which of the following are contained within the thoracic cavity?
    1. lungs
    2. heart
    3. stomach
        a. 1 & 2 only
        b. 1 & 3 only   C^{1016}
        c. 2 & 3 only
        d. 1, 2, & 3

1025. Which of the following articulates with the superior facet of the calcaneus?
        a. navicular
        b. talus
        c. third cuneiform   A^{1017}
        d. cuboid

1026. Which of the following articulates with the trochlea?
    1. radius
    2. ulna
    3. humerus
        a. 1 only
        b. 2 only   B^{1018}
        c. 3 only
        d. 1, 2, & 3

1027. Which of the following best demonstrate the splenic flexure of the colon?
        a. RPO and LAO
        b. LPO and RAO
        c. RPO and LPO
        d. RAO and LAO

1028. What is the proper central ray angulation for a posterior profile A^{1019}
    position (Stenvers method) of the petrous portion of the temporal bone?
        a. 12° cephalad
        b. 15° caudad
        c. 25° cephalad
        d. 37° caudad

                                                B^{1020}

┌ Answer
│ ┌ Question #
↓ ↓

1029. Which of the following describe the parieto-orbital oblique position (Rhese method) for the optic foramen?
    1. the central ray is perpendicular to the image receptor
    2. the acanthiomeatal line is perpendicular to the image receptor
    3. the midsagittal plane forms an angle of 37° with the film
      a. 1 & 2 only
      b. 1 & 3 only
      c. 2 & 3 only
      d. 1, 2, & 3

C^{1041}

1030. Which bone contains the sinus known as the antrum of Highmore?
      a. maxilla
      b. ethmoid
      c. zygoma
      d. frontal

B^{1042}

1031. What term describes the point where the sagittal and lambdoidal sutures meet?
      a. bregma
      b. glabella
      c. nasion
      d. crista galli

C^{1043}

1032. Which portion of the gastrointestinal tract is the longest?
      a. esophagus
      b. stomach
      c. small bowel
      d. colon

1033. Which of the following positions will project the gallbladder free from superimposition of the vertebral column?
      a. AP
      b. PA
      c. LAO
      d. LPO

1034. Which of the following are salivary glands?
    1. sublingual
    2. submandibular
    3. suborbital
      a. 1 & 2 only
      b. 1 & 3 only
      c. 2 & 3 only
      d. 1, 2, & 3

1035. At what angles are the intervertebral foramina of the cervical vertebrae?
  a. 45° posterior and 25° anterior
  b. 45° anterior and 15° inferior
  c. 45° anterior and 15° superior
  d. 35° anterior and 15° inferior

1036. What vertebral body is at the level of the sternal angle?   A^{1024}
  a. C7
  b. T1
  c. T4
  d. T10

1037. Which position is designed for use to demonstrate the humerus B^{1025}
when the arm cannot be rotated or abducted?
  a. axillary
  b. transthoracic
  c. AP internal rotation
  d. AP external rotation

1038. Which of the following comprise the elbow joint?   B^{1026}
  1. humerus
  2. radius
  3. ulna
  a. 1 & 2 only
  b. 1 & 3 only
  c. 2 & 3 only
  d. 1, 2, & 3

1039. Which position will open the interspaces between the medial A^{1027}
carpals?
  a. AP wrist
  b. PA wrist
  c. PA radial flexion
  d. PA ulnar flexion

1040. What is the range of average obliquity required to demonstrate
the sternum as free from vertebral superimposition as possible in A^{1028}
an RAO position?
  a.   5° to 10°
  b. 10° to 15°
  c. 15° to 20°
  d. 20° to 25°

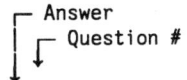

┌ Answer
│ ┌ Question #
↓ ↓

1041. What structures should be palpated on the medial side to locate the knee joint?
    1. femoral epicondyle
    2. femoral condyle
    3. tibial condyle
      a. 1 & 2 only
      b. 1 & 3 only
      c. 2 & 3 only
      d. 1, 2, & 3

B¹⁰⁵⁰

1042. Which of the following involves destructive changes in the small airways with a decrease in the volume of air in the lungs?
      a. pneumonia
      b. emphysema
      c. histoplasmosis
      d. pneumoconiosis

C¹⁰⁵¹

1043. What structure forms the scapular articulation with the head of the humerus?
      a. acromion process
      b. coracoid process
      c. glenoid fossa
      d. scapular notch

D¹⁰⁵²

C¹⁰⁵³

A¹⁰⁵⁴

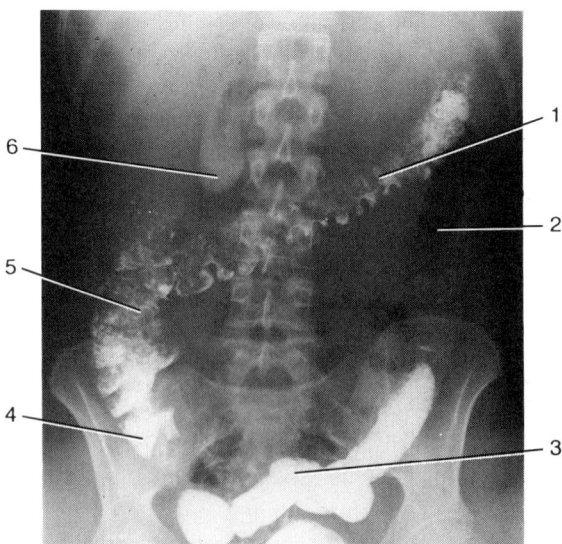

Figure 27

1044. Which number in Figure 27 illustrates the sigmoid colon?
  a. 2
  b. 3
  c. 4
  d. 5

B^{1035}

1045. Which of the following is illustrated by #6 in Figure 27?
  a. hepatic flexure
  b. transverse colon
  c. gall bladder
  d. pancreas

C^{1065}

1046. Which of the following is illustrated by #4 in Figure 27?
  a. cecum
  b. ascending colon
  c. descending colon
  d. sigmoid colon

1047. Which of the following is filled with gas in Figure 27?   B^{1037}
  a. cecum
  b. ascending colon
  c. descending colon
  d. sigmoid colon

1048. Which of the following are critical elements of an operative
  cholangiographic procedure?
    1. minimum exposure time   D^{1038}
    2. film centered to the right upper quadrant of the abdomen
    3. a pressure injector is available if needed
    a. 1 & 2 only
    b. 1 & 3 only
    c. 2 & 3 only
    d. 1, 2, & 3

1049. What is the proper centering point for a PA projection of the C^{1039}
  sinuses?
    a. nasion
    b. acanthion
    c. glabella
    d. inion

C^{1040}

D¹⁰⁶⁰

1050. Which of the following should rest on the image receptor surface for a PA oblique axial position (Law method) of the facial bones?
   1. nose
   2. superorbital ridge
   3. zygoma
      a. 1 & 2 only
      b. 1 & 3 only
      c. 2 & 3 only
      d. 1, 2, & 3

A¹⁰⁶¹

1051. What is the proper position of the orbitomeatal line to the image receptor on a parietoacanthial position (Waters method)?
      a. perpendicular
      b. parallel
      c. 37°
      d. 53°

1052. Which of the following is true regarding the PA axial position of the skull by the Haas method?
   1. the petrous pyramids of the temporal bone are projected symmetrically
   2. the dorsum sellae is projected within the shadow of the forame n magnum
   3. it is essentially a reversed AP axial Townes method position
      a. 1 & 2 only
      b. 1 & 3 only
      c. 2 & 3 only
      d. 1, 2, & 3

1053. Which terms describes the vessel that leaves the renal glomerulus?
   1. Henle's loop
   2. afferent arteriole
   3. efferent arteriole
      a. 1 only
      b. 2 only
      c. 3 only
      d. 1, 2, & 3

C¹⁰⁶²

1054. What is the proper position of the arms for a dorsal decubitus position of the abdomen?
      a. over the head
      b. folded over the upper abdomen
      c. at the sides of the abdomen
      d. extended perpendicular to the midaxillary line

C¹⁰⁶³

Question # ⌐
Answer ⌐ |
↓ |
↓

1055. To which of the following is the liver connected by the portal circulation?
    1. pancreas
    2. spleen
    3. stomach
      a. 1 & 2 only
      b. 1 & 3 only
      c. 2 & 3 only
      d. 1, 2, & 3

B[1044]

1056. What is the purpose of the Valsalva maneuver?
      a. to close the esophagus
      b. to elevate the diaphragms
      c. to distend the trachea
      d. to close the epiglottis

C[1045]

1057. What is accomplished by rotating the palms of the hands upward during a PA position of the chest?
      a. the scapulae are rotated laterally
      b. large breasts are moved laterally
      c. the clavicles are projected below the lung apices
      d. the diaphragms are elevated

A[1046]

1058. At what level should the top of the cassette be placed for an AP pelvis position?
      a. at the iliac crest
      b. 1" to 1.5" above the iliac crest
      c. at the level of the anterior superior iliac spine
      d. half way between the iliac crest and the most lateral portion of the greater trochanter

C[1047]

1059. What is the relationship of the tibia to the fibula?
    1. anterior
    2. lateral
    3. medial
      a. 1 & 2 only
      b. 1 & 3 only
      c. 2 & 3 only
      d. 1, 2, & 3

A[1048]

A[1049]

┌─ Answer
│ ┌─ Question #
↓ ↓

1060. Which of the following positions will demonstrate the axillary border of the scapula best in an AP projection?
    a. arm at the side with hand supinated
    b. arm at the side with hand pronated
    c. arm abducted to a 45° angle with hand toward waist
    d. arm abducted to a right angle with hand by head

C^1070

1061. Which digit is the thumb?
    a. first
    b. second
    c. third
    d. fifth

C^1071

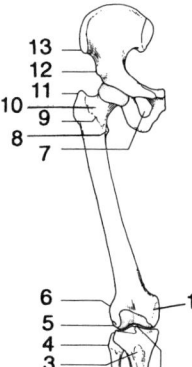

B^1072

Figure 28 (from Akesson EJ, Loeb JA, Wilson-Pauwels L: Thompson's Core Textbook of Anatomy, 2nd ed. Philadelphia, JB Lippincott, 1990)

D^1073

1062. Which number in Figure 28 illustrates the neck of the femur?
    a. 8
    b. 9
    c. 10
    d. 11

D^1074
1063. Which of the following is illustrated by #8 in Figure 28?
    a. greater trochanter
    b. lesser trochanter
    c. intertrochanteric crest
    d. neck of femur

Question # ⌐
Answer ⌐ |
↓ |
↓

1064. Which of the following is illustrated by #5 in Figure 28?
    a. lateral condyle
    b. lateral epicondyle
    c. intercondyloid fossa
    d. tibial tuberosity

1065. What is the proper centering point for the cassette for an AP projection of the abdomen when the patient is supine? D^{1055}
    a. 2" to 3" above the iliac crests
    b. at the iliac crests
    c. at the anterior superior spines
    d. 2" to 3" below the iliac crests

1066. Which of the following is considered to be part of the lymphatic C^{1056}
system?
    a. liver
    b. spleen
    c. gallbladder
    d. pancreas

1067. Which of the following would best demonstrate free air in the A^{1057}
right pleural cavity?
    a. left lateral decubitus chest
    b. right lateral decubitus chest
    c. ventral decubitus chest
    d. dorsal decubitus chest

1068. How is the trachea filled with air to better demonstrate its B^{1058}
position during an AP projection?
    a. the patient slowly inhales during the exposure
    b. the patient slowly exhales during the exposure
    c. the patient holds a deep inspiration
    d. the patient holds a deep expiration

1069. How many segments are fused to form the normal sacrum?
    a. 3
    b. 4
    c. 5
    d. 6 B^{1059}

1070. Which position requires hyperextension of the wrist with the central ray directed 25° to 30° toward the base of the third metacarpal?
    a. PA wrist
    b. lateral wrist
    c. carpal canal Gaynor-Hart method
    d. carpal bridge tangential position

1071. Which of the following describe the anatomic relationship of the lacrimal bones to the orbits?
    1. inferior
    2. anterior
    3. medial
        a. 1 & 2 only
        b. 1 & 3 only
        c. 2 & 3 only
        d. 1, 2, & 3

1072. What term is used to describe the opening between the esophagus and the stomach?
        a. pyloric orifice
        b. cardiac orifice
        c. sphincter of Oddi
        d. pylorus

B^{1079} 1073. Which of the following describe the relationship between the trachea and other thoracic structures?
    1. anterior to the esophagus
    2. anterior to the vertebral column
C^{1080} 3. superior to the heart
        a. 1 & 2 only
        b. 1 & 3 only
        c. 2 & 3 only
        d. 1, 2, & 3

C^{1081} 1074. Which intervertebral foramina is demonstrated only through the specialized Kovacs method PA oblique axial position?
        a. T12-L1
        b. L3-L4
        c. L4-L5
        d. L5-S1

C^{1082}

1075. Which of the following are appropriate centering points for an AP projection of the hip?
    1. at the level of the superior portion of the greater trochanter
    2. at the level of the anterior superior iliac spine
    3. at the level of the most lateral projection of the greater trochanter
      a. 1 only
      b. 2 only
      c. 3 only
      d. 1, 2, & 3

A¹⁰⁶⁴

1076. Which of the following are malignant?
    1. adenoma
    2. sarcoma
    3. adenocarcinoma
      a. 1 & 2 only
      b. 1 & 3 only
      c. 2 & 3 only
      d. 1, 2, & 3

B¹⁰⁶⁵

B¹⁰⁶⁶

1077. Which position of the humerus will demonstrate the humeral head in profile on an AP projection of the shoulder?
    1. neutral
    2. internal rotation
    3. external rotation
      a. 1 only
      b. 2 only
      c. 3 only
      d. 1, 2, & 3

A¹⁰⁶⁷

1078. Which sinuses are visualized through the open-mouth on an open mouth modification of a parietoacanthial projection (Waters method)?
      a. maxillary
      b. sphenoid
      c. ethmoid
      d. frontal

A¹⁰⁶⁸

C¹⁰⁶⁹

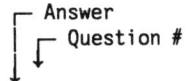

Answer
Question #

B¹⁰⁸⁸

B¹⁰⁸⁹

Figure 29

1079. Which of the following is illustrated by #5 in Figure 29?
    a. ulnar styloid process
    b. radial styloid process
    c. trapezium
    d. lunate

1080. Which number in Figure 29 illustrates the lunate?
    a. 1
    b. 2
    c. 3
    d. 7

1081. Which of the following is illustrated by #6 in Figure 29?
    a. trapezium
    b. lunate
    c. navicular
    d. capitate

1082. What is the proper position of the patient for radiography of the paranasal sinuses?
    a. supine
    b. prone
    c. erect
    d. lateral decubitus

D¹⁰⁹⁰

256

1083. What is the proper centering point for an AP axial position for temporomandibular joints?
    a. glabella
    b. 3" above the glabella
    c. nasion
    d. 3" above the nasion

1084. Which of the following should be superimposed on a lateral position of the facial bones?

A 1075

    1. mandibular rami
    2. orbital roofs
    3. the anterior and posterior walls of the maxillary sinuses
    a. 1 & 2 only
    b. 1 & 3 only
    c. 2 & 3 only
    d. 1, 2, & 3

1085. Which bones form the lambdoidal suture?

C 1076

    1. occipital
    2. parietals
    3. frontal
    a. 1 & 2 only
    b. 1 & 3 only
    c. 2 & 3 only
    d. 1, 2, & 3

1086. Which two portions of bowel meet at the angle of Treitz?

C 1077

    a. duodenum and jejunum
    b. jejunum and ileum
    c. ileum and ascending colon
    d. descending colon and sigmoid

1087. Approximately how much should the knee be flexed for a lateral projection?

B 1078

    a. 10° to 20°
    b. 20° to 30°
    c. 30° to 40°
    d. 40° to 50°

┌ Answer
│ ┌ Question #
↓ ↓

1088. Which of the following methods demonstrate the scapula in a PA oblique position?
   1. Lilienfeld
   2. Lawrence
   3. Lorenz
   a. 1 & 2 only
   b. 1 & 3 only
   c. 2 & 3 only
   d. 1, 2, & 3

B¹⁰⁹⁶

1089. How many bones are there in the hand?
   a. 19
   b. 27
   c. 38
   d. 54

B¹⁰⁹⁷

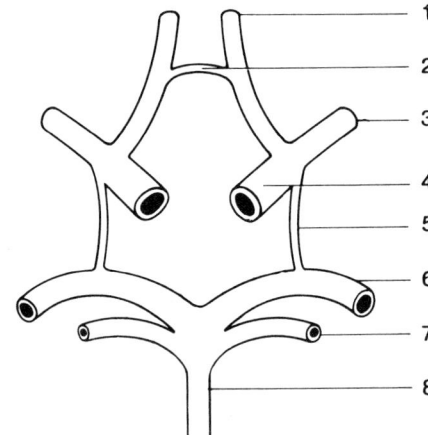

A¹⁰⁹⁸

A¹⁰⁹⁹

Figure 30 (from Akesson EJ, Loeb JA, Wilson-Pauwels L: Thompson's Core Textbook of Anatomy, 2nd ed. Philadelphia, JB Lippincott, 1990)

1090. Which number in Figure 30 illustrates the basilar artery portion of the circle of Willis?
   a. 5
   b. 6
   c. 7
   d. 8

D¹¹⁰⁰

1091. Which of the following is illustrated by #2 in Figure 30?
    a. anterior communicating artery
    b. anterior cerebral artery
    c. posterior communicating artery
    d. superior cerebellar artery

D^{1083}

1092. Which of the following is illustrated by #5 in Figure 30?
    a. anterior communicating artery
    b. posterior communicating artery
    c. internal carotid artery
    d. superior cerebellar artery

1093. What structure is of primary interest on an AP tangential position (modified Hickey method)?
    a. sphenoid sinuses
    b. mastoid process
    c. temporomandibular joints
    d. ethmoid sinuses

A^{1084}

1094. Which of the following structures should be demonstrated on a parietoacanthial position (Waters method) of the facial bones?
    1. maxillary sinuses
    2. sphenoid sinus
    3. frontal sinus
    a. 1 & 2 only
    b. 1 & 3 only
    c. 2 & 3 only
    d. 1, 2, & 3

A^{1085}

1095. Which of the following are auditory ossicles?
    1. incus
    2. stapes
    3. malleus
    a. 1 & 2 only
    b. 1 & 3 only
    c. 2 & 3 only
    d. 1, 2, & 3

A^{1086}

B^{1087}

C¹¹⁰⁶

1096. What is the normal time period from intravenous injection to radiographic appearance of urographic contrast media in the pelvicalyceal system?
  a. 30 to 60 seconds
  b. 2 to 8 minutes
  c. 15 to 20 minutes
  d. 45 to 60 minutes

1097. What is another term for the ensiform process?
  a. gladiolus
  b. xiphoid
B¹¹⁰⁷ c. manubrium
  d. coracoid

1098. Which of the following positions of the foot will cause foreshortening of the femoral neck and the projection of the lesser trochanter beyond the medial edge of the femoral shaft on an AP hip?
  1. external rotation
  2. neutral position
  3. internal rotation
  a. 1 & 2 only
  b. 1 & 3 only
  c. 2 & 3 only
  d. 1, 2, & 3

1099. What is the centering point for an AP projection of the shoulder?
  a. coracoid process
  b. coronoid process
  c. acromion process
  d. glenoid fossa

1100. Which of the following are names for the same carpal?
  1. triquetrum
  2. cuneiform
  3. triangular
  a. 1 & 2 only
  b. 1 & 3 only
  c. 2 & 3 only
  d. 1, 2, & 3

D¹¹⁰⁸

Question # ⌐
Answer ⌐ |
↓ |
↓

1101. Which of the following describe the proper positioning of the skull for a submentovertical (full basal) projection?
   1. the petrous pyramids of the temporal bone are projected symmetrically
   2. the odontoid process of the axis
   3. the sphenoid sinuses
      a. 1 & 2 only
      b. 1 & 3 only
      c. 2 & 3 only
      d. 1, 2, & 3

A[1091]

1102. What term describes the smooth area between the superciliary ridges of the frontal bone?
      a. bregma
      b. glabella
      c. nasion
      d. crista galli

B[1092]

1103. At which margins of the bladder do the ureters enter?
   1. lateral
   2. superior
   3. inferior
      a. 1 & 2 only
      b. 1 & 3 only
      c. 2 & 3 only
      d. 1, 2, & 3

B[1093]

1104. Which of the following are divisions of the stomach?
   1. pylorus
   2. duodenum
   3. fundus
      a. 1 & 2 only
      b. 1 & 3 only
      c. 2 & 3 only
      d. 1, 2, & 3

B[1094]

1105. Where is the liver located?
      a. upper right quadrant
      b. upper left quadrant
      c. lower right quadrant
      d. lower left quadrant

D[1095]

┌─ Answer
│ ┌─ Question #
↓ ↓

1106. How many posterior ribs should be visualized above the diaphragm on a routine PA chest radiograph?
   a. 8
   b. 9
   c. 10
   d. 12

C[1114] 1107. What is the proper central angulation for an AP projection of the knee?
   a. perpendicular
   b. 5° to 7°
   c. 10° to 15°
   d. 25° to 30°

A[1115]

A[1116]

B[1117]

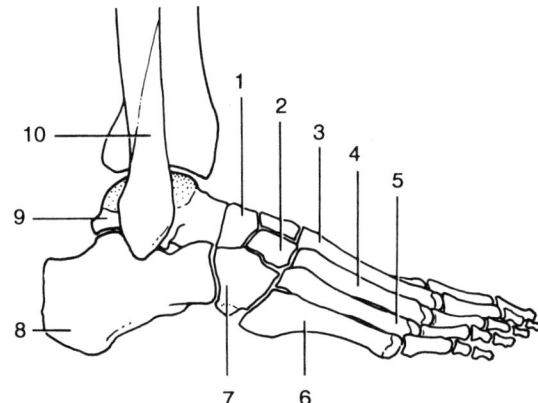

Figure 31 (from Akesson EJ, Loeb JA, Wilson-Pauwels L: Thompson's Core Textbook of Anatomy, 2nd ed. Philadelphia, JB Lippincott, 1990)

C[1118] 1108. Which of the following is illustrated by #5 in Figure 31?
   a. lateral cuneiform
   b. 2nd metatarsal
   c. 3rd metatarsal
   d. 4th metatarsal

1109. Which number in Figure 31 illustrates the cuboid?
    a. 1
    b. 2
    c. 7
    d. 9

1110. Which of the following is illustrated by #9 in Figure 31?
    a. cuboid
    b. talus
    c. calcaneus
    d. navicular

D[1101]

1111. Which of the following is illustrated by #1 in Figure 31?
    a. cuboid
    b. talus
    c. calcaneus
    d. navicular

B[1102]

1112. Which of the following is involved in orthoroentgenologic measurement of leg length?
    1. a single exposure
    2. central ray positioning at the hip, knee, and ankle joints
    3. external rotation of the lower leg
    a. 1 only
    b. 2 only
    c. 3 only
    d. 1, 2, & 3

A[1103]

1113. What is the anatomic term used to describe the winglike lateral mass of the sacral body?
    a. promontory
    b. spine
    c. coracoid process
    d. ala

B[1104]

A[1105]

┌ Answer
│ ┌ Question #

1114. What terms describe the process that fits into the anterior portion of the atlantal ring to act as a pivot for the atlas?
    1. axis
    2. dens
    3. odontoid process
      a. 1 & 2 only
      b. 1 & 3 only
      c. 2 & 3 only
      d. 1, 2, & 3

D[1123]

1115. What names are used to describe the region below the pelvic brim?
    1. true pelvis
    2. lesser pelvis
    3. greater pelvis
      a. 1 & 2 only
      b. 1 & 3 only
      c. 2 & 3 only
      d. 1, 2, & 3

D[1124]

1116. What is the primary bone that is involved in a LeFort fracture?
      a. maxillae
      b. sphenoid
      c. tibia
      d. os calcis

A[1125]

1117. What body part is being examined when the central ray is directed to the long axis of the part, midway between the elbow and shoulder joints?
      a. shoulder
      b. humerus
      c. elbow
      d. forearm

D[1126]

1118. Which position best demonstrates the hepatic flexure of the colon?
      a. PA
      b. lateral
      c. RAO
      d. LAO

C[1127]

D[1128]

Question # ⌐
Answer ⌐ |
↓ |
↓

1119. What is the reason why a patient should be maintained in a left lateral position for 10 to 20 minutes prior to the exposures intended to demonstrate free air in the abdomen?
    1. it allows gas to rise to the right hemidiaphragm   C^{1109}
    2. it allows fluid to accumulate in the retrorenal spaces
    3. it allows gas to distribute evenly under both diaphragms
      a. 1 only
      b. 2 only   B^{1110}
      c. 3 only
      d. 1, 2, & 3

1120. Which of the following is the most accurate verification of rotation on a PA chest radiograph?
      a. symmetrical distance between the lateral-most inner rib margin and the heart shadow
      b. symmetrical distance of the sternoclavicular joints from   D^{1111} the midline
      c. the number of ribs completely visualized above the diaphragm
      d. the length of the clavicle visualized

1121. Which of the following form the bony thorax?
    1. ribs
    2. sternum
    3. thoracic vertebrae
      a. 1 & 2 only   B^{1112}
      b. 1 & 3 only
      c. 2 & 3 only
      d. 1, 2, & 3

1122. What is another name for the ringlike, bodiless, first cervical vertebra?   D^{1113}
      a. atlas
      b. axis
      c. dens
      d. vertebra prominens

1123. Which of the following are contained within the abdominal cavity?
1. liver
2. kidneys
3. stomach
   a. 1 & 2 only
   b. 1 & 3 only
   c. 2 & 3 only
   d. 1, 2, & 3

B^1132   1124. Which of the following are true about the patella?
1. the base is located superior to the apex
2. it is the largest sesamoid bone
3. it lies slightly above the knee joint
   a. 1 & 2 only
B^1133   b. 1 & 3 only
   c. 2 & 3 only
   d. 1, 2, & 3

1125. Which of the following is the more common name for osteitis deformans?
D^1134   a. Paget's disease
   b. rickets
   c. gout
   d. Ewing's sarcoma

1126. Which of the following forms the medial end of the clavicle?
   a. acromion process
   b. acromioclavicular joint
   c. coronoid process
   d. sternoclavicular joint

A^1135   1127. What is the proper angle of the wrist for the oblique position?
   a. 25°
   b. 35°
   c. 45°
   d. 55°

C^1136   1128. What central ray angle should be used to demonstrate the coccyx on an AP projection?
   a. 15° cephalad
   b. 15° caudad
   c. 10° cephalad
   d. 10° caudad

Question # ⌐
Answer ⌐ |
        ↓ |
          ↓

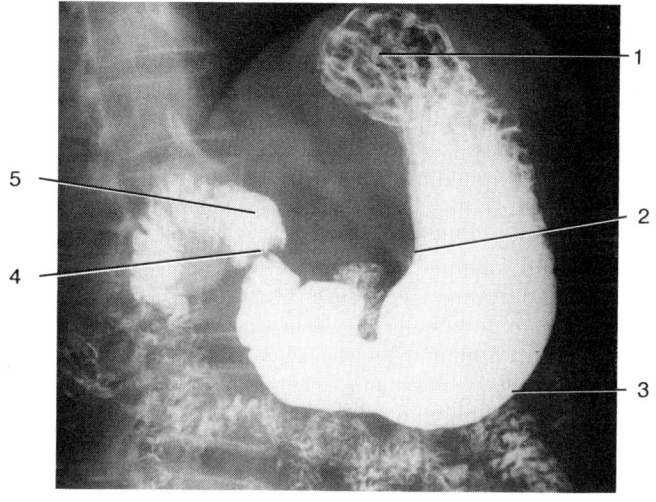

Figure 32

A¹¹¹⁹

B¹¹²⁰

D¹¹²¹

A¹¹²²

1129. Which number in Figure 32 illustrates the pylorus?
     a. 1
     b. 2
     c. 4
     d. 5

1130. Which of the following is illustrated by #2 in Figure 32?
     a. greater curvature
     b. lesser curvature
     c. pylorus
     d. duodenum

1131. Which of the following is illustrated by #5 in Figure 32?
     a. greater curvature
     b. lesser curvature
     c. pylorus
     d. duodenum

┌ Answer
│ ┌ Question #
│ ↓
↓

1132. What structures should be aligned so that a line between them is perpendicular to the image receptor when radiographing the atlas and axis in an AP open mouth position?
    1. inferior tip of the mastoid process
    2. rami of the mandible
    3. occlusal surface of the upper incisors
        a. 1 & 2 only
        b. 1 & 3 only
        c. 2 & 3 only
        d. 1, 2, & 3

C¹¹⁴³

1133. Which of the following is a common cause of ileus?
    a. ingestion of barium
    b. surgery
    c. pneumonia
    d. malignant tumor

A¹¹⁴⁴

1134. Which term describes the loss of blood?
    a. abscess
    b. edema
    c. infarct
    d. hemorrhage

D¹¹⁴⁵   1135. What structure is demonstrated on a transthoracic lateral Lawrence method position?
    1. proximal 2/3 of humerus
    2. glenoid fossa
    3. T2
        a. 1 only
        b. 2 only
        c. 3 only
        d. 1, 2, & 3

B¹¹⁴⁶

1136. What is the proper centering point for a PA axial position (Caldwell method) of the sinuses?
    a. glabella
    b. inion
    c. nasion
    d. acanthion

A¹¹⁴⁷

268

Question # ⌐
Answer ⌐ │
↓ │
↓

1137. What is the primary structure of interest on a tangential position (May method) of the facial bones?
    a. sphenoid sinuses
    b. zygomatic arch
    c. superorbital ridge
    d. nasal bones

1138. How many bones make up the cranium?
    a. 4
    b. 8
    c. 14
    d. 22

1139. What is the proper central ray angulation for an AP axial positi on of the colon?
    a. 10° to 20° caudad
    b. 10° to 20° cephalad
    c. 30° to 40° caudad
    d. 30° to 40° cephalad

1140. Which position produces the best image of the duodenal bulb and pyloric canal during a barium stomach examination?
    a. erect PA
    b. supine PA
    c. prone PA   C^{1129}
    d. semi-prone RAO

1141. To which of the following is the appendix attached?
    a. cecum
    b. duodenum
    c. ileum   B^{1130}
    d. ascending colon

1142. Which of the following are useful in demonstrating air-fluid levels in the abdomen?
    1. dorsal decubitus abdomen
    2. lateral decubitus abdomen   D^{1131}
    3. supine AP abdomen
    a. 1 & 2 only
    b. 1 & 3 only
    c. 2 & 3 only
    d. 1, 2, & 3

1143. Which organ introduces oxygen into, and removes carbon dioxide from, the blood?
      a. spleen
      b. kidney
      c. lung
      d. heart

D^{1151} 1144. In which directions do the ribs move on deep exhalation?
      1. inferiorly
      2. posteriorly
      3. laterally
      a. 1 & 2 only
      b. 1 & 3 only
      c. 2 & 3 only
      d. 1, 2, & 3

A^{1152} 1145. Which of the following make up the hip bone?
      1. ilium
      2. pubis
      3. ischium
      a. 1 & 2 only
      b. 1 & 3 only
      c. 2 & 3 only
      d. 1, 2, & 3

A^{1153} 1146. Which temporal portion will be demonstrated in a posterior profile projection, or Stenvers method, if the head is turned to the right?
      a. right petrous portion
      b. left petrous portion
      c. foramen magnum
      d. palatine plate

A^{1154} 1147. Which of the following are true about the lumbar vertebral bodies?
      1. they are deeper anteriorly than posteriorly
      2. their superior and inferior surfaces are slightly concave
      3. they are connected to the vertebral spines by the lamina
      a. 1 & 2 only
      b. 1 & 3 only
      c. 2 & 3 only
      d. 1, 2, & 3

A^{1155}

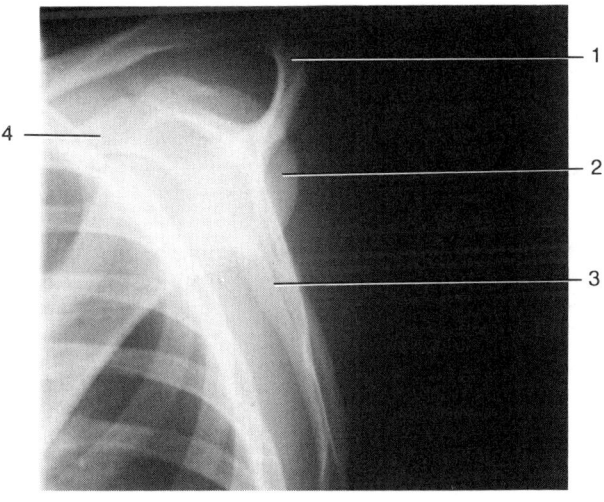

Figure 33

B 1137

B 1138

D 1139

1148. What position is shown in Figure 33?
    a. oblique shoulder
    b. AP scapula
    c. lateral scapula
    d. oblique acromioclavicular joints

D 1140

1149. Which of the following is illustrated by #1 in Figure 33?
    a. acromion process
    b. coracoid process
    c. humerus
    d. scapula

A 1141

1150. Which of the following is illustrated by #2 in Figure 33?
    a. acromion process
    b. coracoid process
    c. humerus
    d. scapula

A 1142

B¹¹⁶²

1151. Which of the following are methods by which malignant neoplasms metastasize?
  1. seeding within body cavities
  2. lymphatic spread
  3. embolistic spread
    a. 1 & 2 only
    b. 1 & 3 only
    c. 2 & 3 only
    d. 1, 2, & 3

C¹¹⁶³

1152. When a patient is unable to extend the elbow for an AP projection, which of the following projections must be obtained?
  1. distal humerus
  2. proximal forearm
  3. distal forearm
    a. 1 & 2 only
    b. 1 & 3 only
    c. 2 & 3 only
    d. 1, 2, & 3

A¹¹⁶⁴

1153. What is the average normal transit time for food to travel from the mouth to the ileocecal valve?
    a. 2 to 3 hours
    b. 10 to 12 hours
    c. 24 hours
    d. 48 hours

C¹¹⁶⁵

1154. Which of the following is examined during endoscopic retrograde cholangiopancreatography?
  1. pancreatic and biliary duct
  2. common bile duct
  3. Wharton's ducts

C¹¹⁶⁶

    a. 1 only
    b. 2 only
    c. 3 only
    d. 1, 2, & 3

D¹¹⁶⁷

1155. What is the proper stress method to delineate the medial side of the knee during vertical ray contrast arthrography?
    a. lateral stress of the lower leg
    b. medial stress of the lower leg
    c. anterior stress of the lower leg
    d. medial stress of the femur

1156. What is the proper centering point for a lateral chest?
    a. T2-T3
    b. T4-T5
    c. T6-T7
    d. T8-T9

1157. What is the relationship of the left upper lobe of the lung to the left lower lobe?
    1. anterior
    2. superior
    3. lateral
      a. 1 & 2 only
      b. 1 & 3 only
      c. 2 & 3 only
      d. 1, 2, & 3

1158. What is another name for the seventh cervical vertebra?
    a. atlas
    b. axis
    c. dens
    d. vertebra prominens

1159. Name the position that is described as the patient is supine with the unaffected leg lifted; the film is positioned with one end above the iliac crest; and the central ray is directed at the neck of the femur entering medially and exiting laterally.
    a. AP hip
    b. axiolateral Danelius-Miller modification of the Lorenz method
    c. AP axial modified Cleaves method
    d. lateral Laurenstein method

C[1148]

A[1149]

1160. How many meniscus/i are there in the knee joint?
    a. 1
    b. 2
    c. 3
    d. 4

C[1150]

1161. Which positions clearly demonstrates all four paranasal sinuses?
    a. parietoacanthial projection (Waters method)
    b. PA axial position (Caldwell method)
    c. axial transoral position (Pirie method)
    d. lateral

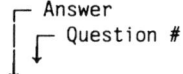

1162. What is the proper central ray angulation for an axiolateral oblique position of the mandible?
 a. 15° cephalad
 b. 25° cephalad
 c. 37° cephalad
 d. 53° cephalad

1163. What is the proper centering point for a lateral position of the facial bones?
 a. external auditory meatus
 b. 3/4" superior and 3/4" inferior to the external auditory meatus
 c. the malar surface of the zygomatic bone
 d. the gonion

1164. Which of the following describes a fistula?
 a. an abnormal passage, usually between two organs
 b. an abnormal passage leading to an abscess
 c. a blocked vein that no longer functions
 d. a blocked artery that no longer functions

A¹¹⁷³ 1165. At which of the following ages would the thymus gland most likely be at its maximum size?
 a. 9 months
 b. 4 years
 c. 14 years
 d. 65 years

A¹¹⁷⁴ 1166. Which of the following is best demonstrated on a left lateral of the lumbar spine?
 a. left apophysial joints
 b. right apophysial joints
 c. 1st to 4th intervertebral foramina
 d. 5th intervertebral foramen

D¹¹⁷⁵ 1167. What structure is at the level of the anterior superior iliac spine?
 a. T12
 b. L2
 c. L4
 d. S1

C¹¹⁷⁶

274

1168. Which of the following are part of the ilium?
    1. greater sciatic notch
    2. posterior inferior spine
    3. anterior superior spine
        a. 1 & 2 only
        b. 1 & 3 only   C^{1156}
        c. 2 & 3 only
        d. 1, 2, & 3

1169. What projection will best demonstrate the tibiofibular
    articulations?
        a. AP lower leg
        b. lateral lower leg
        c. medial (internal) oblique lower leg   A^{1157}
        d. lateral (external) oblique lower leg

1170. Which carpal is also known as the os magnum?
        a. capitatim
        b. unciform
        c. navicular   D^{1158}
        d. pisiform

1171. When a PA axial position (Caldwell method) of the sinuses is
    performed, the central ray can be angled 23° to the glabellomeatal
    line or what equivalent angle to the orbitomeatal line?
        a.   8°
        b. 15°
        c. 23°
        d. 37°

1172. Which of the following sinuses are located anterior to the external   B^{1159}
    auditory meatus?
    1. sphenoid
    2. ethmoid
    3. maxillary
        a. 1 & 2 only
        b. 1 & 3 only   B^{1160}
        c. 2 & 3 only
        d. 1, 2, & 3

                                                D^{1161}

⌐ Answer

⌐ Question #

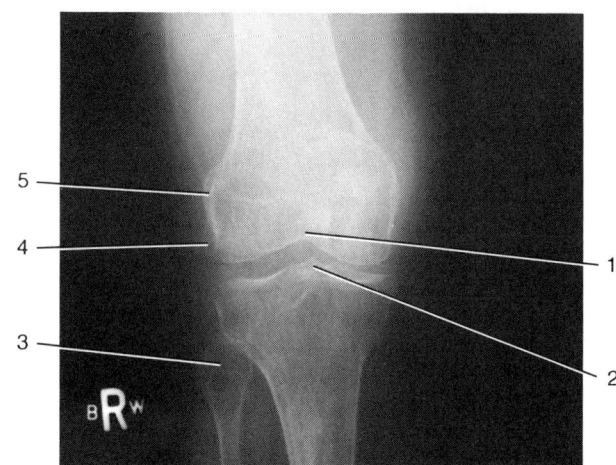

Figure 34

B 1182

B 1183

B 1184

1173. What position is shown in Figure 34?
   a. AP
   b. PA
   c. medial (internal) oblique
   d. lateral (external) oblique

C 1185

1174. Which of the following is illustrated by #5 in Figure 34?
   a. lateral epicondyle
   b. medial epicondyle
   c. lateral condyle
   d. medial condyle

C 1186

1175. Which of the following is illustrated by #1 in Figure 34?
   a. head of tibia
   b. head of fibula
   c. tibial eminence
   d. intercondyloid fossa

1176. Which number in Figure 34 illustrates the head of the fibula?
   a. 1
   b. 2
   c. 3
   d. 4

1177. Which of the following should be positioned parallel to the image receptor for an axiolateral oblique position of the mandible?
   a. rami of the mandible
   b. body of the mandible
   c. zygomatic arch
   d. midsagittal plane

D^{1168}

1178. What is the proper location of the optic foramen on a properly positioned parieto-orbital oblique position (Rhese method)?
   a. inferior medial quadrant of the orbit
   b. superior medial quadrant of the orbit
   c. inferior lateral quadrant of the orbit
   d. superior lateral quadrant of the orbit

C^{1169}

1179. What is the proper positioning of the infraorbitomeatal line for a submentovertical (full basal) projection of the skull?
   a. 37° caudad angle
   b. 15° cephalad angle
   c. parallel to the image receptor
   d. parallel to the central ray

A^{1170}

1180. To which of the following is the renal glomerular capsule connected?
   1. Henle's loop
   2. proximal convoluted tubule
   3. distal convoluted tubule
   a. 1 only
   b. 2 only
   c. 3 only
   d. 1, 2, & 3

B^{1171}

1181. What term describes the sacculations of the colon that are formed between the taeniae coli in the wall?
   a. ligaments
   b. sphincters
   c. haustra
   d. rugae

D^{1172}

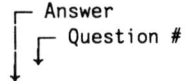

1182. Which of the following occurs that make a second inhalation better than a single breath prior to exposing a routine PA chest radiograph?
1. the heart appears smaller because of less intrathoracic pressure
2. the lungs inflate more without strain
3. large, pendulous breasts are moved laterally away from the lungfields
   a. 1 only
   b. 2 only
   c. 3 only
   d. 1, 2, & 3

B^1192

1183. Which of the following positions will demonstrate the right apophyseal joints of the lumbar spine?
   a. LAO and LPO
   b. LAO and RPO
   c. RAO and LPO
   d. RAO and RPO

A^1193

1184. Although the anterior angle of the neck of the femur varies with age, sex, and body type, what is the approximate range?
   a.   5 to 10°
   b. 15 to 20°
   c. 45 to 50°
   d. 120 to 130°

B^1194

1185. What is the proper central ray angulation to open the joint spaces for an AP position of the foot?
   a.   5° posteriorly
   b. 10° posteriorly
   c. 15° posteriorly
   d. 25° posteriorly

C^1195

1186. What is the proper central ray angle for an axiolateral position by the Lysholm method?
   a. 20° to 25° caudad
   b. 30° to 35° caudad
   c. 30° to 35° cephalad
   d. 40° to 45° cephalad

D^1196

1187. Which of the following are part of the ethmoid bone?
　　　1. perpendicular plate
　　　2. crista galli
　　　3. cribriform plate
　　　　a. 1 & 2 only　　　　　　　　　　　　B^1177
　　　　b. 1 & 3 only
　　　　c. 2 & 3 only
　　　　d. 1, 2, & 3

1188. What is the proper obliquity of the body for an RAO position of the colon?
　　　　a. 45° to 55°　　　　　　　　　　　　C^1178
　　　　b. 35° to 45°
　　　　c. 25° to 35°
　　　　d. 15° to 25°

1189. Which of the following positions will demonstrate esophageal varices by increasing venous pressure during an esophagram?
　　　1. recumbent LPO　　　　　　　　　　C^1179
　　　2. recumbent RAO
　　　3. erect RAO
　　　　a. 1 & 2 only
　　　　b. 1 & 3 only
　　　　c. 2 & 3 only
　　　　d. 1, 2, & 3

1190. What is the approximate length of the human gastrointestinal tract?
　　　　a. 5 feet　　　　　　　　　　　　　B^1180
　　　　b. 10 feet
　　　　c. 30 feet
　　　　d. 75 feet

1191. What is the proper centering point for the cassette for an AP projection of the abdomen when the patient is erect?
　　　　a. 2" to 3" above the iliac crests　　　C^1181
　　　　b. at the iliac crests
　　　　c. at the anterior superior spines
　　　　d. 2" to 3" below the iliac crests

┌ Answer
│ ┌ Question #
↓ ↓

1192. What type of respiration will best demonstrate the lower ribs?
1. inhalation
2. exhalation
D¹²⁰¹
3. shallow breathing
   a. 1 only
   b. 2 only
   c. 3 only
   d. 1, 2, & 3

1193. What term describes the deep depression in the superior aspect of sternum?
   a. manubrial notch
   b. gladiolar notch
   c. sternoclavicular notch
   d. tubercular notch

1194. What is the centering point for a lateral (mediolateral) position of the ankle?
   a. talocalcaneal joint
   b. medial malleolus
   c. 1" proximal to the medial malleolus
   d. talotibial joint

1195. Which of the following is not a malignant tumor?
1. Ewing's sarcoma
2. chondrosarcoma
3. osteochondroma
   a. 1 only
   b. 2 only
A¹²⁰²
   c. 3 only
   d. 1, 2, & 3

1196. Which of the following carpals are not in the distal row?
1. semilunar
2. scaphoid
A¹²⁰³
3. pisiform
   a. 1 only
   b. 2 only
   c. 3 only
   d. 1, 2, & 3

C¹²⁰⁴

1197. Which of the following involves inflammation of the walls of the
   alveoli and supporting structures of the lung?
   a. alveolar pneumonia
   b. bronchopneumonia
   c. interstitial pneumonia
   d. aspiration pneumonia

D¹¹⁸⁷

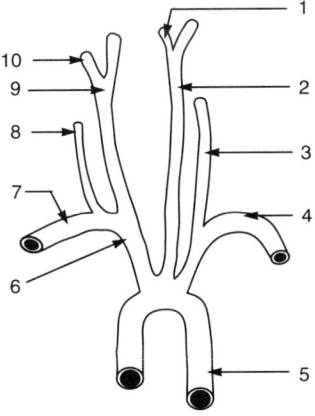

Figure 35

B¹¹⁸⁸

A¹¹⁸⁹

1198. Which of the following is illustrated by #7 in Figure 35?
   a. brachycephalic artery
   b. right subclavian artery
   c. left subclavian artery
   d. right common carotid artery

C¹¹⁹⁰

1199. Which of the following is illustrated by #2 in Figure 35?
   a. right common carotid artery
   b. left common carotid artery
   c. right vertebral artery
   d. left vertebral artery

A¹¹⁹¹

1200. Which number in Figure 35 illustrates the aorta?
   a. 4
   b. 5
   c. 6
   d. 7

1201. Which of the following is illustrated by #8 in Figure 35?
    a. right external carotid artery
    b. right common carotid artery
    c. left common carotid artery
    d. right vertebral artery

D 1209

D 1210

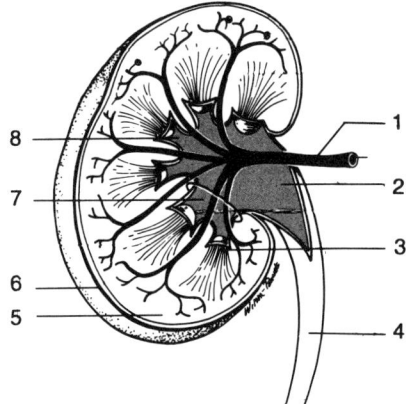

Figure 36 (from Akesson EJ, Loeb JA, Wilson-Pauwels L: Thompson's Core Textbook of Anatomy, 2nd ed. Philadelphia, JB Lippincott, 1990)

B 1211   1202. Which number in Figure 36 illustrates the renal artery?
    a. 1
    b. 3
    c. 4
    d. 8

1203. Which of the following is illustrated by #5 in Figure 36?
B 1212   a. cortex
    b. capsule
    c. renal pyramid (medulla)
    d. minor calyx

1204. Which of the following is illustrated by #7 in Figure 36?
D 1213   a. cortex
    b. renal pyramid (medulla)
    c. major calyx
    d. minor calyx

Question #
Answer

Record Maintenance and Administrative Procedures 1% (14) 1205-1218

1205. Which of the following persons may diagnose from a radiograph?
   1. radiographer
   2. radiologist
   3. nuclear medicine technologist
      a. 1 only
      b. 2 only
      c. 3 only
      d. 1, 2, & 3

C 1197

1206. Which of the following documents are part of the patient's medical record?
   1. record of medications given
   2. consent forms
   3. radiographs
      a. 1 & 2 only
      b. 1 & 3 only
      c. 2 & 3 only
      d. 1, 2, & 3

1207. Which of the following is a valid method of verifying patient identification?
   1. questioning patient
   2. reading wrist identification band
   3. checking bed name plate
      a. 1 only
      b. 2 only
      c. 3 only
      d. 1, 2, & 3

B 1198

1208. What is intended by the abbreviation c̄ ?
      a. with
      b. without
      c. cubic centimeter
      d. centimeter

B 1199

B 1200

┌─ Answer
│ ┌─ Question #
↓ ↓

1209. Which of the following legal concepts apply to radiographers?
  1. failure to carry out professional duties may result in legal action which could result in requirements to pay damages
  2. threatening to perform a procedure that a patient has refused is grounds for legal action against a radiographer
  3. performing a procedure that a patient has refused is grounds fo r legal action against a radiographer
    a. 1 & 2 only
    b. 1 & 3 only
    c. 2 & 3 only
    d. 1, 2, & 3

D^{1219}

C^{1220}

1210. What is the appropriate action if a patient complains of pain in the left wrist, no pain in the right wrist, but the request for examination is for the right wrist?
    a. radiograph the left wrist
    b. radiograph the right wrist
    c. radiograph both left and right wrist
    d. request clarification from the ordering physician

1211. Which of the following persons may prescribe a radiographic procedure?
  1. radiographer
  2. radiologist
  3. nuclear medicine technologist
    a. 1 only
    b. 2 only
    c. 3 only
    d. 1, 2, & 3

C^{1221}

A^{1222}

1212. Which of the following examinations should be suggested if a patient for a knee examination complains of severe pain in the groin when the leg is internally rotated?
    a. abdomen
    b. hip
    c. femur
    d. lower leg

1213. What is intended by the abbreviation prn?
    a. with
    b. without
    c. nothing by mouth
    d. as needed

A^{1223}

1214. Which potential changes could be expected from performing an AP supine chest at 40" instead of a PA erect chest at 72"?
    1. magnified heart
    2. loss of air-fluid levels in the lungs
    3. cervical apical lordosis
        a. 1 & 2 only
        b. 1 & 3 only
        c. 2 & 3 only
        d. 1, 2, & 3

B^{1205}

1215. Which of the following legal principles is violated by discussing patient information with a friend outside the medical setting?
    1. invasion of privacy
    2. professional negligence
    3. assault and battery
        a. 1 only
        b. 2 only
        c. 3 only
        d. 1, 2, & 3

D^{1206}

1216. What is intended by the abbreviation LLQ?
        a. lower left quadrant
        b. locate left quarterly
        c. liquid
        d. nothing by mouth

1217. What legal doctrine, now in decline, holds that the employer is responsible for the acts of the radiographer?
        a. assault and battery
        b. res ipsa loquitur
        c. respondeat superior
        d. habeas corpus

D^{1207}

1218. In which of the following situations would it be possible to proceed with a radiographic procedure although the patient clearly indicates refusal?
    1. the patient is a minor and the parents give permission
    2. the patient is over age 95
    3. the patient is a prisoner in the custody of an officer of the law, who gives permission
        a. 1 & 2 only
        b. 1 & 3 only
        c. 2 & 3 only
        d. 1, 2, & 3

A^{1208}

285

Answer
Question #

Patient Safety and Comfort 1% (14) 1219-1232

1219. Where is the center of gravity for a standing patient?
a. in the cervicothoracic region
b. at the center of the diaphragm
c. at the midline level with the iliac crests
d. in the pelvis near the symphysis pubis

A¹²²⁹ 1220. Which of the following is the preferred method of performing pediatric procedures when it can be achieved?
a. restraint without parental involvement
b. restraint with parental involvement
c. no restraint with parental involvement
d. no restraint without parental involvement

1221. Which of the following are good rules for decreasing the possibility of spinal injury to radiographers when moving patients?
1. the knees should be locked at all times
A¹²³⁰ 2. the feet should be slightly apart to provide a wide base of support for the body
3. the back should be kept as straight as possible
a. 1 & 2 only
b. 1 & 3 only
c. 2 & 3 only
d. 1, 2, & 3

C¹²³¹ 1222. What position places the patient semi-sitting with the head raised from 45° to 60°?
a. Fowler's
b. Sims'
c. supine
d. trendelenburg

1223. Which of the following structures must always be supported when carrying a baby?
1. back
D¹²³² 2. head
3. arms
a. 1 & 2 only
b. 1 & 3 only
c. 2 & 3 only
d. 1, 2, & 3

286

1224. Which of the following are useful indicators of a patient's overall condition?
1. skin color
2. respiratory rate
3. color of the antecubital area
   a. 1 & 2 only
   b. 1 & 3 only
   c. 2 & 3 only
   d. 1, 2, & 3

A¹²¹⁴

A^{1214}

1225. Which of the following is the most effective restraint device for a small child?
   a. sandbags
   b. tape
   c. sheets
   d. lead aprons

1226. Which of the following is a proper element of a wheelchair to x-ray table transfer of a patient who can stand but cannot walk?   A^{1215}
1. the radiographer stands beside the patient with one arm around the patient's waist, the other grasping the patient's opposite forearm
2. the radiographer stands facing the patient and places both hands on the patient's scapulae   A^{1216}
3. the radiographer helps the patient into a standing position then stands behind the wheelchair to prevent it from moving while the patient sits sideways in it
   a. 1 only
   b. 2 only
   c. 3 only
   d. 1, 2, & 3

1227. Which of the following guidelines will effectively protect the radiographer from physical harm while moving a large patient?   C^{1217}
   a. push a weight instead of pulling it
   b. lift with the legs instead of the back
   c. keep the feet as close together as possible
   d. avoid using the patient's moving abilities

1228. What position places the patient flat on his or her back?
   a. Fowler's
   b. Sims'   B^{1218}
   c. supine
   d. trendelenburg

┌ Answer
│ ┌ Question #
└ ↓ └ ↓

1229. Which of the following are elements of a pull sheet transfer of a patient from an x-ray table to a stretcher cart?
   1. roll the sheet as close to the patient's body as possible
   2. when 2 persons are transferring the patient, one should be positioned on each side of the patient
   3. when 3 persons are transferring the patient, all should be on th e same side of the patient
      a. 1 & 2 only
      b. 1 & 3 only
      c. 2 & 3 only
      d. 1, 2, & 3

C¹²³⁸

C[1238]

1230. Which of the following are normal responses of a small child to distress?
   1. crying
   2. kicking
   3. spitting
      a. 1 & 2 only
      b. 1 & 3 only
      c. 2 & 3 only
      d. 1, 2, & 3

B[1239]

1231. Which of the following is most helpful in communicating with very small children?
   a. talking very loud
   b. placing arms or hands around the child immediately
   c. getting down to eye level with the child and maintaining distance
   d. not smiling to avoid showing the teeth

A[1240]

1232. Which of the following conditions are known to cause breakdown of the skin?
   1. immobility in a single position for several hours
   2. prolonged contact with a wet sheet or gown
   3. tension during transfer to an x-ray table
      a. 1 & 2 only
      b. 1 & 3 only
      c. 2 & 3 only
      d. 1, 2, & 3

A[1241]

B[1242]

Question # ⌐
Answer ⌐ |
↓ |
↓

Disinfection and Sterile Technique 2.5% (35) 1233-1267

1233. Which of the following describes reducing the probability of infectious organisms being transmitted to someone who is susceptible?
   a. Disinfection
   b. Medical asepsis
   c. Sterilization
   d. Cleanliness

   A^{1224}

1234. What is the proper action to take if sterilization of an object is in question?
   a. resterilize the object for 50% of original sterilization time
   b. disinfect the object
   c. discard the object
   d. if someone else believes the object is sterile, it may be used

   C^{1225}

1235. Which of the following describes the first stage of an infection?
   a. prodromal phase
   b. full phase
   c. incubation period
   d. convalescent phase

1236. In what position is the patient when the x-ray table is inclined with the patient's head slightly lower than the body?
   a. Fowler's
   b. Sim's
   c. prone
   d. trendelenburg

   B^{1226}

1237. Which of the following are necessary when returning a patient to their room following x-ray examination?
   1. lower the bed to the lowest position
   2. report the return of the patient to the appropriate nursing station
   3. take the patient's medical chart to the radiology department to add the report from the x-ray examination
   a. 1 and 2 only
   b. 1 and 3 only
   c. 2 and 3 only
   d. 1, 2, & 3

   B^{1227}

   C^{1228}

1238. Which of the following are most resistant to aseptic techniques?
    a. yeasts
    b. streptococci bacteria
    c. bacillic spore bacteria
    d. moving protozoa

D^{1248}

1239. Which of the following can help a patient feel more comfortable and relaxed prior to a radiological examination?
    1. specifying exactly what clothing should be removed
    2. leaving the patient to discover how to wear a patient gown
    3. explaining the radiographic procedure
        a. 1 & 2 only
        b. 1 & 3 only
        c. 2 & 3 only
        d. 1, 2, & 3

A^{1249}

1240. Which of the following is the appropriate method for cleaning a contaminated x-ray table?
    a. start with the least contaminated area and work into the higher contamination
    b. start with the higher contamination and work out toward the least contaminated areas
    c. soak the entire area with a disinfectant for 2 to 3 minutes and then wipe dry
    d. use only dry wipes to clean the area to prevent contaminants from entering the waste disposal system

A^{1250}

A^{1251}

1241. What term describes the destruction of pathogens by using chemicals?
    a. disinfection
    b. medical asepsis
    c. sterilization
    d. cleanliness

1242. Which of the following are forms of fungi?
    1. yeasts
    2. protozoa
    3. molds
        a. 1 & 2 only
        b. 1 & 3 only
        c. 2 & 3 only
        d. 1, 2, & 3

B^{1252}

1243. Which items are often required for entry into an operating room?
    1. cap
    2. face mask
    3. shoe covers
        a. 1 & 2 only
        b. 1 & 3 only
        c. 2 & 3 only
        d. 1, 2, & 3

B[1233]

1244. Which method of sterilization is the most effective and convenient for items that can withstand high temperatures?
        a. gas
        b. steam
        c. chemicals
        d. dry heat

C[1234]

1245. What is the primary reason why hand lotion should be used by persons who must wash their hands often?
        a. it retains infectious materials that may reach the skin so they can be washed away later
        b. it produces a pH that serves as a mild antiseptic
        c. it prevents cracking of the skin surface, which would provide access to infectious materials
        d. it contains infection-fighting microorganisms

C[1235]

1246. Which of the following are one of the basic groups of microorganisms that can cause infections in humans?
    1. bacteria
    2. viruses
    3. protozoa
        a. 1 & 2 only
        b. 1 & 3 only
        c. 2 & 3 only
        d. 1, 2, & 3

D[1236]

1247. Which of the following are recommended for communicating with mentally impaired patients?
    1. speak in a loud voice
    2. talk to them as adults
    3. give simple instructions
        a. 1 & 2 only
        b. 1 & 3 only
        c. 2 & 3 only
        d. 1, 2, & 3

A[1237]

Answer

Question #

1248. What capabilities have been lost by a paraplegic patient?
   a. the right or left side of the body is paralyzed
   b. the upper or lower part of the body is paralyzed
   c. the right side of the body is paralyzed
   d. the lower part of the body is paralyzed

B[1258]   1249. Which of the following instances should require the filing of an incident report?
   1. pricking of the skin by a used needle
   2. failure to wear a face mask in a respiratory isolation unit
   3. failure to use hand lotion after hand washing
   a. 1 & 2 only
   b. 1 & 3 only
   c. 2 & 3 only
   d. 1, 2, & 3

B[1259]   1250. Which of the following describes the process where as many microorganisms as possible are eliminated, although spores are seldom destroyed?
   a. disinfection
   b. medical asepsis
   c. sterilization
   d. cleanliness

1251. What is a nosocomial infection?
   a. an infection acquired by a patient while in a health-care institution
B[1260]   b. an infection of the upper nasal passages
   c. an infection of the inferior nasal conchae
   d. a virulent microorganism that resists sterilization

1252. Which of the following are recommended when discarding needles?
   1. never recap a needle before discarding
   2. break all needles to prevent reclamation from trash
   3. consider all needles to be contaminated
   a. 1 & 2 only
B[1261]   b. 1 & 3 only
   c. 2 & 3 only
   d. 1, 2, & 3

1253. Which of the following are recommended for communicating with geriatric patients?
   1. speak in a normal voice unless indications of hearing difficulties are given by the patient
   2. talk to them as children
   3. give simple instructions
      a. 1 & 2 only
      b. 1 & 3 only
      c. 2 & 3 only
      d. 1, 2, & 3

D[1243]

1254. Which method of sterilization is the most effective and convenient for items that cannot withstand high temperatures?
      a. gas
      b. steam
      c. chemicals
      d. dry heat

B[1244]

1255. Which of the following are means of transporting infectious diseases from one person to another?
   1. insect vectors
   2. airborne droplets
   3. indirect contact fomites
      a. 1 & 2 only
      b. 1 & 3 only
      c. 2 & 3 only
      d. 1, 2, & 3

C[1245]

1256. If a sterile tray has been opened, but the procedure is delayed for an hour, what should be done with the tray?
      a. it should be watched to guarantee that no one contaminates it
      b. it should be covered and then watched to guarantee that no one contaminates it
      c. it should be discarded
      d. it should be returned to its original container

D[1246]

1257. Which of the following is a physical method of disinfecting that does not sterilize items?
      a. gas
      b. steam
      c. boiling
      d. ionizing radiation

C[1247]

1258. Which of the following sterilization methods can be used on electronic equipment?
1. boiling
2. gas
3. pressurized steam
   a. 1 only
   b. 2 only
   c. 3 only
   d. 1, 2, & 3

C¹²⁶⁷

1259. What is the proper method of painting the skin with antiseptic as part of surgical skin preparation?
   a. begin at the outside of the area and move in a circular motion toward the center
   b. begin at the center of the area and move in a circular motion toward the outside
   c. begin at one corner and move in a linear pattern
   d. begin at one corner and move in a linear pattern, followed by a second linear pattern perpendicular to the first

D¹²⁶⁸

1260. When a cassette transfer is performed using a sterile cassette bag to permit the cassette to be positioned in a sterile area under the patient, which of the following is a sterile area?
1. the inside of the cassette bag
2. the hands of the person holding the cassette bag
3. the cassette
   a. 1 only
   b. 2 only
   c. 3 only
   d. 1, 2, & 3

C¹²⁶⁹

1261. Which of the following is not an airborne infection?
1. measles
2. acquired immunodeficiency syndrome (AIDS)
3. tuberculosis
   a. 1 only
   b. 2 only
   c. 3 only
   d. 1, 2, & 3

D¹²⁷⁰

1262. Which of the following methods are capable of removing all microorganisms and their spores from an article?
    1. dry heat
    2. ionizing radiation
    3. gas
        a. 1 & 2 only
        b. 1 & 3 only
        c. 2 & 3 only
        d. 1, 2, & 3

B ^{1253}

1263. Which of the following can transmit infectious disease?
    1. contact with blood
    2. contact with feces
    3. breathing droplets from coughing
        a. 1 & 2 only
        b. 1 & 3 only
        c. 2 & 3 only
        d. 1, 2, & 3

A ^{1254}

1264. When dressing for a sterile operating room procedure, which of the following should be done last?
        a. shoe covers
        b. face mask
        c. gloves
        d. gown

1265. Which of the following describes the stage of an infection where the person appears most sick?
        a. prodromal phase
        b. full phase
        c. incubation period
        d. convalescent phase

D ^{1255}

1266. What term is used to describe a device designed to sterilize items with steam under pressure?
        a. gas chamber
        b. laminar flow device (LFD)
        c. autoclave
        d. steam packer

B ^{1256}

C ^{1257}

1267. Which of the following requires sterile technique procedures?
   1. cleaning of an ileus
   2. insertion of a naso-gastric tube
   3. insertion of a urinary catheter
     a. 1 only
     b. 2 only
     c. 3 only
     d. 1, 2, & 3

C^{1277}

Isolation Techniques 1% (14) 1268-1281

1268. Which of the following diseases require blood and body fluid precautions?
   1. acquired immunodeficiency syndrome (AIDS)
   2. hepatitis B
   3. syphilis
     a. 1 & 2 only
     b. 1 & 3 only
     c. 2 & 3 only
     d. 1, 2, & 3

D^{1278}

1269. When undressing from an isolation procedure, which of the following should be removed first?
     a. shoe covers
     b. face mask
     c. gloves
     d. gown

C^{1279}

1270. When performing mobile radiography of a patient in a strict isolation unit, under what circumstances can the x-ray controls be touched?
   1. before the patient or items in the room have been touched
   2. by another radiographer who has not touched the patient or items in the room
   3. after the patient or items in the room have been touched as long as new gloves are put on first
     a. 1 & 2 only
     b. 1 & 3 only
     c. 2 & 3 only
     d. 1, 2, & 3

D^{1280}

1271. Which of the following is the primary concern during respiratory isolation procedures?
    a. blood
    b. airborne droplets
    c. fecal material
    d. semen

1272. Which of the following is the primary concern during enteric isolation procedures? D^{1262}
    a. blood
    b. airborne droplets
    c. fecal material
    d. semen

1273. Which of the following must be worn in strict isolation?
    1. gown $\qquad\text{D}^{1263}$
    2. mask
    3. gloves
        a. 1 & 2 only
        b. 1 & 3 only
        c. 2 & 3 only
        d. 1, 2, & 3

1274. Which of the following is a recommended procedure for C^{1264} transferring a patient with a communicable disease?
    a. wrap the patient completely in a plastic bag with sealed ends
    b. wrap the patient completely in a plastic sheet
    c. wrap the patient completely in a cotton sheet
    d. cover the patient, including the head, in a cotton sheet

1275. What is the most common method of the spread of B^{1265} microorganisms?
    a. touching with hands
    b. brushing with clothing
    c. sneezing and coughing
    d. normal breathing

1276. Which of the following is the appropriate technique for medically C^{1266} aseptic hand washing?
    a. keep elbows lower than the hands
    b. keep hands lower than the elbows
    c. keep hands and elbows at the same level
    d. wash hands first, then elbows

┌─ Answer
│ ┌─ Question #
│ ↓
↓

B^1287 1277. Which of the following diseases require only contact isolation precautions?
1. acquired immunodeficiency syndrome (AIDS)
2. *staphylococcus aureus* drainage
3. herpes simplex
   a. 1 & 2 only
   b. 1 & 3 only
   c. 2 & 3 only
   d. 1, 2, & 3

B^1288 1278. Which of the following are primary concerns for avoiding contamination of the radiographer's eyes when working with isolation patients?
1. spattering of blood
2. spattering of body waste
3. rubbing eyes with hands
   a. 1 & 2 only
B^1289 b. 1 & 3 only
   c. 2 & 3 only
   d. 1, 2, & 3

1279. Which of the following is an acceptable reason for not rinsing bedpans and urinals immediately after use?
   a. the patient is likely to use again within 1 hour
   b. the patient is in protective isolation
A^1290 c. a specimen is required
   d. the volume of waste is less than 100 cc

1280. Which of the following are basic principles for dealing with patients who have a communicable disease?
1. frequent hand washing
2. placement of needles in puncture-resistant receptacles
3. bagging and labeling contaminated materials for laundry and waste handling
   a. 1 & 2 only
   b. 1 & 3 only
A^1291 c. 2 & 3 only
   d. 1, 2, & 3

1281. Why is it recommended that a second person be available to assist during radiography of a patient with a communicable disease who is in an isolation unit?
    a. to get help in the event of accidental contamination
    b. to document all handling procedures
    c. to advise the radiographer on procedures
    d. to assist in handling items to and from contaminated areas

B^{1271}

Monitoring Vital Signs 1% (14) 1282-1295

C^{1272}

1282. What is the range of normal adult respiration?
    a. 2 to 5 breaths per second
    b. 2 to 5 breaths per minute
    c. 10 to 20 breaths per minute
    d. 40 to 50 breaths per minute

1283. Which artery is most commonly used to measure blood pressure?
    a. brachial
    b. axillary
    c. coronary
    d. carotid

D^{1273}

1284. What biophysical measurement is made during an electrocardiogram?
    a. electrical activity
    b. physical activity
    c. biochemical interactions
    d. muscle movement

C^{1274}

1285. Where is an apical pulse taken?
    a. at the posterior surface of the knee
    b. over the carotid artery
    c. over the heart
    d. at the antecubital fossa of the elbow

A^{1275}

1286. What is the normal adult oral temperature?
    a. 36.2° C
    b. 36.4° C
    c. 37.0° C
    d. 37.5° C

B^{1276}

1287. What is the range of normal adult resting pulse rates?
 a. 30 to 50 beats per minute
 b. 60 to 90 beats per minute
 c. 90 to 100 beats per minute
 d. 110 to 120 beats per minute

B^1297 1288. Which of the following methods of temperature monitoring is the most accurate?
 a. orally
 b. rectally
 c. axillary
 d. all are equally effective

A^1298 1289. Which of the following are types of sphygmomanometers?
 1. mercury
 2. barometric
 3. aneroid
 a. 1 & 2 only
B^1299 b. 1 & 3 only
 c. 2 & 3 only
 d. 1, 2, & 3

1290. Which of the following blood pressure readings indicates the patient is hypertensive?
 a. 160/100
 b. 120/100
 c. 120/80
 d. 100/50

A^1300 1291. Systolic pressure is best described by which of the following:
 a. top number of a blood pressure reading measures the pumping action of the heart
 b. bottom number of a blood pressure reading which measures the pumping action of the heart
 c. top number of a blood pressure reading which measures the ability of the arterial system to accept the pulse of blood
A^1301 d. bottom number of a blood pressure reading which measures the ability of the arterial system to accept the pulse of blood

1292. Which of the following are proper terms to describe variations in respiratory patterns?
    1. labored
    2. shallow
    3. rapid
      a. 1 & 2 only
      b. 1 & 3 only   D^{1281}
      c. 2 & 3 only
      d. 1, 2, & 3

1293. Which of the following constitutes bradycardia?
      a. 120 beats per minute
      b. 100 beats per minute
      c. 80 beats per minute
      d. 40 beats per minute

1294. Which of the following is the most common location for detecting C^{1282}
the pulse?
      a. radial
      b. apical
      c. popliteal
      d. femoral

1295. What is the normal range of adult diastolic blood pressure?   A^{1283}
      a. 30 to 50 mm Hg
      b. 60 to 80 mm Hg
      c. 110 to 140 mm Hg
      d. 140 to 180 mm Hg

Contrast Media 4% (56) 1296-1351   A^{1284}

1296. Why are contrast media reactions more severe during venous injection than during arterial injection?
      a. because the blood must flow through the heart before it is C^{1285}
         collected by the kidneys
      b. because the blood must flow through the kidneys before it
         reaches the heart
      c. because the blood must flow through the spleen before it
         reaches the kidneys   C^{1286}
      d. because the lining of the veins is more susceptible to
         irritation

1297. What causes positive contrast material to produce an area of reduced image density?
    a. scatter of primary photons
B^1307
    b. absorption of primary photons
    c. scatter of secondary photons
    d. absorption of secondary photons

1298. Which of the following is the more toxic cation that is incorporated into the organic iodide contrast media?
C^1308
    a. sodium
    b. meglumine
    c. iodine
    d. calcium

1299. What term describes a thick contrast medium that is resistant to free
A^1309
    flow?
    a. water soluble
    b. viscous
    c. residual
    d. oily

A^1310   1300. Which of the following are used as the high-pressure mechanism in an automatic angiographic pressure injector?
    1. electromechanical
    2. compressed air
    3. magnetic resonance
    a. 1 & 2 only
B^1311
    b. 1 & 3 only
    c. 2 & 3 only
    d. 1, 2, & 3

1301. What is the most common route of administration for radiologic contrast media?
    a. intravenous
    b. intramuscular
B^1312
    c. intradermal
    d. subcutaneous

1302. Which of the following are possible adverse effects of contrast material?
1. headaches
2. aphasia
3. unconsciousness
   a. 1 & 2 only
   b. 1 & 3 only
   c. 2 & 3 only
   d. 1, 2, & 3

D^{1292}

1303. What are the purposes of connecting an intravenous line to the vessel being used for injection during an angiogram?
1. to provide an open line for medications
2. for additional contrast material
3. to remove blood samples for arterial gasses
   a. 1 & 2 only
   b. 1 & 3 only
   c. 2 & 3 only
   d. 1, 2, & 3

D^{1293}

1304. Which of the following drugs would relax vascular walls to permit greater blood flow?
   a. stimulant
   b. diuretic
   c. vasodilator
   d. anticoagulant

A^{1294}

1305. What is a normal injection time for ethiodolized oil injection of the lymph vessels?
   a. 3 to 5 sec
   b. 10 to 20 sec
   c. 1 to 2 min
   d. 45 to 90 min

B^{1295}

1306. What type of adverse reaction is characterized by an exaggerated response to a substance which had previously sensitized the organism?
   a. hypotension
   b. anaphylactic reaction
   c. pitressin reaction
   d. generalized convulsion

A^{1296}

```
 ┌ Answer
 │ ┌ Question #
 │ │
 ↓ ↓
```

1307. Which of the following decreases viscosity?
    a. cooling
    b. warming
    c. maintaining at a constant temperature
    d. decreasing pressure

D^{1319} 1308. Which of the following is a vasodilator?
    a. reserpine
    b. vasopressin
    c. nitroglycerin
    d. glucagon

B^{1320} 1309. Why is anaphylactic shock the type of shock most often seen in angiography?
    a. it is caused by contrast material use
    b. most angiography patients are very weak
    c. its effects are enhanced by radiation
    d. many angiography patients are hypertensive

A^{1321} 1310. Which type of contrast media studies should be performed first?
    a. iodine
    b. barium
    c. iodinated oil
    d. air

1311. What is the correct level for an intravenous set to be raised above the vein?
    a. 10" to 16"
    b. 18" to 24"

A^{1322} c. 26" to 30"
    d. 32" to 48"

1312. Approximately how far should an enema tip be inserted into the rectum of an adult?
    a. 1" to 2"
    b. 3" to 4"
    c. 5" to 6"
    d. 7" to 8"

D^{1323}

Question #
Answer

1313. How long should anticoagulants be withheld prior to angiography?
    a. 4 hours
    b. 12 hours
    c. 24 hours
    d. 48 hours

1314. What type of shock is caused by the pooling of blood due to the failure of arterial resistance? D^1302
    a. hypovolemic
    b. cardiogenic
    c. neurogenic
    d. anaphylactic

1315. What type of drug should be considered for a patient who complains of having "tongue thickness?" A^1303
    a. antihistamine
    b. sedative
    c. anesthetic
    d. anticoagulant

1316. Which is used for visualization of the gastrointestinal tract?
    a. barium sulfite
    b. barium sulfate C^1304
    c. potassium sulfite
    d. potassium sulfate

1317. What is the most appropriate action if resistance is encountered when inserting an enema tip for a barium enema?
    1. retract the tip and try from a different angle until the tip has been inserted completely D^1305
    2. request assistance from a physician
    3. cancel the examination
    a. 1 only
    b. 2 only
    c. 3 only
    d. 1, 2, & 3

1318. Which of the following is not an acceptable method of cleansing the bowel for a barium enema? B^1306
    a. castor oil
    b. bismuth laxative
    c. saline enema
    d. soap suds enema

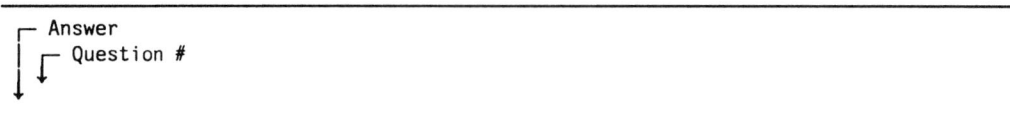

1319. Which organs can be examined with iodinated contrast media?
 1. gallbladder
 2. kidneys
 3. adrenal glands
 a. 1 & 2 only
 b. 1 & 3 only
D¹³²⁹ c. 2 & 3 only
 d. 1, 2, & 3

1320. Why is fluid run to an enema tip prior to inserting it in the rectum?
 a. venous emboli are avoided
 b. the instillation of air into the colon is avoided
 c. air left in the tubing will slow the flow of fluid
 d. air emboli are avoided

B¹³³⁰ 1321. What is the most common route of administration of contrast media for a cystogram?
 a. urinary catheter
 b. intravenous
 c. intramuscular
 d. oral

A¹³³¹ 1322. Why should geriatric patients be advised to increase fluid intake following a barium enema examination?
 1. barium absorbs fluid from the bowel
 2. barium may solidify into an impaction
 3. barium becomes toxic if not flushed from the bowel within 48 hours
 a. 1 & 2 only
 b. 1 & 3 only
 c. 2 & 3 only
 d. 1, 2, & 3

D¹³³² 1323. Which of the following is true regarding the hemodynamic consequences of iodinated contrast material?
 1. causes vasodilation
 2. increases cardiac output
 3. increases heart rate
 a. 1 only
 b. 2 only
A¹³³³ c. 3 only
 d. 1, 2, & 3

1324. Which type of cleansing enema removes interstitial fluid from the bowel, thus promoting peristalsis?
    a. normal saline
    b. hypertonic saline
    c. oil retention
    d. soap suds

A[1313]

1325. Which of the following are necessary to begin an intravenous infusion?
    1. tourniquet
    2. alcohol wipes
    3. adhesive tape
    a. 1 & 2 only
    b. 1 & 3 only
    c. 2 & 3 only
    d. 1, 2, & 3

C[1314]

1326. Which of the following minimizes electrolyte balance problems and cardiac insufficiency following a barium enema?
    1. mixing barium with normal saline solution
    2. decreasing the barium solution temperature
    3. hydrating patients well prior to examination
    a. 1 only
    b. 2 only
    c. 3 only
    d. 1, 2, & 3

A[1315]

B[1316]

1327. Toward what landmark should the enema tip be directed as it is inserted into the anus?
    a. symphysis pubis
    b. L5-S1 joint
    c. sacral canals
    d. umbilicus

1328. Within what period of time do most reactions to iodinated contrast media occur?
    a. 0 to 1 minute
    b. 2 to 10 minutes
    c. 15 to 30 minutes
    d. 1 to 2 hours

B[1317]

B[1318]

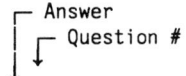

D¹³³⁸

1329. Which of the following patients require priority over other patients f or examination of the gastrointestinal system?
    1. pediatric
    2. diabetic
    3. geriatric
        a. 1 & 2 only
        b. 1 & 3 only
        c. 2 & 3 only
        d. 1, 2, & 3

1330. What is a cathartic?
        a. a special enema tip used for the instillation of air into the colon
        b. a laxative
        c. a hypertonic enema solution
        d. a special tip used for colostomy patients

A¹³³⁹

1331. Which of the following is a common cause of a spasm of the colon during an enema?
    1. when 200 to 400 ml have been administered
    2. when a RAO position is assumed
    3. if more than 50 ml of air have been administered

C¹³⁴⁰
        a. 1 only
        b. 2 only
        c. 3 only
        d. 1, 2, & 3

1332. Which describes a percutaneous transhepatic cholangiogram?
    1. a long, thin needle is used
    2. insertion is through the liver into the biliary ducts

C¹³⁴¹
    3. peritonitis is a potential side effect
        a. 1 & 2 only
        b. 1 & 3 only
        c. 2 & 3 only
        d. 1, 2, & 3

B¹³⁴²

1333. What is the purpose of an inflatable balloon cuff on an enema tip?
    1. retention of barium
    2. expansion of the rectal sphincter for easier evacuation
    3. increased sphincter pressure to slow the defecation urge
        a. 1 only
        b. 2 only
        c. 3 only
        d. 1, 2, & 3

1334. Which of the following contrast media can be used to visualize the colon?
    1. air
    2. iodine
    3. barium
       a. 1 & 2 only
       b. 1 & 3 only
       c. 2 & 3 only
       d. 1, 2, & 3

B [1324]

1335. Which are potential complications of barium leaking into the peritoneal cavity or bloodstream during a gastrointestinal examination?
    1. peritonitis
    2. venous embolism
    3. carcinoma
       a. 1 & 2 only
       b. 1 & 3 only
       c. 2 & 3 only
       d. 1, 2, & 3

D [1325]

1336. What type of shock is caused by an abnormally low volume of circulating blood?
       a. anaphylactic
       b. neurogenic
       c. hypovolemic
       d. cardiogenic

A [1326]

1337. Which of the following are possible causes of bowel perforation?
    1. gastric ulcer
    2. polyps of the colon
    3. trauma to the abdomen
       a. 1 & 2 only
       b. 1 & 3 only
       c. 2 & 3 only
       d. 1, 2, & 3

D [1327]

B [1328]

1338. Which of the following are signs of anaphylactic shock?
1. sneezing and coughing
2. itching at the site of injection, eyes, and nose
3. apprehensiveness
   a. 1 & 2 only
   b. 1 & 3 only
   c. 2 & 3 only
   d. 1, 2, & 3

A^{1348}

1339. Which of the following are true concerning non-ionic iodinated contrast media?
1. they are less likely to cause anaphylactic shock
2. they are considerably more expensive
3. they produce higher quality images
   a. 1 & 2 only
   b. 1 & 3 only
   c. 2 & 3 only
   d. 1, 2, & 3

B^{1349}

1340. What is the recommended temperature range for barium solution that will be used for rectal administration?
   a. 68° to 72° F
   b. 98° to 100° F
   c. 102° to 105° F
   d. 110° to 115° F

B^{1350}

1341. What is the approximate quantity of barium required for an average normal adult barium enema examination without air contrast techniques?
   a. 120 to 180 ml
   b. 400 to 500 ml
   c. 1,200 to 1,500 ml
   d. 3,000 to 4,000 ml

B^{1351}

1342. What is the most efficient route for administration of medications to counteract adverse reactions?
   a. subcutaneous
   b. intravenous
   c. intramuscular
   d. oral

A^{1352}

1343. Which of the following is a recommended sequence of contrast media studies?
    a. upper GI, lower GI, urinary, biliary
    b. biliary, urinary, lower GI, upper GI
    c. urinary, biliary, lower GI, upper GI
    d. biliary, urinary, upper GI, lower GI

1344. Which contrast medium is indicated for a gastrointestinal procedure when a perforation of the bowel is possible?   D[1334]
    1. barium
    2. iodine
    3. air
    a. 1 only
    b. 2 only
    c. 3 only
    d. 1, 2, & 3

1345. Which of the following must be scheduled prior to a barium examination of the colon?   A[1335]
    1. barium upper gastrointestinal examination
    2. gastroscopy
    3. thyroid iodine uptake
    a. 1 & 2 only
    b. 1 & 3 only
    c. 2 & 3 only   C[1336]
    d. 1, 2, & 3

1346. Which of the following constitutes a fasting order?
    a. NPO
    b. prn
    c. gts
    d. c/o

1347. Which of the following may occur if the barium solution bag is too high during a barium enema examination?   B[1337]
    1. severe abdominal cramping
    2. excessive pressure on the anal veins
    3. rupture of diverticula in the colon
    a. 1 & 2 only
    b. 1 & 3 only
    c. 2 & 3 only
    d. 1, 2, & 3

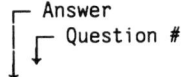

1348. Which of the following stool materials is an indication of upper gastrointestinal bleeding?
    1. black, tarry blood
    2. fresh, red blood
    3. white mucous
      a. 1 only
D^{1358} b. 2 only
      c. 3 only
      d. 1, 2, & 3

1349. Which of the following best describes the examination of the urinary system that is accomplished by intravenous injection of iodinated contrast media?
      a. KUB
      b. urogram
D^{1359} c. pyelogram
      d. cystogram

1350. Why should barium be administered orally with a straw?
      a. to avoid ingesting air
      b. to avoid coating the mouth with barium
      c. to slow the ingestion rate
      d. to increase the ingestion rate

A^{1360} 1351. In what position should a patient be placed for insertion of an enema tip?
      a. Fowler's
      b. Sims
      c. trendelenburg
      d. prone

B^{1361} 1352. Which of the following should not be ingested 24 hours prior to a barium examination of the gastrointestinal tract?
    1. whole grain cereals
    2. carbonated beverages
    3. clear gelatin
      a. 1 only
C^{1362} b. 2 only
      c. 3 only
      d. 1, 2, & 3

Emergency Situations 3% (42) 1353-1393

1353. What is the proper action during the first five seconds of rescue activity when an unwitnessed cardiac arrest has occurred?   C^{1343}
    a. palpate carotid pulse
    b. open the airway
    c. thump the chest
    d. establish unresponsiveness

1354. What is the most common cause of airway obstruction in the unconscious victim of an unwitnessed collapse?
    a. food
    b. mucous
    c. dentures   B^{1344}
    d. tongue

1355. What is the proper treatment for a patient experiencing hypoglycemia?
    a. administration of insulin
    b. administration of sugar
    c. cardiopulmonary resuscitation
    d. move to a Sims position and administer water

1356. Artificial circulation is produced during cardiopulmonary C^{1345}
resuscitation when the chest is compressed by squeezing the heart between which two structures?
    a. clavicle and the scapula
    b. sternum and the spine
    c. clavicle and ribs
    d. sternum and xiphoid process

1357. What are the primary functions of an intravenous line during A^{1346}
angiographic studies of the circulatory system?
    1. to establish a direct route for introducing medication
    2. to establish the primary route for contrast media injection
    3. to establish a secondary route for the injection of additional contrast media
    a. 1 & 2 only
    b. 1 & 3 only
    c. 2 & 3 only   B^{1347}
    d. 1, 2, & 3

1358. Which of the following drugs are considered essential for CPR?
    1. oxygen
    2. lidocaine
    3. epinephrine
       a. 1 & 2 only
       b. 1 & 3 only

D^{1368} c. 2 & 3 only
       d. 1, 2, & 3

1359. If several acute emergency orders are received at once, what procedure should determine which is done first by the radiographer?
       a. the order on top should be done first

D^{1369} b. the patient whose surname begins with the first letter of the alphabet should be done first
       c. the ordering physicians should be contacted to determine which patient is done first
       d. the procedure that can be completed in the shortest length of time should be done first

C^{1370} 1360. Which of the following is the most likely cause of one-sided muscle weakness and eye deviation with difficult speech and a sudden stiff neck?
       a. cerebral vascular accident
       b. convulsive seizure
       c. cardiac arrest
       d. septic shock

1361. What is the proper number of ventilations for every 15 cardiac compressions during adult cardiopulmonary resuscitation?

C^{1371} a. 1
       b. 2
       c. 7
       d. 15

1362. What is the maximum length of time cardiac compressions may be interrupted once cardiopulmonary resuscitation has begun?
       a. 1 second
       b. 3 seconds
       c. 7 seconds

B^{1372} d. 10 seconds

1363. Which of the following are symptoms of a partially obstructed airway?
    a. flushed warm skin, confusion, seizures
    b. noisy breathing, wheezing, labored breathing
    c. clammy cold skin, pallor, weakness
    d. itching, sneezing, dilated pupils

1364. Into what positions should a patient be moved to avoid aspiration of vomitus?   D^{1353}
    1. lateral recumbent
    2. sitting
    3. supine
    a. 1 & 2 only
    b. 1 & 3 only
    c. 2 & 3 only   D^{1354}
    d. 1, 2, & 3

1365. Which drug will resolve an acute asthmatic episode?
    a. sodium bicarbonate
    b. epinephrine
    c. Benadryl (diphenhydramine)   B^{1355}
    d. hydrocortisone

1366. How far should the sternum be compressed during cardiopulmonary resuscitation of an adult?
    a. 0.5"
    b. 1.5" to 2"
    c. 3" to 5"   B^{1356}
    d. 6"

1367. Which of the following is part of the Heimlich maneuver?
    1. quick forceful pressure upward against the diaphragm
    2. clearing the mouth with two fingers
    3. mouth-to-mouth resuscitation
    a. 1 only
    b. 2 only
    c. 3 only
    d. 1, 2, & 3

    B^{1357}

B¹³⁷⁸ 1368. Which of the following are valid artificial ventilation methods?
1. tracheal intubation
2. cricothyreotomy
3. bag-valve-mask
   a. 1 & 2 only
   b. 1 & 3 only
   c. 2 & 3 only
   d. 1, 2, & 3

C¹³⁷⁹ 1369. What term describes labored or difficult breathing?
   a. epistaxis
   b. diaphoresis
   c. eclampsia
   d. dyspnea

A¹³⁸⁰ 1370. Which drug will assist in resolving a mild reaction to iodinated contrast medium?
   a. sodium bicarbonate
   b. epinephrine
   c. benadryl (diphenhydramine)
   d. hydrocortisone

C¹³⁸¹ 1371. Which of the following is not a correct action to take for a patient experiencing a seizure?
1. assist the patient into a supine position on the floor
2. move objects out of the patient's reach
3. hold the patient's tongue with your fingers
   a. 1 only
C¹³⁸²   b. 2 only
   c. 3 only
   d. 1, 2, & 3

1372. Which of the following is a correct procedure for sealing the airway during cardiopulmonary resuscitation?
1. placing the fingers in the external auditory meatus
2. clamping the nose with the fingers
3. hyperextending the chin
   a. 1 only
   b. 2 only
D¹³⁸³   c. 3 only
   d. 1, 2, & 3

Question # ⌐
Answer ⌐ |
↓ |
↓

1373. What condition results from an excess amount of insulin in the bloodstream of a patient with diabetes mellitus?
    a. hypoglycemia
    b. ketoacidosis   B ^{1363}
    c. cardiac arrest
    d. hyperosmolar coma

1374. Which of the following are considered essential drugs for CPR?
    1. sodium bicarbonate
    2. morphine sulfate
    3. nitroglycerine
    a. 1 & 2 only
    b. 1 & 3 only
    c. 2 & 3 only   A ^{1364}
    d. 1, 2, & 3

1375. Which of the following are required for effective cardiac compression during cardiopulmonary resuscitation?
    1. patient supine
    2. a clear airway   B ^{1365}
    3. a hard surface under the patient
    a. 1 & 2 only
    b. 1 & 3 only
    c. 2 & 3 only
    d. 1, 2, & 3

1376. Which of the following is an appropriate action if a patient is not B ^{1366} breathing but the carotid pulse can be detected?
    1. cardiac compressions
    2. ingestion of sugar
    3. ventilations
    a. 1 only
    b. 2 only
    c. 3 only
    d. 1, 2, & 3

1377. Which of the following are potentially life-threatening?   A ^{1367}
    1. asthmatic attack
    2. diabetic reactions
    3. anaphylaxis
    a. 1 & 2 only
    b. 1 & 3 only
    c. 2 & 3 only
    d. 1, 2, & 3

1378. Which term describes profuse sweating?
a. epistaxis
b. diaphoresis
c. eclampsia
d. dyspnea

B¹³⁸⁹

1379. Which of the following is a nosebleed?
a. anaphylaxis
b. syncope
c. epistaxis
d. ataxia

B¹³⁹⁰

1380. When cardiopulmonary resuscitation is performed, where should the second hand of the person performing the compressions be placed?
a. on top of the first hand
b. superior to the first hand
c. inferior to the first hand
d. to the patient's left side from the first hand

A¹³⁹¹

1381. What is the recommended location to take a pulse reading prior to beginning resuscitation?
a. radial
b. brachial
c. carotid
d. femoral

B¹³⁹²

1382. What is the recommended rate of external cardiac compressions for one-rescuer CPR of an adult?
a. 5
b. 60
c. 80
d. 100

B¹³⁹³

1383. Which of the following are important during cardiopulmonary resuscitation?
1. locked elbows
2. check carotid pulse every minute
3. call for assistance
a. 1 & 2 only
b. 1 & 3 only
c. 2 & 3 only
d. 1, 2, & 3

C¹³⁹⁴

1384. Which part of the hand should be placed on the sternum to initiated cardiac compression during cardiopulmonary resuscitation?
    a. the fingertips
    b. the palm
    c. the heel
    d. the medial side

A[1373]

1385. What is meant by a "stat" order?
    a. it is to be performed after all other orders
    b. it is to be performed as soon as possible after other orders
    c. it is to receive highest priority
    d. a postmortem examination

A[1374]

1386. What is the function of a triage procedure?
    a. efficient handling of cardiopulmonary resuscitation
    b. efficient handling of large numbers of trauma patients
    c. proceedings for determining priority when a single patient requires numerous examinations
    d. institutional method of contacting large numbers of employees at one time

1387. What is the proper action to take if no pulse is obtained while ventilating a patient with an airway obstruction?
    1. terminate ventilations
    2. begin cardiac compression
    3. sharply compress the abdomen just below the ribs
    a. 1 only
    b. 2 only
    c. 3 only
    d. 1, 2, & 3

B[1375]

1388. What is the proper number of cardiac compressions for every two ventilations during adult cardiopulmonary resuscitation?
    a. 1
    b. 2
    c. 7
    d. 15

C[1376]

C[1377]

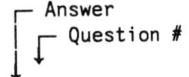

1389. After what period of time does irreparable brain damage occur during cardiac arrest?
    a. 30 to 60 seconds
    b. 3 to 5 minutes
    c. 8 to 10 minutes
    d. 15 to 20 minutes

A^{1400} 1390. What is the recommended rate of external cardiac compressions for two-rescuer CPR of an adult?
    a. 5
    b. 60
    c. 80
    d. 100

1391. What is the most common cause of respiratory arrest?
    a. aspiration of food
    b. aspiration of drink
    c. laughing
    d. severe coughing

1392. What term describes defective muscular coordination?
    a. epistaxis
    b. ataxia
    c. dyspnea
    d. diaphoresis

1393. What condition results from the mobilization of fatty acids when insufficient insulin is available to metabolize glucose?
    a. hypoglycemia
    b. ketoacidosis
    c. cardiac arrest
    d. hyperosmolar coma

Monitoring of Medical Equipment 0.5% (6) 1394-1400

1394. What is the function of a T-tube that is surgically implanted in the biliary ducts?
    a. release of bile to an external drain
    b. admission of contrast media into the biliary system
    c. drainage of bile
    d. mixing of bile with outside air for smoother flow

1395. Which of the following may be reconnected by the radiographer if they are accidently disconnected?
    1. Swan-Ganz catheter line
    2. oxygen line
    3. urinary catheter line
        a. 1 & 2 only
        b. 1 & 3 only
        c. 2 & 3 only
        d. 1, 2, & 3

C[1384]

1396. From what location does a cystostomy tube drain fluid?
        a. urinary bladder
        b. heart
        c. colon
        d. bile ducts

C[1385]

1397. Which of the following require surgical procedures during insertion?
    1. closed chest drainage tube
    2. nasogastric
    3. tracheostomy
        a. 1 & 2 only
        b. 1 & 3 only
        c. 2 & 3 only
        d. 1, 2, & 3

B[1386]

1398. Which of the following are tissue drains?
    1. Cantor
    2. Penrose
    3. Hemovac
        a. 1 & 2 only
        b. 1 & 3 only
        c. 2 & 3 only
        d. 1, 2, & 3

B[1387]

1399. Which of the following deliver the highest concentration of oxygen?
        a. nonrebreathing mask
        b. partial rebreathing mask
        c. venturi mask
        d. aerosol mask

D[1388]

321

1400. Which of the following are types of gastric tubes?
    1. Cantor
    2. Levin
    3. Penrose
        a. 1 & 2 only
        b. 1 & 3 only
        c. 2 & 3 only
        d. 1, 2, & 3

C^{1395}

A^{1396}

B^{1397}

C^{1398}

A^{1399}

Patient Care and Management

┌─ Answer
│ ┌─ Question #
↓ ↓

RADIATION PROTECTION
Patient Protection
8% (112) 1-112

1. (D) There are three acute radiation syndromes: hemopoietic, gastrointestinal, and central nervous system. **syndromes (Travis, Bushong)**

2. (C) Medical radiation exposure such as radiation therapy is not part of the natural background radiation received by everyone. **radiation, background (Noz, Bushong, Selman)**

3. (C) A single, half value layer (HVL) reduces the exposure to one half its original energy by definition. Therefore, one HVL reduces the original intensity to 50%, the second HVL reduces it to 25%, the third to 12.5%, and the fourth to 6.25%, which is less than 10%. **filtration, half value layer (Cullinan, Carlton, Bushong)**

4. (B) A shadow shield casts a shadow in the primary beam light field which indicates where it will protect the gonads from primary beam exposure. **radiation protection, gonad shielding (Bushong, Noz, Selman, Carlton)**

5. (A) The term genetic describes inherited traits, which, in this case, would be the effects of radiation exposure to the ancestors. **radiation effects, genetic (Bushong, Travis)**

6. (B) This is the classic definition of the genetically significant dose (GSD) that is used to gauge the total radiation exposure of large populations. **genetically significant dose, GSD (Travis, Bushong)**

7. (A) Because of the undifferentiated nature of the duodenal membrane cells, it is the most sensitive. **radiosensitivity, tissue (Travis, Noz, Bushong)**

8. (B) Because damage to a base can cause the DNA to continue with incorrect information, and because damage to a double strand can halt information flow within the cell, these can both have serious consequences for the cell. A single-strand break has a greater likelihood of repair. **radiation effects, DNA (Travis, Bushong)**

9. (A) Grids absorb some of the exit radiation in the interspace material. The lack of a grid for an air-gap technique permits a slight reduction in mAs while maintaining the same image density. **grids, air-gap (Curry, Carlton, Bushong, Cullinan)**

10. (D) The filter material is designed to absorb the low-energy photons that are not strong enough to penetrate the patient. If these photons were allowed to reach the patient, they would contribute to the exposure dose but could not reach the image receptor to contribute to the image. **filtration (Bushong, Noz, Selman, Carlton)**

11. (C) Because the glass window is a part of the tube, the term inherent is used to describe filtration that occurs there. **filtration, inherent (Bushong, Noz, Selman, Carlton)**

12. (C) Positive beam limitation is a defined term. **collimation, positive beam limitation (Carlton, Bushong, Noz, Selman)**

13. (C) The definition of a half value layer is the amount of filtration required to reduce the primary beam to half its original intensity. **half value layer, filtration (Bushong, Noz, Selman, Carlton)**

14. (B) The positive beam limitation device automatically limits the primary beam field size to the size of the cassette in the bucky tray. **positive beam limitation, collimation, beam restriction (Carlton, Bushong, Cullinan, Curry)**

15. (C) As a general rule a, lower mAs value produces less patient exposure dose, although kVp level must also be considered. In this problem, A and C are close answers; however, a reduction of half the mAs probably would be more effective than a 10% kVp reduction. **radiation protection, kilovoltage (Carlton, Bushong)**

16. (A) MAs, kVp, and filtration have a definite effect on patient dose; however, focal spot size is primarily a geometric/recorded detail factor and has little, if anything, to do with patient dose. **radiation protection, focal spot (Carlton, Bushong)**

17. (D) Higher speed screens require less mAs to achieve density. A lower mAs value decreases the patient exposure dose. **intensifying screens, film/screen combinations, radiation protection (Bushong, Cullinan, Selman, Carlton)**

18. (A) Younger persons who are likely to live longer and persons who are likely to reproduce increase GSd. Although the 12-year-old male is likely to make a similar GSD contribution, the 4-year-old female would have all her eggs exposed, while the male's sperm for reproduction would be produced at a later date. **genetically significant dose, GSD (Bushong, Noz, Selman, Travis)**

19. (C) U.S. government recommendations. **radiation protection, fluoroscopy (Carlton, Bushong, Selman)**

20. (C) NCRP Report #33, 1968. **filtration (Curry, Bushong, Selman)**

21. (C) The PA projection places the eye the greatest distance from the entrance beam, thus permitting attenuation of the beam in the head to reduce the intensity of the beam before it reaches the eye. **radiation protection (Carlton)**

22. (B) A nonlinear curve is not a straight line. A nonthreshold effect represents a response without a dose; consequently, the curve must intersect the vertical axis at no dose. **dose effect (Travis, Bushong)**

23. (A) A linear curve is a straight line. A nonthreshold effect represents a response without a dose; consequently, the curve must intersect the vertical axis at no dose. **dose effect (Travis, Bushong)**

24. (A) Because a back-up time is less than the tube overload, when it is activated, it safeguards against the patient receiving a tube overload range exposure, which would cause a repeated exposure in addition to the overexposed image. **automatic exposure control, phototiming (Carlton, Cullinan)**

25. (B) Nonspecific indicates that no particular set of symptoms or pathologies can be identified for accelerated and premature life shortening. **nonspecific, life shortening (Travis, Bushong)**

26. (D) Somatic effects are seen in the effected individual. **somatic effects, radiation effects (Travis, Bushong)**

27. (B) According to the graph, a dose at this time occurs during organogenesis, which includes bone development. Spontaneous abortions are prenatal deaths that occur during preimplantation. Cancer is a long-term effect that occurs during the fetal stages of development or later. Note that all these are 1st trimester effects. **radiation effects, embryo, pregnancy (Travis, Bushong)**

28. (C) The backup time is usually set to approximately 1.5 X the expected maximum mAs to safeguard against accidental or excessive patient exposure. **automatic exposure control, phototimer, backup time (Curry, Carlton)**

29. (A) The least amount of filtration would permit the maximum low-energy photons to reach the entrance skin, thus resulting in the highest exposure dose to the patient. **filtration (Curry, Carlton, Bushong, Selman)**

30. (D) Low-ripple generator configurations produce higher average x-ray photon energies. This permits a reduction in mAs values and decreases patient exposure dose. **generator types (Curry, Carlton, Bushong)**

31. (C) The lowest mAs value produces the lowest patient exposure dose. The highest grid ratio would absorb the most radiation, thus producing the lowest patient exposure dose. **radiation protection of the patient, grids (Carlton, Curry, Bushong)**

32. (A) Contact shields can be placed directly over the breasts and gonads when they are not within areas of diagnostic interest. Shadow shields can be used to absorb radiation before it reaches the patient under similar conditions. **radiation protection, shielding (Carlton, Bushong, Selman)**

33. (D) Lethality and congenital abnormalities occur during the 1st trimester of embryologic development. Long-term effects may begin at any time but are not seen until the late fetal stages of development or even later in life. **radiation effects, embryo, pregnancy (Travis, Bushong)**

34. (A) This is a definition of a stochastic (or random) effect. **stochastic, late effects, radiation effects (Travis)**

35. (B) Doubling dose is the term that describes the dose that will produce a doubling of mutations in experiments. **radiation effects, genetic effects, doubling dose (Travis)**

36. (A) The bone marrow, circulating blood, and lymphoid organs (spleen, thymus, and lymph nodes) comprise the hemopoietic system. **hemopoietic, bone marrow (Travis, Bushong)**

37. (D) The acute radiation syndromes all exhibit a prodromal, latent, and manifest illness stage. **radiation effects, acute radiation effects, radiation syndromes (Bushong, Travis)**

38. (C) Damage to the red bone marrow will be seen as anemia in the circulating blood as red blood cells die and fail to be replaced. **radiation effects, acute radiation effects, radiation syndromes (Bushong, Travis)**

39. (B) Skin cancer is believed to have a threshold response, and the early radiologist as well as groups of patients who were treated for ringworm and acne all exhibited dramatically increased incidence of the disease. **radiation effects, skin cancer (Bushong, Travis)**

40. (A) The mature spermatozoa are dividing slowly and are well-differentiated as they have evolved from immature spermatogonia. According to the Law of Bergonie and Tribondeau, low mitotic rate and well differentiated cell populations are more radioresistant. **reproductive system, gonads (Bushong, Travis)**

41. (C) The curve in Figure 3 shows damage without any dose; therefore, it is non-threshold. Because the curve is a straight line it shows a linear relationship. **radiation effects, thyroid (Bushong, Travis)**

42. (B) Research has established the approximate dose for male sterility at 5 to 6 Gy. **reproductive system, gonads (Bushong, Travis)**

43. (B) Erythema is a reddening of the skin. **radiation effects, skin (Bushong, Travis)**

44. (A) Because of the rapid growth of the embryo and the large number of undifferentiated and highly mitotic cells present, the 1st trimester is the most radiosensitive portion of a pregnancy. **radiation effects, pregnancy, fetus, embryo (Bushong, Travis)**

45. (C) It is generally considered that avoidance of high radiation dose areas such as surgery, mobile, and fluoroscopic procedures is a reasonable approach for the pregnant radiographer. **pregnancy (Bushong)**

46. (D) Younger patients, especially females, have more undifferentiated and rapidly dividing cells; therefore, they are often considered slightly more radiosensitive. **radiosensitivity, acute effects of radiation (Bushong, Travis)**

47. (B) A single half value layer (HVL) reduces the exposure to one half its original energy by definition. Therefore, one HVL reduces the original intensity to 50%, the second HVL reduces it to 25%, the third to 12.5%, the fourth to 6.25%, the fifth to 3.13%, the sixth to 1.57%, and the seventh to 0.79%, which is less than 1%. **filtration, half value layer (Carlton, Bushong, Selman)**

48. (B) Faster film/screen combinations permit lower technical factors to be used while maintaining image density, thus decreasing patient dose. **intensifying screens, film/screen combinations (Carlton, Cullinan, Curry, Bushong)**

49. (B) Linear energy transfer relates to the amount of energy transferred as a photon travels through tissue. It is measured in keV/μm. **linear energy transfer (Bushong, Travis)**

50. (A) The Law of Bergonie and Tribondeau states that highly specialized and highly mitotic cells are more radiosensitive. **Law of Bergonie and Tribondeau (Bushong, Travis)**

51. (B) Interphase death refers to the death of the cell before it can reproduce. In other words, the cell remains in interphase, the step before the mitotic phases, until it dies. **interphase death, biological factors (Bushong, Travis)**

52. (D) Positive beam limitation (PBL) is required by law for all diagnostic units. **positive beam limitation, collimation, beam restriction (Carlton, Bushong, Curry, Selman)**

53. (A) A reciprocating grid will absorb approximately 10% more radiation than the same grid when it is stationary. **grids (Bushong, Selman, Cullinan)**

54. (B) A collimator eliminates off-focus, secondary scattered radiation and restricts the primary beam to the area of interest. Although it adds a small amount of inherent filtration, added aluminum filtration must be added to control filtration. **beam restriction, collimation (Bushong, Curry, Carlton, Selman)**

55. (D) Oxygen is the primary chemical cell radiosensitizer. **radiosensitizers, oxygen, chemical factors, biological factors (Bushong, Travis)**

56. (A) The ovaries are located within the primary beam of an AP abdomen but outside the primary beam for the other procedures. **reproductive system, radiation effect (Travis, Bushong)**

57. (D) As a general rule, a lower mAs value produces less patient exposure dose, although kVp level must also be considered. In this problem, D uses the least mAs because it has the highest kVp. All four exposure techniques would produce the same image density. **radiation protection, kilovoltage (Carlton, Bushong)**

58. (C) The PA projection places the breast the greatest distance from the entrance beam, thus permitting attenuation of the beam in the chest to reduce the intensity of the beam before it reaches the breast. **radiation protection (Carlton)**

59. (A) Increased filtration reduces the quantity and increases the quality of the primary beam photons thus requiring an increase in the exposure factors (mAs and kVp) to maintain image density. However, entrance skin exposure dose is reduced, resulting in an overall decrease in patient dose. This holds true from approximately 0.5 to 3.5 mm Al/Eq. **filtration (Curry, Carlton)**

60. (A) Relative biological effect is used to compare various types of radiation to a given biologic result. **relative biological effect (Bushong, Travis)**

61. (A) Inherent filtration is that which is already present in the normal equipment structures. **filtration (Carlton, Bushong, Cullinan, Curry, Selman)**

62. (D) Film/screen combinations affect the amount of mAs, and, therefore, the patient exposure dose. Filtration affects the amount of low-energy photons that would add to patient dose without contributing to the image. Beam restriction affects the primary beam that adds to patient exposure without contributing diagnostic information. **film/screen combinations, filtration, beam restriction (Carlton, Bushong, Selman)**

63. (B) The primary field would include male gonads and possibly female gonads during a lateral hip; however, the gonads lie so that they could be shielded. **gonads, radiation protection (Carlton, Bushong)**

64. (A) Off-focus radiation occurs because photons can be created within the x-ray tube but away from the x-ray tube focal spot. **off-focus (Cullinan, Carlton, Bushong)**

65. (C) The central nervous syndrome occurs at 50 Gy and more. **radiation syndromes, radiation effects, central nervous syndrome (Bushong, Travis)**

66. (D) By definition, carcinogenis is the creation of cancer. **radiation effects, carcinogenis (Bushong, Travis, Noz)**

67. (D) The prodromal stage of all three acute radiation syndromes includes these symptoms. **acute radiation syndromes, prodromal (Bushong, Travis)**

68. (B) Most humans exposed to 1 to 2 Gy will recover within 90 days. **acute radiation, syndromes, hemopoietic syndrome (Bushong, Travis)**

69. (B) Mucosal cells are undifferentiated and rapidly dividing and are therefore the most radiosensitive of those listed. **cell response, tissue response, Law of Bergonie and Tribondeau (Bushong, Travis)**

70. (C) Because its cells are highly differentiated and have a low mitotic rate, the central nervous system is the most radioresistant system. **central nervous system, Law of Bergonie and Tribondeau (Bushong, Travis)**

71. (A) Skin cancer and leukemia have been proven to be caused by radiation exposure. Diabetes has not been directly linked to radiation exposure. **late effects, leukemia, skin cancer (Bushong, Travis)**

72. (A) Figure A is not diagnostic for the public bones because a male gonad shield has been used and is superimposed over them. **shielding (Carlton, Bushong)**

73. (A) The gonads should be shielded when they lie within 5 cm of the edge of the primary beam field. **radiation protection, shielding (Bushong, Travis, Carlton, Selman)**

74. (A) Sublethal damage describes radiation effects that are below the levels needed to kill a cell. **sublethal damage (Bushong, Travis)**

75. (B) The ability to reduce the primary beam field size has no bearing on decisions to use gonad shielding. The field size should be reduced as much as possible whether or not gonad shielding is used. **radiation protection, shielding, gonad shielding (Carlton, Bushong, Selman)**

76. (A) NCRP Report #33, 1968. **filtration (Curry, Bushong, Selman)**

77. (C) The testes are located within the primary beam of a lateral hip but outside the primary beam for the other procedures. **reproductive system, radiation effect (Travis, Bushong)**

78. (A) Desquamation is a loss of skin cells that can lead to ulceration, necrosis, and cancer. **radiation effects, skin (Bushong, Travis)**

79. (D) The linear energy transfer increases as the radiation mass and energy increase. **linear energy transfer (Bushong, Travis)**

80. (B) The greatest area, 84"^{2}, is produced by the 6" x 14" field. **beam restriction, collimation (Carlton, Bushong, Selman, Cullinan)**

81. (A) The presence of abdominal bowel gas presents the possibility of it being located over activated ion chambers, thus reducing image density to an unsatisfactory level. **automatic exposure controls, phototiming (Carlton, Cullinan, Bushong, Curry)**

82. (D) Free radicals are extremely volatile chemicals that are toxic to normal physiology. **free radical (Bushong, Travis)**

83. (C) The kidneys are located more posterior than the liver, stomach, or bladder. **urinary system, gastrointestinal system, liver (Ballinger)**

84. (C) With the possible exception of a cone, an extended cylinder would remove the most off-focus scatter. **beam restriction, collimation (Carlton, Bushong, Selman)**

85. (A) Because attenuation of the beam as it travels through the subject reduces the beam's intensity, the entrance skin surface would receive the maximum reduction in exposure when filtration is increased. **filtration, attenuation (Bushong, Curry, Carlton)**

86. (D) Higher atomic number, greater thickness, and higher density all contribute to the shielding ability of a material. **shielding (Noz, Bushong, Selman)**

87. (B) Patients receive diagnostic radiation exposure in acute doses. **early effects, acute exposure (Bushong, Selman, Travis)**

88. (C) Because it is critical to cell function, DNA is the most likely focus of the target theory. **target theory (Bushong, Travis)**

89. (A) The higher the grid ratio and the higher the grid frequency, the more radiation is absorbed, thus requiring more radiation to enter the patient to maintain adequate image density. **grids (Carlton, Bushong, Selman, Cullinan, Curry)**

90. (B) Indirect effects of ionizing radiation occur in locations distant from the site of damage and are often metabolic and physiologic in nature. **indirect effect (Bushong, Travis)**

91. (B) Because linear energy transfer is a measurement of photon travel in tissue, it is measured in terms of photon energy (keV) and distance in tissue on a microscopic scale (μm). **linear energy transfer (Bushong, Travis)**

92. (A) Contact shields can be placed directly on the eyes. Because of the potential for slight movement of the head, shadow shields are not effective for protection of the lens of the eye. **radiation protection, shielding (Bushong)**

93. (D) The AP projection places the kidney the greatest distance from the entrance beam, thus permitting attenuation of the beam in the abdomen to reduce the intensity of the beam before it reaches the kidney. **radiation protection (Carlton)**

94. (A) Tissues and organs with more undifferentiated and rapidly dividing cells are more radiosensitive. Therefore, the fetus would be the most radiosensitive. **Law of Bergonie and Tribondeau (Bushong, Travis)**

95. (B) This is the definition of radiolysis, the first event in the formation of free radicals. **radiolysis, free radicals (Bushong, Travis)**

96. (C) A collimator is the only beam restrictor listed that is capable of a square field. The circular fields would expose additional tissue beyond the edges of the film to assure corner coverage. **beam restrictors, collimation (Curry, Carlton, Bushong)**

97. (D) All three factors work to produce more light photons which increase image density, thus permitting a decrease in the energy of the primary beam that controls patient exposure dose. **intensifying screens (Carlton, Bushong, Curry, Cullinan, Selman)**

98. (C) Low-energy photons are absorbed within the first few centimeters of tissue. This is the highest patient dose that filtration is used to eliminate. **filtration (Curry, Carlton, Selman, Bushong)**

99. (B) As all four sets of technical factors would produce similar image density, the higher kVp (120) permits less mAs to be used, and therefore reduces patient exposure dose. Of the two 120 kVp techniques, the higher relative film/screen speed (400) permits a further reduction in mAs therefore, producing the greatest reduction in patient exposure dose. **intensifying screens, film/screen combinations (Carlton, Bushong, Cullinan, Curry)**

100. (B) Film/screen mammography performed with low ratio grids has been shown to have a significantly lower patient exposure dose. **mammography (Ballinger)**

101. (C) Because oxygen makes tissues more radiosensitive, any condition that produces a hypoxic state, as does vasoconstriction, would make a tissue more radioresistant. **oxygen enhancement ratio (Bushong, Travis)**

102. (A) Grid ratio and frequency determine the intensity of the primary beam necessary to satisfactorily penetrate the grid and form an image. Therefore, they have a major impact on patient exposure dose. The grid type does not have this type of effect. **grids (Carlton, Bushong, Selman, Curry, Cullinan)**

103. (C) Carbon graphite attenuates very little of the primary beam thus permitting a reduction in primary beam intensity. This reduces patient exposure dose. **equipment, graphite, radiation protection (Carlton, Bushong, Curry)**

104. (A) The film/screen combination speed determines the intensity of the primary beam. This can permit reductions in patient exposure dose. However, the focal spot size affects only geometric factors such as recorded detail and distortion. **focal spot, film/screen combinations (Carlton, Bushong, Curry)**

105. (A) Penetrating ability increases as the radiation mass decreases. X-rays have no mass while electrons, neutrons, and alpha particles have increasing mass in the order given. **linear energy transfer (Bushong, Travis)**

106. (B) Hydrogen peroxide can be produced by the reaction of a free radical hydrogen atom with a free oxygen atom, although this is an unlikely combination. **free radical (Bushong, Travis)**

107. (B) Research has established the approximate dose for female sterility at 5 to 6 Gy. **reproductive system, gonads (Bushong, Travis)**

108. (B) NCRP Report #33, 1968. **filtration (Curry, Bushong, Selman)**

109. (B) Genetic effects are seen in the offspring of the effected individual. **genetic effects, radiation protection (Travis, Bushong)**

110. (C) Epilation is a loss of hair. **radiation effects, skin (Bushong, Travis)**

111. (C) As all four sets of technical factors would produce similar image density, the higher kVp (92) permits less mAs to be used and therefore reduces patient exposure dose. Of the two 92 kVp techniques, the higher relative film/screen speed (400) permits a further reduction in mAs therefore producing the greatest reduction in patient exposure dose. **intensifying screens, film/screen combinations (Carlton, Bushong, Cullinan, Curry)**

112. (B) RBE is calculated as the dose of a standardized radiation (usually 250 kVp x-rays) required to produce the biological effect divided by the dose of the subject radiation required to produce the same effect. In this case: 5.2/4.0 = 1.3. **relative biological effect (Bushong, Travis)**

RADIATION PROTECTION
Personnel Protection
4% (56) 113-168

113. (C) The percentage of time a beam is directed at a barrier is the use factor. **use factor (Bushong)**

114. (B) NCRP Report #102. **leakage (Travis, Noz, Carlton, Bushong)**

115. (D) According to the inverse square law, (200 mR/wk/25 mR/wk) x 100 cm^2 = 80,000 cm. The square root of 80,000 cm is 282.8 cm; 400 cm is the only distance that would be less than 25 mR/wk. **inverse square law (Travis, Noz, Bushong)**

116. (B) NCRP Report #91. **effective dose equivalent limit, maximum permissible dose (Carlton, Curry)**

117. (D) Occupational exposure is calculated from only exposure received while engaging in the occupation. Background radiation and medical exposures are not included in occupational totals. **effective dose equivalent limit, maximum permissible dose (Travis, Bushong, Noz, Carlton)**

118. (C) NCRP Report #91. **effective dose equivalent limit, maximum permissible dose (Carlton, Curry)**

119. (D) NCRP Report #102. **exposure switch, dead-man switch (Carlton, Bushong, Curry)**

120. (C) NCRP Report #91. **effective dose equivalent limit, maximum permissible dose (Carlton, Curry)**

121. (A) NCRP Report #102. **fluoroscopy, protective curtain (Bushong, Noz)**

122. (C) NCRP Report #102. **tabletop (NCRP #102)**

123. (B) NCRP Report #102. **radiation protection (Bushong, Noz, Carlton)**

124. (D) All of the diagnostic range interactions produce scattered radiation. Although photoelectric effect interactions absorb the incident photon, they produce characteristic photons. **interactions, photoelectric, coherent, classical, Compton (Carlton, Bushong, Travis, Curry)**

125. (B) Fluoroscopic x-ray tubes operate at much lower mA values than diagnostic tubes because they are in operation for relatively long periods of time (minutes instead of seconds). **fluoroscopy, x-ray tubes (Carlton, Bushong, Selman)**

126. (C) NCRP Report #102. **radiation protection, mobile, portable (Carlton, Selman, Bushong)**

127. (C) NCRP Report #102. **fluoroscopy, filtration (Bushong, Noz)**

128. (D) NCRP Report #91. **effective dose equivalent limit, maximum permissible dose (Carlton, Curry)**

129. (C) NCRP Report #102. **fluoroscopy, bucky (Carlton, Bushong, Selman)**

130. (B) NCRP Report #102. **fluoroscopy, timer (Carlton, Bushong, Curry)**

131. (B) Increases in kVp and generator phase both increase the average photon energy. An increase in mAs, while increasing the total number of photons, will not increase the average photon energy. **x-ray production, x-ray emission spectrum (Carlton, Bushong)**

132. (A) Only persons that are necessary to the examination are permitted in a fluoroscopic room during a procedure. This would normally eliminate a hospital administrator. **NCRP Report #102 fluoroscopy (Carlton, Bushong, Curry)**

133. (B) NCRP Report #102. **radiation protection, fluoroscopy (Carlton, Selman, Bushong)**

134. (B) To distinguish it from other ejected electrons, the Compton interaction electron is called a recoil electron. The name Compton electron also has been used. **Compton effect (Carlton, Bushong, Curry, Selman)**

135. (B) Secondary barriers are designed to shield areas from secondary scattered radiation. **shielding, secondary barrier (Bushong, Noz, Selman)**

136. (A) Because of their mass, the two electrons, the photoelectron and recoil electron, are most likely to interact with nearby atoms or become free electrons. A characteristic photon may have sufficient energy to exit the body as scattered radiation. **interactions, photoelectric, Compton, characteristic (Carlton, Bushong, Selman, Curry)**

137. (A) The automatic brightness control is essentially a fluoroscopic automatic exposure control. **fluoroscopy, automatic brightness control (Carlton, Bushong, Curry)**

138. (B) NCRP Report #91. **effective dose equivalent limit, maximum permissible dose (Carlton, Curry)**

139. (B) The inverse square law reduces the dose to 25% if the distance is doubled. **inverse square law (Carlton, Bushong, Selman, Curry, Cullinan)**

140. (A) NCRP Report #102. **fluoroscopy, bucky (Carlton, Bushong, Selman)**

141. (D) NCRP Report #102 (2.1 R/mA min is recommended, 3.2 R/mA min is mandated). **fluoroscopy (Carlton, Bushong, Noz)**

142. (C) Because of binding energy levels, Compton interactions are most likely with 50 keV and greater photons in bone. **interactions, Compton (Carlton, Bushong, Curry)**

143. (A) Primary barriers are designed to shield areas from the primary beam. **shielding, primary barrier (Bushong, Noz, Selman)**

144. (B) NCRP Report #102. **fluoroscopy, shielding, barrier (Bushong, Noz)**

145. (D) Occupational workers, such as a student radiographer, should be avoided, as should radiology department employees, such as an aide. Although a nurse is a better choice because he or she is not regularly occupationally exposed, a parent would be the least likely to be exposed in the future and is, therefore, the best choice. **radiation protection (Carlton, Bushong)**

146. (D) The pair production annihilation reaction produces the two 0.51 MeV photons. **interactions, pair production (Carlton, Bushong, Curry, Selman)**

147. (D) All three terms describe systems that maintain the brightness of the fluoroscopic image automatically. **fluoroscopy, brightness control (Carlton, Curry, Bushong)**

148. (C) Because it is ejected during a photoelectric interaction, the electron is given the name photoelectron to describe how it was ejected. **photoelectric effect (Carlton, Bushong, Curry, Selman)**

149. (B) NCRP Report #102. **fluoroscopy, aprons (Carlton, Bushong, Selman, Noz)**

150. (A) Because of binding energy levels, photoelectric interactions are most likely with 40 keV and lower photons in bone. **interactions, photoelectric (Carlton, Bushong, Curry)**

151. (D) NCRP Report #102. **radiation protection (Carlton, Bushong)**

152. (C) NCRP Report #39. **maximum permissible dose (Bushong, Selman)**

153. (B) Coherent scatter simply changes the direction of travel of the incident photon. No energy is exchanged, and no ionization occurs. **interactions, coherent scatter (Carlton, Bushong, Curry, Selman)**

154. (C) NCRP Report #91. **effective dose equivalent limit, maximum permissible dose (Carlton, Curry)**

155. (B) The inverse square law demonstrates a dramatic reduction in radiation intensity as distance increases. Several example problems amply demonstrate this fact. **inverse square law (Bushong, Cullinan, Curry, Travis, Carlton)**

156. (B) Secondary barriers are designed to protect against scattered radiation. They are not designed to protect against the primary beam or exit radiation. **radiation protection, secondary barriers, shielding (Carlton, Bushong, Noz)**

157. (D) Although greater energy can be present, Compton effect interactions occur when less than 1.02 MeV is available. **interactions, pair production (Carlton, Bushong, Curry, Selman)**

158. (B) NCRP Report #102. **fluoroscopy, aprons (Carlton, Bushong, Selman, Noz)**

159. (A) NCRP Report #91. **effective dose equivalent limit, maximum permissible dose (Carlton, Curry)**

160. (A) Federal regulations limit the distance to 12" (30 cm). **radiation protection, fluoroscopy (Bushong, Selman, Noz)**

161. (C) NCRP Report #39. **effective dose equivalent limit, maximum permissible dose (Bushong, Selman)**

162. (A) Photoelectric interactions occur when the incident photon energy is slightly higher than the binding energy of the inner shell electron. In this case, only the 33.2 keV binding energy is likely to be involved with the 35 keV photon. **photoelectric (Carlton, Bushong, Selman, Curry)**

163. (B) NCRP Report #102. **radiation protection, mobile, portable (Carlton, Selman, Bushong)**

164. (B) According to the isodose curve shown in Figure 5, moving from a point 1 ft from the image intensifier to a point 1.5 ft away would reduce the total scatter exposure by 50% (from 200 mR/hr to 100 mR/hr). At 1.5 ft the exposure is 100 mR/hr. To reduce this exposure by 50% the scatter level must be reduced to 50 mR/hr. According to Figure 5 this occurs at a point 2.5 ft from the image intensifier. **radiation protection, scatter, interactions (Carlton, Bushong, Curry)**

165. (D) Although the top view shows 3 ft to be far enough to avoid the 50 mR/hr line, the end view requires 4 ft to avoid the same line. **fluoroscopy, inverse square law (Carlton, Bushong, Curry, Selman)**

166. (B) The dose rate at 1 to 2 ft is 100 mR/hr. 20 minutes = 0.33 hr. 100 mR/0.33 = 33 mR. **fluoroscopy, dose rates, dose calculation (Carlton, Bushong, Curry, Selman)**

167. (C) Due to binding energy levels, Compton interactions are most likely with 30 keV and greater photons in water. **interactions, Compton (Carlton, Bushong, Curry)**

168. (D) NCRP Report #91. **effective dose equivalent limit, maximum permissible dose (Carlton, Curry)**

RADIATION PROTECTION
Radiation Exposure and Monitoring
4% (56) 169-224

169. (C) Only film uses silver halides to record a latent image. **personnel monitoring, film, (Bushong, Noz, Carlton)**

170. (A) A digital dosimeter is used to measure radiation dose but is too large and expensive to be an effective personnel monitor. **personnel monitoring, dosimeter (Carlton, Bushong, Selman)**

171. (C) During fluoroscopic work, the waist is at the level of the patient, which is the primary source of scattered radiation. The monitor at this level outside the apron would receive the highest dose. **personnel monitoring (Carlton, Bushong)**

172. (D) Scintillation counters are used primarily in imaging equipment, pocket dosimeters are not precise for accurate measurement, and thermoluminescent dosimeters do not produce instant readings. Ionization chambers are accurate and produce instant readings to terminate exposures. **ionization chambers (Carlton, Bushong, Selman)**

173. (D) Any unit expressing dose per time measures exposure rate. **exposure rate (Carlton, Bushong, Selman)**

174. (B) A dosimeter is a dose meter. A densitometer is a density meter. A galvanometer measures electrical current, and a sensitometer produces a sensitized optical wedge on a film. **radiation measurement, dosimetry (Carlton, Bushong, Selman)**

175. (C) The roentgen measures radiation exposure in air and is represented by the symbol R. **radiation units (Carlton, Bushong)**

176. (B) The inverse square law gives (14 mrem/X) = $(48"^2/24"^2)$, which is (14 mrem/X) = (2304/576), which is 3.5 mrem. **inverse square law (Carlton, Bushong, Selman, Noz)**

177. (B) Within the diagnostic range of x-ray energies, rad and rem are essentially equal. **radiation units (Carlton, Bushong, Selman)**

178. (A) The gray (Gy) replaces the rad (radiation absorbed dose) in the SI system. **radiation units (Carlton, Bushong, Selman)**

179. (C) Although a film badge will measure exposure accumulations as low as 10 mrem, a thermoluminescent dosimeter is capable of measuring doses as low as 0.1 mrem. **personnel monitoring, thermoluminescent dosimeter (Carlton, Bushong, Selman)**

180. (A) According to the inverse square law, $I_1/I_2 = D_2^2/D_1^2$, so $1.1\ R/x = 72"^2/40"^2$, or $1.1\ R/x = 0.340\ R = 340\ mR$. **inverse square law (Selman, Carlton, Bushong)**

181. (C) NCRP Report #91. **dose equivalent limits, radiation protection, pregnancy (Carlton, Bushong, Noz)**

182. (B) NCRP Report #91. **dose equivalent limit, radiation protection (Carlton, Bushong, Noz)**

183. (C) One gray = 100 rad, so 1 rad = 0.01 gray. **radiation units (Carlton, Bushong, Curry)**

184. (A) The ALARA concept is an acronym representing "as low as reasonably achievable," and it has been applied to all exposure to radiation. **ALARA, radiation protection (Carlton, Bushong, Travis, Noz)**

185. (C) It is generally accepted that quarterly reports are too long. Nearly all film badges are reported on a monthly basis. **radiation protection, personnel monitoring, film badge (Carlton, Bushong, Selman)**

186. (C) The control film badge travels and is stored with a series of film badges to measure base-plus-fog level accumulations for the entire series. **radiation protection, personnel monitoring, film badge (Carlton, Bushong, Selman)**

187. (C) Film badges can be worn for about 1 to 2 months, thermoluminescent dosimeters can be worn for up to 3 months. **radiation protection, personnel monitoring (Carlton, Bushong, Selman, Noz)**

188. (C) Only personnel who are assigned duties in radiation areas and expected to be exposed to 25% of the dose limit are required to wear monitors. **radiation protection, personnel monitoring (Carlton, Bushong, Selman)**

189. (C) The quality factor accounts for the biological effectiveness of various types of radiation. Because alpha particles have a high mass, their biological effectiveness is high, and their quality factor has been determined to be 20. **quality factor, dose equivalence (Carlton, Bushong, Noz)**

190. (A) Both collar and waist are appropriate locations. Because the front of a film badge must face the direction in which scattered radiation is emitted, a pants pocket does not assure that the badge is facing the same direction for an entire month. **personnel monitoring, film badge (Carlton, Bushong, Selman, Noz)**

191. (C) Because the fetal dose limit is 50 mrem per month, non-radiation area duties must be assigned (NCRP Report #91). **dose equivalent limits, pregnancy, radiation protection (Carlton, Bushong, Noz)**

192. (C) Exposure dose estimates are calculated from an mR/mAs chart by multiplying the mAs by the mR/mAs for the kVp used. In this example because 80 kVp produces 3.1 mR/mAs the answer is found as 22.5 mAs x 3.1 mR = 69.75 mR. Because the problem requires the entrance skin dose, the inverse square law must be applied to calculate the increase in exposure because the entrance skin is closer to the source than the mR/mAs given in Figure 6. Because the patient measures 24 cm, the entrance skin is located 76 cm from the source (100 cm to 24 cm). The inverse square law is then (69.75 mR/X) = (76 cm^2/100 cm^2) which is 120.8 mR. **radiation units, mR/mAs (Carlton, Bushong)**

193. (D) Exposure dose estimates are calculated from an mR/mAs chart by multiplying the mAs by the mR/mAs for the kVp used. In this example because 70 kVp produces 1.9 mR/mAs the answer is found as 37 mAs x 1.9 mR = 70.3 mR x 4 AP exposures = 281.2 mR. To this is added the two oblique exposures as 44 mAs x 1.9 mR = 83.6 mR x 2 exposures = 167.2 The total now stands as 281.2 + 167.2 = 448.4 mR. Because the patient measures 32 cm, the entrance skin is located 68 cm from the source. The inverse square law is then (448.4 mR/X) = (68 cm^2/100 cm^2), which is 969.7 mR. **radiation units, mR/mAs (Carlton, Bushong)**

194. (D) The monitor placed closest to the gonads. **personnel monitoring (Carlton, Bushong)**

195. (A) The sievert measures exposure in biologic systems and is the best unit for reporting human exposure. **personnel monitoring, rem (Carlton, Bushong, Noz, Selman)**

196. (C) Compton interactions are most likely to produce scattered radiation because they occur at the higher energies. **interactions between x-rays and matter (Carlton, Bushong, Selman)**

197. (C) Scatter would be greater at the waist outside protective devices. **radiation protection, personnel monitoring (Carlton, Bushong, Selman, Noz)**

198. (D) Because the fetal dose limit is 50 mrem per month, only a warning is necessary (NCRP Report #91). **dose equivalent limits, pregnancy, radiation protection (Carlton, Bushong, Noz)**

199. (C) NCRP Report #91. **dose equivalent limits, radiation protection, pregnancy (Carlton, Bushong, Noz)**

200. (D) NCRP Report #91. **dose equivalent limit, radiation protection (Carlton, Bushong, Noz)**

201. (A) Personnel monitoring devices are for measuring occupational exposure only. They are not to be worn during personal examinations. **personnel monitoring devices (Carlton, Bushong, Selman)**

202. (B) The quality factor accounts for the biological effectiveness of various types of radiation. Because they are roughly equivalent within the diagnostic range, rad and rem both have been given a quality factor of 1. **quality factor, dose equivalence (Carlton, Bushong, Noz)**

203. (B) Film badges can be worn for 1 to 2 months before being read. **radiation protection, personnel monitoring (Carlton, Bushong, Selman)**

204. (A) A nurse is classified as a non-occupational worker. However, because there are regular duties with radiation-producing equipment, the limit for non-occupational continuous or frequent exposure applies, which is 0.1 rem per year (NCRP Report #91). **dose equivalent limit, radiation protection (Carlton, Bushong, Noz)**

205. (B) The quality factor accounts for the biological effectiveness of various types of radiation. Because they are roughly equivalent within the diagnostic range, grays and sieverts have both been given a quality factor of 1. **quality factor, dose equivalence (Carlton, Bushong, Noz)**

206. (B) The gray replaces the rad for radiation absorbed dose measurements. **radiation units (Carlton, Bushong)**

207. (A) Lithium fluoride is the thermoluminescent material used in dosimeters. **thermoluminescent dosimeters (Bushong, Selman, Noz, Carlton)**

208. (B) NCRP Report #102. **radiation protection (Bushong, Selman, Noz)**

209. (A) NCRP Report #91. **dose equivalent limits, radiation protection, personnel monitoring (Carlton, Bushong, Noz, Selman)**

210. (A) 1,338 mrad = 1.338 rad = 0.01338 Gy. **radiation units (Carlton, Bushong, Selman, Noz)**

211. (B) Film badges can be worn for about 1 to 2 months, pocket ionization chambers should be read daily. **radiation protection, personnel monitoring (Carlton, Bushong, Selman, Noz)**

212. (A) NCRP Report #91. **dose equivalent limits, radiation protection, pregnancy (Carlton, Bushong, Noz)**

213. (A) $(X/180.4 \text{ mR}) = (18"^2/40"^2)$, which is $(X/180.4 \text{ mR}) = (324/1600)$, which is 36.5 mR at 40". 36.5.4 mR/15 mAs = 2.4 mR/mAs at 40". **radiation protection, mR/mAs (Carlton, Bushong)**

214. (C) Because 0.01 millisievert (mSv) = 0.00001 Sv = 0.001 rem = 1.0 mrem. **radiation units (Carlton, Bushong, Noz)**

215. (B) During fluoroscopic work the waist is at the level of the patient, which is the primary source of scattered radiation. The monitor at the neck inside the apron would receive the lowest dose. **personnel monitoring (Carlton, Bushong)**

216. (C) One Gy = 100 rad. **radiation units (Carlton, Bushong)**

217. (B) High kVp and low mAs have a significant effect on reducing total patient dose, thus adhering to the "as low as reasonably achievable" concept. **ALARA, fixed kVp systems, kVp (Carlton, Bushong, Selman)**

218. (C) As the name implies, secondary barriers are designed to protect against secondary scattered radiation. **radiation protection, secondary scatter (Carlton, Bushong, Selman)**

219. (B) Only the desk drawer is a safe environment away from excessive heat and all ionizing radiation. **personnel monitor, film badge (Noz, Selman, Carlton, Bushong)**

220. (A) Photoelectric effect interactions result in complete absorption of the incident photon's energy. **interactions between x-rays and matter (Carlton, Bushong, Selman)**

221. (A) The inverse square law gives $(22 \text{ mrem}/X) = (36"^2/12"^2)$, which is $(22 \text{ mrem}/X) = (1296/144)$, which is 2.4 mrem. **inverse square law (Carlton, Bushong, Selman, Noz)**

222. (C) 12.75 mSv = 12,750 Sv = 127.5 rem. **radiation units (Carlton, Bushong, Selman, Noz)**

223. (B) Most film badges use copper, cadmium, and aluminum filters for this purpose. **personnel monitors, film badge (Noz, Carlton, Bushong, Selman)**

224. (D) These exposures are well under the annual occupational limit of 5 rem per year, so the lifetime occupational limits also are not a problem. Only the current year limit applies to calculating the current year maximum remaining exposure (5,000 mrem to 350 mrem = 4,650 mrem)(NCRP Report #91). **dose equivalent limit, radiation protection (Carlton, Bushong, Noz)**

EQUIPMENT OPERATION AND MAINTENANCE
Radiographic Equipment
11% (154) 225-378

225. (C) Because fluoroscopic tubes operate for minutes instead of seconds, as do diagnostic tubes, they must operate at lower mA levels to reduce heat levels. **fluoroscopy, x-ray tubes (Carlton, Bushong, Selman, Curry)**

226. (B) Electrons must travel at nearly half the speed of light, with kilovolts of energy, and then be suddenly stopped at a target to produce x-rays. **x-ray production (Carlton, Bushong, Selman, Curry)**

227. (C) 0.4 + 0.8 + 2.4 = 3.6 ohm. **resistance (Carlton, Bushong, Selman)**

228. (B) Tungsten is heated at both the filament and anode focal track to the point where it vaporizes. Some of the free tungsten atoms that are thus released form a thin layer on the inside of the tube envelope. **x-ray tube (Carlton, Bushong, Selman)**

229. (D) The sine waves of a three-phase, twelve-pulse generator have less ripple than a wave with fewer pulses. A single-phase, half-wave form has one pulse. A single-phase, full-wave form has two pulses. **generators, waveform (Carlton, Bushong, Selman, Cullinan)**

230. (C) The sound of damaged rotor bearings on the rotor cuff which spins at high speed to rotate the anode disk, is often a grinding noise. **x-ray tubes, rotors (Carlton, Bushong)**

231. (B) A large-diameter conductor decreases resistance because a greater outside surface area along which the electrons may move is available. **resistance (Carlton, Bushong, Selman)**

232. (B) Ohm's Law is V=IR (voltage = current x resistance). **Ohm's Law (Carlton, Bushong, Selman)**

233. (B) (1/8.6) + (1/12) + (1/114) = 1/R, which is 0.11 + 0.08 + 0.009 = 1/R, which is 0.199 = 1/R, which is = 5.03 ohm. **resistance. (Carlton, Bushong, Selman)**

234. (C) The anode has a positive charge, the cathode a negative. The filament is part of the cathode assembly. **x-ray tube, cathode (Carlton, Bushong, Selman, Curry)**

235. (C) Most rotating anode x-ray tubes operate at 2,000 to 3,000 revolutions per minute. **x-ray tube, anode rotation (Carlton, Bushong, Selman, Curry)**

236. (A) A 80 kilovoltage peak represents the maximum possible voltage. **generators, kVp (Carlton, Bushong, Selman, Cullinan)**

237. (D) Materials such as iron, cobalt, and nickel strongly repel all magnetic fields. **magnetism (Carlton, Bushong, Selman)**

238. (D) Most diagnostic x-ray tube anode disks are alloys of tungsten, molybdenum, and rhenium. **x-ray tubes, anode (Carlton, Bushong, Selman, Cullinan)**

239. (B) The cathode assembly includes the filament. The focal track is part of the anode disk, the rotor surrounds the shaft of the anode, and the stator surrounds the rotor outside the glass envelope. **x-ray tubes, cathode (Carlton, Bushong, Cullinan, Selman)**

240. (B) The negative charge on the focusing cup causes the negatively charged electrons to focus into a more narrow beam. **x-ray tubes, cathode (Carlton, Bushong, Cullinan, Selman, Curry)**

241. (B) The volt, which measures potential difference or electromotive force, is named for the Italian physicist Alessandro Volta (1745-1827). **volt, electricity (Carlton, Bushong, Selman)**

242. (B) Generator armatures always produce alternating current, which can be either transmitted as AC or converted into DC by a commutator ring. **generators (Carlton, Bushong, Selman)**

243. (D) In a series circuit, resistances are added, voltage is added, and amperage is the same. In a parallel circuit, resistances are the sum of the reciprocals (less than in a series circuit), voltage is the same, and amperage is added. **series circuits, parallel circuits, circuits (Carlton, Bushong, Selman)**

244. (B) An ion is an atom with extra or missing electrons. Therefore, the process of creating an ion is known as ionization. **ionization (Carlton, Bushong, Selman)**

245. (B) Both the star and delta wye secondary transformer coil windings permit the use of three-phase power to the x-ray tube. **transformers, generators, three-phase windings, delta wye, star (Carlton, Bushong, Selman)**

246. (C) The thumb indicates the movement of the conductor, the index finger indicated the direction of the magnetic lines of force, and the middle and other fingers indicate the direction of current or electron flow. **electromagnetism, hand rules (Carlton, Selman, Bushong)**

247. (C) The gauss and tesla are the units of magnetic field strength. 10,000 gauss = 1 tesla. **units of measurement, magnetism (Carlton, Bushong, Curry, Selman)**

248. (B) The diagnostic range of useful wavelengths is 0.1 to 0.5 angstroms. **x-ray production (Bushong, Selman, Cullinan, Curry, Carlton)**

249. (A) Only electrons are capable of moving easily from atom to atom to produce a flow of electrical current. **electricity (Carlton, Bushong, Selman)**

250. (C) Current is equal to voltage divided by resistance. **Ohm's Law (Carlton, Bushong, Selman)**

251. (A) The maximum number of electrons that can occupy a shell is determined by the formula $2n^2$. Therefore, the first shell, the K shell, can be occupied by a maximum of 2 electrons. **atomic structure, valence (Bushong, Curry, Selman, Carlton)**

252. (A) Heat units are determined by kV x mA x seconds x generator phase constant. The phase constant for a single-phase generator is 1.00, so 75 kVp x 100 mA x 0.4 sec x 1.00 = 3,000 HU. **heat units (Bushong, Cullinan, Selman, Carlton)**

253. (D) The oil that surrounds the x-ray tube is enclosed within the tube housing and not only dissipates heat but also assists in preventing shock and adds a slight amount of filtration to the primary beam. **x-ray tube (Bushong, Selman, Cullinan, Carlton)**

254. (B) Electricity can be generated by moving a conductor through a stationary, unchanging strength magnetic field; moving magnetic lines of force through a stationary conductor; or by varying magnetic field strength through a stationary conductor. **electromagnetism (Carlton, Bushong, Selman)**

255. (D) P=IV, so P=50x10 = 500 W. **power formula, watt (Carlton, Bushong, Selman)**

256. (A) Adding loops to a helix coil of wire will increase the induced magnetic field, causing the lines of force to move closer together, thus intensifying the magnetic field strength. **electromagnetism (Carlton, Bushong, Selman)**

257. (B) Frequency is measured in cycles per second (cps) or Hertz (Hz). **frequency, Hertz, cycles per second (Carlton, Bushong, Selman)**

258. (B) The valence describes the number of electrons in the outermost shell of an atom according to the octet rule. **atomic structure, valence (Carlton, Bushong, Selman)**

259. (A) The autotransformer is located between the incoming line and exposure switch. The mA selector is located in the filament circuit between the incoming line and step-down transformer. The timer circuit is located between the exposure switch and step-up transformer. The rotor switch is a separate circuit to the stator of the anode motor. **basic x-ray circuit, autotransformer (Carlton, Bushong, Selman)**

260. (B) Single-phase, half-wave rectification produces 1 pulse, full-wave produces 2 pulses. Three-phase, full-wave rectified units produce 6 or 12 pulses depending on their multiphase configurations. **rectification, full-wave (Bushong, Selman, Curry, Carlton)**

261. (A) Thermionic emission is the heat caused ionic emission of electrons from the surface of a metal. **thermionic emission, filament (Carlton, Bushong, Selman, Curry)**

262. (C) Rectification circuits convert alternating to direct current. **rectification (Carlton, Bushong, Selman)**

263. (B) Step-up transformers have more turns on their secondary coils. **transformers (Carlton, Bushong, Selman)**

264. (A) Only 90 kVp at 0.6 seconds is located over the 600 mA line. All other techniques are located on or under the mA lines. **tube rating charts (Bushong, Selman, Curry, Cullinan, Carlton)**

265. (B) Only 110 kVp at 0.02 seconds is located under the 600 mA line. All other techniques are located over the mA lines. **tube rating charts (Bushong, Selman, Curry, Cullinan, Carlton)**

266. (B) (80 V/X) = (10,000/100), which is 10,000 X = 80 x 100, which is X = 8,000/10,000, which is 0.8 V. **transformers (Carlton, Bushong, Selman)**

267. (D) Only videotape can record dynamic images. The others are all static imaging systems for single images. **fluoroscopy, videotape (Bushong, Curry, Carlton)**

268. (C) No current reaches the x-ray tube of a mobile unit except during an exposure; therefore, there is no danger of leakage radiation when the unit is not in use. Mobile units will not produce exposures when insufficiently charged to prevent partial exposure of a patient. Exposures occur immediately when the exposure switch is activated. **mobile units, portable units, capacitor discharge units (Carlton, Bushong, Selman)**

269. (C) Automatic exposure controls affect only time. The mA and kVp must still be set by the radiographer. **automatic exposure control, phototiming (Carlton, Bushong, Cullinan, Curry)**

270. (A) Because the secondary side has fewer turns of wire, this is a step-down transformer which means the voltage will decrease and the amperage increase. **transformers (Carlton, Bushong, Selman)**

271. (B) A meter measures voltage when it is wired in parallel, and amperage when it is wired in series. **galvanometer, meter, voltage, amperage (Carlton, Bushong, Selman)**

272. (B) The thumb indicates the movement of the conductor, the index finger indicated the direction of the magnetic lines of force, and the middle and other fingers indicate the direction of current or electron flow. **electromagnetism, hand rules (Carlton, Selman, Bushong)**

273. (B) A few materials, such as beryllium, bismuth, and lead weakly repel all magnetic fields. **magnetism (Carlton, Bushong, Selman)**

274. (B) Normal rotating anodes usually spin at 3,200 to 3,600 revolutions per minute (rpm). **rotating anode, anode (Carlton, Bushong, Cullinan, Curry, Selman)**

275. (B) The anode-heel effect is caused by the heel of the anode absorbing more of the isotropically emitted radiation, thus permitting more radiation emitted in the direction of the cathode to exit the tube housing. This results in a slightly more intense beam at the cathode end of the x-ray tube. **anode-heel effect (Carlton, Bushong, Selman, Cullinan, Curry)**

276. (A) A falling load generator begins each exposure at the highest mA possible and then drops the mA as the heat units build toward a given percentage of the x-ray tube's capacity. **falling load generators (Carlton, Curry)**

277. (D) The output phosphor converts the electrons back into light. **fluoroscopy, image intensification tube (Carlton, Bushong, Curry, Selman)**

278. (A) A meter measures voltage when it is wired in parallel, and amperage when it is wired in series. **galvanometer, meter, voltage, amperage (Carlton, Bushong, Selman).**

279. (A) The slip rings permit the armature to turn while maintaining contact with the external circuit connections. **generators, slip rings (Carlton, Bushong, Selman)**

280. (C) Electromagnets exist only when an electrical current is flowing. When the current ceases, their magnetic properties also cease. **magnetism, electromagnets (Carlton, Bushong, Selman)**

281. (D) In a series circuit, resistances are added, voltage is added, and amperage is the same. In a parallel circuit, resistances are the sum of the reciprocals (less than in a series circuit), voltage is the same, and amperage is added. **series circuits, parallel circuits, circuits (Carlton, Bushong, Selman)**

282. (A) The ohm, which measures simple resistance, is named for the German physicist Georg Ohm (1787-1854). **ohm, electricity (Carlton, Bushong, Selman)**

283. (A) Housing cooling and anode cooling charts are designed to avoid overheating the x-ray tube and housing. There is no such thing as a cable heating chart for x-ray units. **x-ray tubes, anode cooling charts, housing cooling charts (Carlton, Bushong, Selman, Cullinan, Curry)**

284. (A) The dielectric oil in the housing electrically insulates the x-ray tube and helps dissipate heat. It has no effect on filtration of the x-ray beam because the tube window is usually sealed to the housing, thus eliminating oil between the window and the exit to the housing. **x-ray tube housing, protective housing (Carlton, Bushong, Selman)**

285. (C) Grid-biased tubes have an extra wire to permit reversing the charge on the focusing cup. When the focusing cup is positive, the grid wire repels the thermionic cloud. When the grid wire is negative, it permits the thermionic cloud to travel to the anode, thus producing x-rays. Rapid alternating of the grid wire produces a pulsed x-ray beam that can be used to advantage during cine-fluorography. **cathode, focusing cup, grid-biased tube (Carlton, Bushong, Selman, Curry, Cullinan)**

286. (B) The autotransformer is located between the incoming line and exposure switch. The mA selector is located in the filament circuit between the incoming line and step-down transformer. The timer circuit is located between the exposure switch and step-up transformer. The rotor switch is a separate circuit to the stator of the anode motor. **basic x-ray circuit, mA selector (Carlton, Bushong, Selman)**

287. (A) The low-voltage side usually includes the autotransformer, exposure switch, timer circuit, mA indicator, and primary side of the high-voltage transformer. The high-voltage side usually includes the secondary side of the high-voltage transformer, the rectification circuit, and the x-ray tube. The filament circuit usually includes an amperage control and step-down transformer. **x-ray circuit (Carlton, Bushong, Selman, Cullinan)**

288. (A) The great danger of failing to warm up an x-ray tube is heating a small area with the first exposure causing it to expand too rapidly, thus cracking the anode disk. **x-ray tubes, anode, warm-up procedure (Carlton, Bushong, Selman)**

289. (C) This is a definition of a capacitor. **capacitor (Carlton, Bushong, Selman)**

290. (B) Generator armatures always produce alternating current, which can be either transmitted as AC or converted into DC by a commutator ring. **generators (Carlton, Bushong, Selman)**

291. (A) #1 is the image intensification tube output screen. **fluoroscopy (Bushong, Curry, Carlton, Selman)**

292. (B) #2 is the image intensification tube anode. **fluoroscopy (Bushong, Curry, Carlton, Selman)**

293. (C) #3 is the image intensification tube's electrostatic focusing lenses. **fluoroscopy (Bushong, Curry, Carlton, Selman)**

294. (B) In a series circuit, resistances are added, voltage is added, and amperage is the same. In a parallel circuit, resistances are the sum of the reciprocals (less than in a series circuit), voltage is the same, and amperage is added. **series circuits, parallel circuits, circuits (Carlton, Bushong, Selman)**

295. (A) High temperature increases resistance because there are more electrons moving at higher speed (the definition of heat) which interfere with the movement of electrons that is electricity. **resistance (Carlton, Bushong, Selman)**

296. (A) Potential difference, electromotive force, and voltage are the same force. **electricity, voltage, potential difference (Carlton, Bushong, Selman)**

297. (C) Because a three-phase, twelve-pulse generator produces more energy than a single-phase unit, it will cause 41% more heat. **heat units (Bushong, Curry, Cullinan, Carlton)**

298. (C) The electron gun produces the electron stream which is directed by the deflecting coils. **video monitors, cathode ray tubes, video display tube (Bushong, Curry, Selman, Carlton)**

299. (C) The glass window is a thin portion of the glass envelope designed not to filter exiting photons. **x-ray tube (Cullinan, Curry, Carlton, Bushong)**

300. (A) The filament is the tungsten wire from which the thermionic cloud of electrons is produced. **x-ray tube (Cullinan, Curry, Carlton, Bushong)**

301. (B) The actual focal spot is larger than the effective focal spot, and it comes from the cathode. **x-ray tube (Cullinan, Curry, Carlton, Bushong)**

302. (D) The stator is located outside the glass envelope, surrounding the rotor. **x-ray tube (Cullinan, Curry, Carlton, Bushong)**

303. (C) The rotor is located inside the glass envelope inside the stator. **x-ray tube (Cullinan, Curry, Carlton, Bushong)**

304. (A) The effective focal spot is smaller than the actual focal spot, and it comes from the anode. **x-ray tube (Cullinan, Curry, Carlton, Bushong)**

305. (C) The autotransformer is located between the incoming line and exposure switch. The mA selector is located in the filament circuit between the incoming line and step-down transformer. The timer circuit is located between the exposure switch and step-up transformer. The rotor switch is a separate circuit to the stator of the anode motor. **basic x-ray circuit, timer (Carlton, Bushong, Selman)**

306. (D) These are three of the more important recommendations for prolonging x-ray tube life. **x-ray tubes, x-ray tube life (Carlton, Bushong, Selman, Cullinan, Curry)**

307. (D) All three terms have been used to describe the anode target area. **anode, target, focal spot (Bushong, Selman, Curry, Carlton, Cullinan)**

308. (C) Below 2,200°C, a tungsten x-ray tube filament does not exhibit thermionic emission. 10,000°C is well above the melting point of tungsten. **filament (Carlton, Bushong, Curry, Selman)**

309. (A) A falling load generator begins each exposure at the highest mA possible and then drops the mA as the heat units build toward a given percentage of the x-ray tube's capacity. **falling load generators (Carlton, Curry)**

310. (C) The low-voltage side usually includes the autotransformer, exposure switch, timer circuit, mA indicator, and primary side of the high-voltage transformer. The high-voltage side usually includes the secondary side of the high-voltage transformer, the rectification circuit, and the x-ray tube. The filament circuit usually includes an amperage control and step-down transformer. **x-ray circuit (Carlton, Bushong, Selman, Cullinan)**

311. (D) Modern electronic timers are capable of exposure times as short as 1 ms (0.001 s). **timers (Carlton, Bushong, Selman)**

312. (A) Both audible and visible indicators are required on x-ray exposure switches. **exposure switch, basic x-ray circuit (Carlton, Bushong, Selman)**

313. (D) The electrostatic lenses focus the electrons, increase their speed, and condense them to brighten the image. **fluoroscopy, image intensification tube (Bushong, Curry, Selman, Carlton)**

314. (B) The terms generator and dynamo are interchangeable, although generator is more common. **generators, dynamos (Carlton, Bushong, Selman)**

315. (C) Electrons move from negative cathode to positive anode to produce x-rays in an x-ray tube. **x-ray production, x-ray tube (Bushong, Selman, Curry, Carlton)**

316. (D) This is a definition of induction. **induction (Carlton, Bushong, Selman)**

317. (B) The charge on the focusing cup repels the electrons, forcing them into a more narrow beam to strike the anode focal spot. **x-ray tube (Carlton, Bushong, Selman, Cullinan, Curry,)**

318. (C) Ohm's Law is V=IR (voltage = current x resistance). **Ohm's Law (Carlton, Bushong, Selman)**

319. (A) Anode target angles of less than 45° will produce effective focal spots that are smaller than the actual focal spots. **anode angle, target angle, anode (Carlton, Bushong, Curry, Selman, Cullinan)**

320. (C) Power ratings are determined by V x A = W, so 120,000 V x 0.8 A = 96,000 watts. **power, generators (Carlton, Bushong, Curry, Selman)**

321. (C) A falling load generator permits the mA to decrease as the tube load increases as a method of protecting the tube from overloading. **falling load generators (Carlton, Curry)**

322. (D) The autotransformer is located between the incoming line and exposure switch. The mA selector is located in the filament circuit between the incoming line and step-down transformer. The timer circuit is located between the exposure switch and step-up transformer. The rotor switch is a separate circuit to the stator of the anode motor. **basic x-ray circuit, rotor, anode (Carlton, Bushong, Selman)**

323. (A) Step-up transformers have more turns in their secondary coils. **transformers (Carlton, Bushong, Selman)**

324. (C) The autotransformer is the primary device for varying the x-ray tube circuit current to the high-voltage step-up transformer. This also controls the kVp to the x-ray tube. **autotransformer (Carlton, Bushong, Selman)**

325. (B) The input phosphor converts the incident x-ray beam to light photons. **fluoroscopy, image intensification tube (Carlton, Bushong, Curry, Selman)**

326. (C) A galvanometer measures voltage when it is wired in parallel, and amperage when it is wired in series. Induction motors use multiple stators with a divided rotor winding to generate powerful torque. **motors, induction motors (Carlton, Bushong, Selman)**

327. (A) The induction motor is the most powerful because its rotor is driven by numerous powerful electromagnets. **motors (Carlton, Selman, Bushong)**

328. (B) The cosine symbol, ϕ, is used to designate power phase. **three-phase, single-phase (Carlton, Bushong, Selman)**

329. (C) American generators operate at 60 Hz (cps). **generators (Carlton, Bushong, Selman)**

330. (B) The commutator ring essentially switches the contacts as the armature turns to maintain a single direction of outgoing current flow, thus producing direct current. **generators, commutator ring (Carlton, Bushong, Selman)**

331. (B) This is a definition of self induction, which occurs only in alternating currents. **electromagnetism, self induction (Carlton, Bushong, Selman)**

332. (B) Electricity can be generated by moving a conductor through a stationary, unchanging strength magnetic field; moving magnetic lines of force through a stationary conductor; or by varying magnetic field strength through a stationary conductor. **electromagnetism (Carlton, Bushong, Selman)**

333. (A) According to the right-hand thumb rule (for current flow), the arrows would go right if the thumb is pointing down the wire in the direction of the current flow. The left hand thumb rule is used for electron flow, which would be the opposite direction for the flow, but still results in the arrows pointing right. **electricity, hand rules (Carlton, Selman, Bushong)**

334. (A) A long conductor increases resistance because the same force must move more electrons a greater distance. **resistance (Carlton, Bushong, Selman)**

335. (C) Electrical charge, which is composed of negative electrons that constantly repel from one another, will concentrate where curvature of a conductor is greatest because that surface permits them to satisfy the attraction-repulsion law while collecting closer together. **electricity, laws of electrical charge (Carlton, Bushong, Selman)**

336. (B) Most rotating anode x-ray tubes operate at 10,000 to 12,000 revolutions per minute. **x-ray tube, anode rotation (Carlton, Bushong, Selman, Curry)**

337. (A) The positive charge attracts the negative electrons, thus accelerating them toward the anode and output phosphor screen. **fluoroscopy, image intensification tube (Carlton, Bushong, Selman, Curry)**

338. (B) Backup times should be set 1.5X the anticipated maximum time for the procedure and serve as a patient exposure dose protection by terminating the exposure in case of improper control settings. **automatic exposure control, phototiming, backup time (Bushong, Cullinan, Carlton)**

339. (A) Multiphase power (such as three-phase) is produced by using multiple generator armatures. In an x-ray circuit, it can be transmitted by multiple secondary coils adjacent to the primary, high-voltage transformer coil in a delta wye or star configuration. **generators, multiphase, three-phase (Carlton, Selman, Bushong)**

340. (B) Electromotive force (voltage) is equal to amperage times resistance. **Ohm's Law (Carlton, Bushong, Selman)**

341. (A) (1/0.4) + (1/0.8) + (1/2.4) = 1/R, which is 2.5 + 1.25 + 0.4 = 1/R, which is 4.15 = 1/R, which is = 0.24 ohm. **resistance (Carlton, Bushong, Selman)**

342. (D) The glass envelope is isolated from all charge during x-ray production. **x-ray tube, glass envelope (Carlton, Bushong, Curry)**

343. (A) Both half and self rectification suppress half the incoming sine wave. Full-wave rectification converts one-half of the wave to produce twice as many pulses. **rectification, half-wave rectification (Bushong, Selman, Curry, Carlton)**

344. (C) (220 V/X) = (1,000/12,000), which is 1,000 X = 220 x 12,000, which is X = 2,640,000/1,000, which is 2,640 V. **transformers (Carlton, Bushong, Selman)**

345. (B) Only 80 kVp at 0.3 seconds is located over the 600 mA line. All other techniques are located on or under the mA lines. **tube rating charts (Bushong, Selman, Curry, Cullinan, Carlton)**

346. (A) Only 90 kVp at 0.3 seconds is located over the 500 mA line. All other techniques are located on or under the mA lines. **tube rating charts (Bushong, Selman, Curry, Cullinan, Carlton)**

347. (C) Only 110 kVp at 0.4 seconds is located under or on the 400 mA line. All other techniques are located over the mA lines. **tube rating charts (Bushong, Selman, Curry, Cullinan, Carlton)**

348. (A) Hysteresis loss occurs when the constantly changing magnetization and re-magnetization from the alternating current begins to leave residual magnetism in the transformer core, thus reducing transformer efficiency and causing current loss. **transformers, eddy currents (Carlton, Bushong, Selman)**

349. (D) These are the three primary determinants of resistance. **resistance (Carlton, Bushong, Selman)**

350. (B) The maximum number of electrons that can occupy a shell is determined by the formula, $2n^2$. Therefore, the second shell, the L shell, can be occupied by a maximum of 8 electrons. **atomic structure, valence (Bushong, Curry, Selman, Carlton)**

351. (D) Ohm's Law is V=IR (voltage = current x resistance). **Ohm's Law (Carlton, Bushong, Selman)**

352. (D) X-ray production is an extremely inefficient process with more than 99% of the energy used being emitted as heat. **x-ray production, bremsstrahlung, characteristic (Selman, Bushong, Cullinan, Carlton)**

353. (B) The electron gun produces the electron stream from the incoming pulsed signal. **video monitors, cathode ray tubes, video display tube (Bushong, Curry, Selman, Carlton)**

354. (D) Plumbicon (TM), orthicon, and vidicon tubes all have been used successfully in fluoroscopic imaging systems. Most modern systems use plumbicon (TM) tubes. **fluoroscopy, video tubes, plumbicon (TM) tubes (Bushong, Curry, Carlton, Selman)**

355. (D) Brightness gain is calculated as flux gain x minification gain. Any increase in input phosphor intensity, which comes from the incident primary beam, will also add to the quantity of electrons available to the image intensification tube. **fluoroscopy, image intensification, brightness gain (Carlton, Bushong, Curry, Selman)**

356. (B) In a series circuit, resistances are added, voltage is added, and amperage is the same. In a parallel circuit, resistances are the sum of the reciprocals (less than in a series circuit), voltage is the same, and amperage is added. **series circuits, parallel circuits, circuits (Carlton, Bushong, Selman)**

357. (A) Copper is the most common conducting material used in electrical wiring. **electricity, conductors (Carlton, Bushong, Selman)**

358. (C) Because a single-phase unit is the standard for heat unit calculations, its constant is 1. **heat units (Bushong, Curry, Cullinan, Carlton)**

359. (D) The output waveform for a high-frequency unit has very little ripple, unlike the generator-produced sine waves of the single and three-phase units, which do not hold the maximum voltage at all times. **generators, waveform (Carlton, Bushong, Selman, Cullinan)**

360. (A) The negative end is the cathode, the positive end is the anode. **x-ray tubes (Bushong, Selman, Curry, Carlton)**

361. (A) The ampere, which measures the amount of current, is named for the French scientist Andrè Ampere (1775-1836). **ampere, electricity (Carlton, Bushong, Selman)**

362. (A) A charge-coupled device (CCD) is a more efficient and higher resolution light converter tube that can replace a plumbicon (TM) video camera tube in an image intensification system. **image intensification, video cameras (Carlton, Bushong, Curry)**

363.   (A) Single-phase, half-wave rectification produces 1 pulse; full-wave produces 2 pulses.   Three-phase full-wave rectified units produce 6 or 12 pulses depending on their multiphase configurations.   **rectification, full-wave (Bushong, Selman, Curry, Carlton)**

364.   (D) The farad measured capacitance. **capacitors (Carlton, Bushong, Selman)**

365.   (A) Step-down transformers have more coils in their primary coils. **transformers (Carlton, Bushong, Selman)**

366.   (B) Eddy currents swirl in opposing directions to the primary magnetic lines of flux, thus reducing transformer efficiency and causing current loss. **transformers, eddy currents (Carlton, Bushong, Selman)**

367.   (A) The raster pattern is the left-to-right indexing used in video display terminals. **fluoroscopy, raster pattern, video display (Carlton, Bushong, Curry, Selman)**

368.   (C) The photocathode converts light to electrons. **fluoroscopy, image intensification tube (Carlton, Bushong, Curry, Selman)**

369.   (D) Increasing strength, speed, angle, and number of coil turns all will increase the voltage produced by an electrical generator. **electromagnetism, generators (Carlton, Bushong, Selman)**

370.   (B) Electricity can be generated by moving a conductor through a stationary unchanging strength magnetic field, moving magnetic lines of force through a stationary conductor, or by varying magnetic field strength through a stationary conductor. **electromagnetism (Carlton, Bushong, Selman)**

371.   (A) The thumb indicates the movement of the conductor, the index finger indicated the direction of the magnetic lines of force, and the middle and other fingers indicate the direction of current or electron flow. **electromagnetism, hand rules (Carlton, Selman, Bushong)**

372.   (A) Most materials that lock atoms into crystalline or molecular patterns are nonmagnetic.   This classification includes both rubber and plastic. **magnetism (Carlton, Bushong, Selman)**

373.   (D) This is a definition of an insulator. **electricity, insulators (Carlton, Bushong, Selman)**

374.   (C) The maximum number of electrons that can occupy a shell is determined by the formula $2n^2$. Therefore, the third shell, the M shell, can be occupied by a maximum of 18 electrons. **atomic structure, valence (Bushong, Curry, Selman, Carlton)**

375.   (A) Resistance is equal to voltage divided by current. **Ohm's Law (Carlton, Bushong, Selman)**

376. (B) While characteristic radiation produces approximately 10% of the primary beam, the remainder consists of bremstrahlung radiation. **target interactions, bremstrahlung, characteristic (Bushong, Selman, Cullinan, Carlton)**

377. (B) More electrons flow the the same force when amperage is increased and all other factors remain the same. **electricity, amperage, voltage (Carlton, Bushong, Selman)**

378. (B) The low-voltage side usually includes the autotransformer, exposure switch, timer circuit, mA indicator, and primary side of the high-voltage transformer. The high-voltage side usually includes the secondary side of the high-voltage transformer, the rectification circuit, and the x-ray tube. The filament circuit usually includes an amperage control and step-down transformer. **x-ray circuit (Carlton, Bushong, Selman, Cullinan)**

EQUIPMENT OPERATION AND MAINTENANCE
Maintenance and Malfunctions of Radiographic Unit and Accessories
4% (56) 379-434

379. (A) Both a pinhole camera and star resolution test tool can be used to evaluate focal spot size. A dosimeter is a radiation exposure measuring tool. **quality control, focal spot size (Gray, Carlton, Bushong)**

380. (C) Linearity refers to a straight line graph that would result as the mAs level is increased if all mA stations were accurate. **quality control, linearity (Gray, Selman, Carlton, Bushong)**

381. (A) The collimator light beam must be within 1 to 2% of the primary beam field. **quality control, collimator accuracy (Gray, Carlton, Bushong)**

382. (C) The gyroscopic effect, which can be strong enough to pull a piece of the anode disk apart, occurs when the centrifugal force pulling on the rapidly spinning anode is counteracted by a pulling force in the opposite direction. **x-ray tube, anode (Carlton, Bushong, Curry)**

383. (B) Because radiographic film is matched to the color of the light emissions from the intensifying screen, mismatched film and screens will result in not as much light being absorbed by the film emulsion. This produces a lighter image. **intensifying screens (Carlton, Bushong)**

384. (C) An upside-down focused grid will absorb more of the primary beam at the outer margins where it is more severely angled toward the central ray. This produces a lighter image. **grids (Carlton, Bushong, Cullinan)**

385. (B) Higher kVp increases the x-ray to light conversion efficiency of intensifying screens. **intensifying screens (Bushong, Selman, Curry)**

386. (D) This is a definition of quality control. **quality control (Gray, Carlton, Bushong)**

387. (D) Radiographing a wire mesh permits edge-to-edge evaluation of the geometrically recorded detail of the wires, thus evaluating the film/screen contact. **quality control, film/screen contact (Gray, Carlton, Bushong, Selman)**

388. (A) A collimator test tool evaluates the congruence of the collimator light field with the primary beam field. **collimator test tool, quality control (Gray, Carlton, Bushong)**

389. (C) Quantum mottle occurs when insufficient mA is used to produce enough photons to completely fill in the visual image. **quantum mottle (Carlton, Bushong, Curry, Cullinan, Selman)**

390. (B) A dosimeter measures radiation dose. **dosimeter, quality control, radiation measurements (Selman, Carlton, Bushong)**

391. (B) Tints decrease speed but increase resolution. **intensifying screens (Bushong, Curry, Selman)**

392. (C) Photons do not damage intensifying screen phosphors. Decreased efficiency is primarily due to the abrasion of films over their surface many times. **intensifying screens (Curry, Bushong)**

393. (C) Resolution is not affected by phosphor sensitivity, speed in increased, and conversion efficiency is increased with a more sensitive intensifying screen phosphor. **intensifying screens (Bushong, Selman, Curry, Carlton, Cullinan)**

394. (B) The conversion efficiency of an intensifying screen measures its ability to create the maximum number of light photons for each incident x-ray photon. **intensifying screens, conversion efficiency (Carlton, Bushong, Curry)**

395. (B) The timer should be within 5% of the stated values. **quality control, kVp accuracy (Gray, Carlton, Bushong)**

396. (A) Both patient exposure dose and image quality are directly affected by filtration, which is measured by half value layer. The x-ray tube life is not affected. **x-ray tubes, filament, tube life (Carlton, Bushong, Selman, Carroll)**

397. (B) A radiographic room log is designed to maintain information on equipment problems and service. **quality control, room log (Gray, Carlton)**

398. (A) Flexibility and the ability to be inert chemically are important characteristics of intensifying screen base material. It does not have to be transparent, although it must be uniformly radiolucent. **intensifying screens (Bushong, Curry, Selman, Carlton, Cullinan)**

399. (A) Lower temperatures increase intensifying screen phosphor emissions. **intensifying screens (Bushong, Curry, Selman)**

400. (B) Resolution is increased, speed is decreased, and conversion efficiency is decreased with smaller intensifying screen phosphor crystals. **intensifying screens (Bushong, Selman, Curry, Carlton, Cullinan)**

401. (A) Isotropical emissions occur in all directions from the source. **intensifying screens, isotropical emission (Carlton, Bushong, Selman, Curry, Cullinan)**

402. (A) Higher atomic number phosphors produce more interactions with the incident x-ray photons, which increases their ability to emit light. This increases the intensifying screen's conversion efficiency. **intensifying screens, phosphors (Carlton, Bushong, Selman, Curry, Cullinan)**

403. (D) Viewboxes require reproduceability checks, and cassettes require periodic cleaning and film/screen contact evaluations. **quality control, viewboxes, cassettes, film/screen contact (Gray, Carlton, Bushong)**

404. (B) Only primary beam field size reductions are possible with positive beam limitation (PBL) activated. **positive beam limitation, beam restriction, collimators (Carlton, Bushong, Selman, Cullinan)**

405. (A) Quantum mottle occurs when insufficient mA is used to produce enough photons to completely fill in the visual image. **quantum mottle (Carlton, Bushong, Curry, Cullinan, Selman)**

406. (C) This describes an image receptor speed and linearity test. **image receptor speed, quality control (Gray, Carlton)**

407. (A) Resolution is increased, speed is increased, and conversion efficiency is increased with a more densely packed layer of intensifying screen phosphor crystals. **intensifying screens (Bushong, Selman, Curry, Carlton, Cullinan)**

408. (C) The phosphor layer is the layer of active crystals that emit light when struck by x-ray photons. **intensifying screens (Carlton, Bushong, Selman, Curry, Cullinan)**

409. (B) The thickness of the plastic controls the transmission of light from the bulb. The brightness level controls the light available to be transmitted. **quality control, viewbox uniformity (Gray, Carlton, Bushong)**

410. (B) kVp stations should be within 5% of their stated values. **quality control, kVp accuracy (Gray, Carlton, Bushong)**

411. (D) Angulator accuracy, collimator congruence, and mA linearity are all appropriate quality control evaluations. **quality control (Bushong, Gray, Carlton)**

412. (B) This is a definition of half value layer. **half value layer (Bushong, Selman, Cullinan, Carlton)**

413. (A) A pinhole camera provides the most accurate estimation of focal spot size. **quality control, focal spot size (Gray, Carlton, Bushong)**

414. (A) Intensifying screens need to be cleaned on a regular basis to remove dust and dirt particles that will produce artifacts on the radiographs. **intensifying screens (Carlton, Bushong, Selman, Curry, Cullinan)**

415. (B) Intensifying screens average about 10 to 12 lp/mm as compared to film, which is capable of up to 100 lp/mm. **intensifying screens (Carlton, Bushong, Curry, Selman)**

416. (B) Discoloration of intensifying screens causes absorption of emitted light photons which reduces the film density. **intensifying screens (Carlton, Selman, Cullinan)**

417. (A) Fluorescence occurs when a phosphor emits light within one electron orbit of the affected shell. It is essentially instantaneous emission, unlike phosphorescence, which has a delay between absorption and emission. **luminescence (Carlton, Bushong, Selman)**

418. (B) Exposure reproduceability is the ability of the x-ray unit to reproduce within acceptable limits the same image density for several consecutive exposures. **quality control, automatic exposure controls (Gray, Carlton, Bushong)**

419. (D) Timer, mA station, and kVp accuracy are the primary generator quality control tests. **quality control, timer accuracy, mA linearity, kVp accuracy (Gray, Carlton, Bushong)**

420. (B) Exposures should never be repeated until verification has been obtained that no exposure occurred. This is accomplished by viewing the processed film. **radiographic equipment (Carlton, Selman)**

421. (B) Backscatter from the primary beam bouncing back toward the film can be eliminated by a thin lead sheeting behind the rear intensifying screen. **cassettes (Bushong, Selman, Curry, Carlton, Cullinan)**

422. (C) Resolution is decreased, speed is increased, and conversion efficiency is increased with a thicker intensifying screen phosphor layer. **intensifying screens (Bushong, Selman, Curry, Carlton, Cullinan)**

423. (A) A collimator test tool evaluates the congruence of the collimator light field with the primary beam field. It can also be used to verify central ray alignment. **collimator test tool, quality control (Gray, Carlton, Bushong)**

424. (C) A spinning top test permits evaluation of timer accuracy by imaging a hole in a spinning top as a dot on a film. The number of dots for a particular time can then be calculated and verified with the film for timer accuracy. **quality control, timer accuracy (Gray, Carlton, Bushong)**

425. (B) Because half value layer is a measurement of the filtration in the beam, an increase in primary beam filtration would increase the half value layer. **quality control, filtration (Gray, Carlton, Bushong, Curry, Selman)**

426. (B) A spinning top test is valid only with single-phase equipment. It is made by spinning a metal disk with a single hole on top of a cassette during an exposure. Because each Hz of half-wave rectified current has one point where no radiation is being emitted, each pulse will produce a dot on the film as it images the hole in the disk. Because 60 Hz current is being used, a full second of exposure will produce 60 dots (60 Hz x 1 pulse). 60 dots x 0.2 sec = 12 dots. **quality control, spinning top, timer accuracy (Carlton, Bushong, Selman)**

427. (D) Patient dose is reduced dramatically by the use of intensifying screens. **intensifying screens (Selman, Carlton, Bushong, Curry, Cullinan)**

428. (A) Flexibility and uniform radiolucency are important characteristics of intensifying screen base material. It does not have a high atomic number. **intensifying screens (Bushong, Curry, Selman, Carlton, Cullinan)**

429. (D) Gadolinium, lanthanum, and yttrium are rare earths that have been used as intensifying screen phosphors. Calcium tungstate, zinc sulfide, and barium lead sulfate are not rare earths, although they also have been used as intensifying screen phosphors. **intensifying screens (Bushong, Curry, Selman, Carlton, Cullinan)**

430. (B) The reflective layer reflects the isotropically emitted light back toward the film, thus increasing the efficiency of the intensifying screens. **intensifying screens (Carlton, Bushong, Cullinan, Selman, Curry)**

431. (A) NEMA focal spot standards are focal spots smaller than 0.8 mm may be 50% larger than stated, focal spots between 0.8 and 1.5 mm may be 40% larger than stated, and focal spots larger than 1.5 mm may be 30% larger than stated. **focal spot size (Bushong, Curry, Carlton)**

432. (B) Calcium tungstate has been used for intensifying screens since their first introduction soon after Roentgen's discovery of x-rays. **intensifying screens (Selman, Curry, Carlton, Bushong, Cullinan)**

433. (C) White specks appear when dirt in the cassette prevents light from the intensifying screens from reaching the film. Cleaning the cassette will remove these artifacts. Half moon marks are produced by bending of the film and is corrected by more careful handling of the film when loading and unloading cassettes. Branching tree artifacts are produced by static electricity discharges during loading and unloading of cassettes, and are prevented by increasing humidity, grounding the loading bench, and having film handlers avoid high-static clothing such as nylon. **artifacts, intensifying screen cleaning (Carlton, Bushong, Gray)**

434. (D) Section thickness, uniformity and completeness of motion, and section depth indicator accuracy are the three most important tomography quality control measurements. **tomography, quality control (Gray, Carlton)**

435. (B) Increasing OFD increases image magnification and decreases recorded detail. **recorded detail, detail, magnification (Carlton, Bushong, Cullinan, Selman)**

436. (C) Increasing the film/screen speed will increase density. **density, film/screen combinations (Carlton, Bushong, Cullinan, Selman)**

437. (B) Reducing beam size will decrease density because less scatter produces less overall image density. **beam restriction, density (Carlton, Bushong, Cullinan, Selman)**

438. (A) Increasing the grid ratio results in more primary beam being absorbed by the grid. This produces less density. Increasing the grid ratio also results in more absorption of scattered radiation. This produces higher contrast. **grids, contrast (Carlton, Bushong, Cullinan, Selman,)**

439. (A) When no other factors are considered, the lowest kVp always produces the highest, or shortest, scale of contrast. **contrast, kVp (Carlton, Bushong, Cullinan, Selman)**

440. (A) Photoelectric interactions result in complete absorption of the incident photon, thus preventing it from reaching the image receptor. This lack of information, when combined with nearby information from photons that did not undergo photoelectric interactions, results in contrast permitting the image to become visible. **contrast, photoelectric interaction (Carlton, Bushong, Cullinan, Selman)**

441. (B) The magnification factor is calculated by dividing the FFD by the FOD (FFD/FOD). **magnification factor, distortion, size distortion (Cullinan, Carroll, Carlton, Bushong, Selman, Curry)**

442. (D) Because distance and film/screen combinations are identical, they are not a factor. The mAs values are: A=75, B=75, C=75, D=75, so they are not a factor. Only kVp and grid must be considered in this problem. The lowest ratio grid (6:1) far outweighs the 2 kVp differences, so D is the correct answer. **density (Carlton, Cullinan)**

443. (C) Because grid ratios are identical they are not a factor. The mAs values are: A=50, B=50, C=75, D=15, so they must be considered. kVp and distance differences are minimal, therefore they need to be considered only if mAs and film/screen combinations are very close. If the mAs level is adjusted to compensate for the film/screen combinations by using a 100 relative speed for all the new mAs, the results are: A=25, B=50, C=75, D=30. Because C is 50% darker than the next darkest (B), neither the slight kVp or distance difference will predominate. Thus C is the correct answer. **density (Carlton, Cullinan)**

444. (D) Because kVp and grid ratios are identical, they are not a factor. The mAs values are: A=150, B=75, C=120, D=100, thus they must be considered. Distance differences are minimal, thus they need to be considered only if mAs and film/screen combinations are very close. If the mAs level is adjusted to compensate for the film/screen combinations by using a 100 relative speed for all the new mAs, the results are: A=150, B=150, C=120, D=200. Because D is 25% darker than the next darkest (A&B), the slight distance difference can be ignored. Thus D is the correct answer. **density (Carlton, Cullinan)**

445. (B) Because distance and grid ratios are identical, they are not a factor. The mAs values are: A=25, B=25, C=25, D=25. If the mAs level is adjusted to compensate for the film/screen combinations by using a 100 relative speed for all the new mAs, the results are: A=25, B=100, C=25, D=13. If mAs is adjusted to compensate for the kVp differences by using the 15% rule to use 76 kVp for all the new mAs results are: A=25, B=100, C=13, D=7. Because B is 4X the mAs of the next darkest (A), the correct answer is B. **density (Carlton, Cullinan)**

446. (B) An automatic exposure device controls only the exposure time, therefore, a decrease in mA will result in increased exposure time. **automatic exposure control, phototiming (Carlton, Cullinan, Curry, Selman)**

447. (A) mAs is the primary controller of image density. **density, mAs (Carlton, Cullinan, Selman, Bushong, Carroll)**

448. (C) Focal spot size has its major effect on recorded detail. **detail, recorded detail, focal spot size (Carlton, Cullinan, Carroll, Bushong, Selman)**

449. (C) A compression band will decrease the thickness of the abdomen, which decreases subject density, increases subject contrast, and increases radiographic density. **density, subject density, subject contrast, compression bands (Carlton, Cullinan, Carroll)**

450. (A) The 15% rule accomplishes changes in contrast while maintaining density. A 15% increase in kVp while halving the mAs value or a 15% decrease in kVp while doubling the mAs value will maintain the density. **15% rule, contrast, density (Carlton, Cullinan, Carroll)**

451. (D) kVp, primary beam field size, and grid ratio all produce changes in radiographic density. **density, kVp, collimation, grids (Carlton, Cullinan, Carroll)**

452. (B) X-ray tube output, and therefore, image density, is increased by a high vacuum inside the glass envelope, a smooth anode focal track, and decreased added filtration. **x-ray tubes (Cullinan, Carlton, Bushong, Selman, Carroll)**

453. (C) kVp, mAs, and subject density have no effect on recorded detail. Recorded detail is reduced dramatically by subject motion. **recorded detail, definition, motion (Carlton, Cullinan, Carroll)**

454. (B) 68 kVp produces the maximum number of photons at the keV energy that is slightly higher than the binding energy of the inner shell electrons of iodine. This increases the probability of photoelectric interactions, which increases the image contrast. **contrast media, iodine, photoelectric interactions (Carlton, Curry, Carroll, Cullinan)**

455. (B) Depending on the author, the minimum mAs difference required to produce a visible density change is given as 25%, 30%, or 33%. Choices 1 and 3 change the time by at least these percentages, while choice 2 does not. **density, mAs (Carlton, Carroll, Cullinan)**

456. (D) The maximum mA permits the minimum time to reduce patient motion. **mAs, motion (Carlton, Cullinan, Carroll)**

457. (C) The silver bromide that is formed is photosensitive and will begin latent image formation if struck by photons (i.e., heat, light, x-rays). **film production (Carlton, Bushong, Selman, Cullinan, Curry, Carlton)**

458. (B) The curve that describes the relationship between exposure and density is called a D log E, H & D, sensitometric, or characteristic curve. **sensitometry, characteristic curves, H&D curve, D log E curve (Cullinan, Carlton, Bushong, Selman, Curry)**

459. (A) This is a definition of a latent image. **latent image formation (Carlton, Bushong, Selman, Curry, Cullinan, Carlton)**

460. (B) Hydroquinone and phenidone are the reducing agents. Potassium bromide is the restrainer. Metol replaces phenidone in manual processing. **processing, developer (Carlton, Bushong, Cullinan, Selman, Curry)**

461. (C) Glutaraldehyde is the hardener in the developer. **processing, developer (Carlton, Bushong, Cullinan, Carlton, Selman)**

462. (A) An open processor top permits warm air to escape as the solutions cool down, preventing cross-contamination of developer and fixer from condensation. **automatic film processors (Carlton, Gray)**

463. (A) Developer replenishment must occur at a higher rate than fixer in most automatic processors. **automatic film processors (Carlton, Gray)**

464. (D) A fixed kVp system uses as few mAs changes as possible. **fixed kVp, exposure systems (Carlton, Cullinan, Carroll)**

465. (A) Electrolytic silver recovery units are most efficient in average radiology department use. Low use situations often are more efficient with metallic replacement units. **silver recovery (Carlton)**

466. (A) A finger is normally imaged between 30 to 40 kVp. **kVp, contrast, technique factors, technical factors (Carlton, Cullinan)**

467. (A) Radiographic density would increase with increased developer temperature and high temperature in film storage area. Fixing time has minimal effect on radiographic density. **density, film processing, film storage (Carlton, Bushong, Selman, Cullinan)**

468. (C) Average gradient is a measurement of the slope of the straight line portion of the D log E (H&D or characteristic) curve. Wide latitude films typically exhibit low contrast, low speed, and low average gradients. A typical wide latitude film is shown as film C in Figure 13. **D log E curves, sensitometry, characteristic curves, H&D curves (Cullinan, Bushong, Selman, Curry, Carlton)**

469. (B) Pleural effusion and congestive heart failure increase beam attenuation, thus requiring increased technical factors. Pneumothorax decreases beam attenuation, thus requiring decreased technical factors. **pathology, tissue density, density (Carlton, Cullinan, Bushong)**

470. (C) Both density and contrast are affected by the use of a grid, which changes the amount of scattered radiation reaching the film. Although a change may be seen in the visibility of recorded detail, the recorded detail itself does not vary with grid changes. **grids, density, contrast, recorded detail (Carlton, Bushong, Selman, Curry)**

471. (A) Increasing the FOD will increase the magnification, decrease the recorded detail, and decrease contrast. **recorded detail, magnification, contrast, air-gap (Cullinan, Carlton, Carroll, Bushong, Selman, Curry)**

472. (B) Changing from a 200 to a 100 relative speed film/screen combination requires a halving of the mAs value to maintain the same density. Changing from 12 to 6 mAs accomplishes this compensation, thus maintaining the density. **film/screen combinations (Cullinan, Carlton, Carroll)**

473. (D) Increasing the size of the primary beam field will increase the amount of scattered radiation produced, thus decreasing contrast and increasing density. In addition, it increases the exposure dose to the patient. **beam restriction, collimation, contrast (Cullinan, Carlton, Carroll)**

474. (D) Decreasing the distance will increase the intensity of the primary beam, thus increasing density. Although the increased density will affect the visibility of recorded detail, the geometric factors controlling recorded detail itself will not change. **grids, density, contrast (Cullinan, Carlton, Carroll)**

475. (A) When no other factors are considered, the lowest kVp always produces the highest, or shortest, scale of contrast. **contrast, kVp (Carlton, Bushong, Cullinan, Selman, Carlton)**

476. (C) Figure 12B exhibits lower contrast but a similar density. It could only have been produced with higher (92 kVp) and half the mAs (15 mAs) to maintain density. **contrast, kVp (Carlton, Cullinan, Carroll)**

477. (A) Figure 12B exhibits lower (longer scale) contrast than Figure 12A. The densities of both images are identical (they were produced by a digital radiography system with a set density exposure point at the center of the straight line portion of the curve). There is no apparent magnification or other indication that the FFD was changed. **contrast, density (Carlton, Cullinan, Carroll)**

478. (B) Because the distance and film/screen combinations are identical, they are not a factor. The mAs values are: A=8, B=8, C=8, D=8, so they are not a factor. Only kVp and grid must be considered in this problem. The lowest ratio grid (10:1) and highest kVp (120) would produce the darkest image. Thus, B is the correct answer. **density (Carlton, Cullinan)**

479. (D) Because the grid ratios are identical, they are not a factor. The mAs values are: A=15, B=15, C=16, D=15, which are essentially identical, so they need not be considered. kVp and distance differences are minimal and actually balance one another (lower kVp values are paired with shorter distances), so they need not be considered either. Film/screen combinations are the only variable factor. Therefore, the 400 speed system would produce the darkest image. Thus, D is the correct answer. **density (Carlton, Cullinan)**

480. (A) Because the distance and grid ratios are identical, and the kVp values are very close, they are not a factor. The mAs values are: A=36, B=36, C=48, D=36, so they must be considered. If the mAs level is adjusted to compensate for the film/screen combinations by using a 100 relative speed for all, the new mAs results are: A=90, B=72, C=48, D=72. Thus, A is the correct answer. **density (Carlton, Cullinan)**

481. (B) Because the distances are identical they are not a factor. The mAs values are: A=33, B=16, C=33, D=32. If the mAs level is adjusted to compensate for the film/screen combinations by using a 100 relative speed for all the new mAs results are: A=33, B=64, C=33, D=64. If the mAs level is adjusted to compensate for the kVp differences by using the 15% rule to use 90 kVp for all, the new mAs results are: A=33, B=128, C=33, D=128. A and C can be ruled out because they are only 25% of the density of B and D. Because B has a lower grid ratio than D, the correct answer is B. **density (Carlton, Cullinan)**

482. (D) The ion chamber will produce a diagnostic range density for the structures positioned over it. In this instance, the normal density would be achieved for the bowel gas positioned over the ion chamber, thus leaving the entire abdomen too light. **automatic exposure control, phototiming (Carlton, Bushong, Cullinan)**

483. (D) Film/screen combination affects density, contrast, and recorded detail. It does not affect distortion. **film/screen combinations, density, contrast, recorded detail (Carlton, Carroll, Cullinan)**

484. (C) Focal spot size does not affect density to any degree of measurement. Although some authors hold that focal spot blooming may add density, all agree that the effect would not be visible and, in fact, would be difficult to measure. **focal spot size, density (Carlton, Cullinan, Carroll)**

485. (D) Alignment of tube-part-image receptor determines shape distortion. **distortion, alignment (Carlton, Cullinan, Carroll)**

486. (D) Conditions that have increased tissue attenuation require greater quantity or quality of the incident x-ray beam. Increased mAs, increased kVp, and decreased distance all achieve this effect. **pathology, tissue density, density (Carlton, Cullinan, Bushong)**

487. (A) Abdominal compression reduces the thickness of the part, thus increasing density and contrast. It has no appreciable effect on recorded detail. **compression, density, contrast (Carlton, Cullinan)**

488. (C) Magnification is calculated as FFD/FOD, so 100/93.8 = 1.07. **magnification, size distortion, distortion (Carlton, Cullinan, Curry, Bushong, Selman)**

489. (C) This is a definition of grid frequency. **grids (Carlton, Cullinan, Bushong, Curry, Selman)**

490. (A) When no other factors are considered, the highest kVp always produces the lowest, or longest, scale of contrast. **contrast, kVp (Carlton, Bushong, Cullinan, Selman, Carlton)**

491. (D) This is a definition of foreshortening. **distortion, foreshortening (Carlton, Cullinan)**

492. (C) This is a definition of density. **density (Carlton, Cullinan, Bushong)**

493. (B) The primary function of a radiographic grid is to increase contrast. Its use also decreases image density and, when compensation is made to maintain density, the result is an increase in patient exposure dose. **grids (Carlton, Bushong, Cullinan, Carlton, Selman, Curry)**

494. (B) Attenuation of the primary beam results in fewer photons reaching the image receptor, which produces less image density. **density, attenuation (Carlton, Curry, Bushong, Cullinan)**

495. (B) This is a definition of distortion. **distortion (Carlton, Cullinan, Bushong)**

496. (A) Incorrect alignment of central ray, part of interest, and film will produce distortion of the joint. However, incorrect centering of the film will not distort the joint. It will simply not image the distal 2" of the knee. **alignment, distortion (Carlton, Cullinan)**

497. (A) Magnification is calculated as FFD/FOD. **magnification, size distortion, distortion (Cullinan, Curry, Carlton, Bushong, Selman)**

498.   (D) Patient motion is decreased with increased mA, increased kVp, increased film/screen speed, and decreased FFD. **motion, recorded detail, detail (Carlton, Cullinan)**

499.   (C) All of the examples given would increase recorded detail, except decreased FFD, which will decrease it. **recorded detail, detail, distance, OFD (Carlton, Bushong, Selman, Cullinan)**

500.   (C) High contrast film will provide the high speed desired. Wide latitude film tends to have lower contrast and speed, while increased patient exposure dose requirements result from slower speed film. **film/screen combinations, film, intensifying screens (Carlton, Bushong, Cullinan)**

501.   (D) Grid ratio is determined by lead strip height divided by interspace width, so: grid ratio = 3.2 mm/0.20 mm = 16:1. **grids, grid ratio (Cullinan, Curry, Selman, Carlton, Bushong)**

502.   (A) Tumor and edema increase beam attenuation, thus requiring increased technical factors. Atrophy decreases beam attenuation, thus requiring decreased technical factors. **pathology, tissue density, density (Carlton, Cullinan, Bushong)**

503.   (A) Depending on the author, the minimum mAs difference required to produce a visible density change is given as 25%, 30%, or 33%. Choices 1 & 2 only change more than these percentages, while choice 3 does not. **density, mAs (Carlton, Carroll, Cullinan)**

504.   (D) Distance, filtration, and anatomic part size all affect density. **density, distance, filtration, part size or thickness (Carlton, Cullinan, Carroll)**

505.   (C) old mAs/X = old distance^2/new distance^2, which is 20 mAs/X = 40"^{2}/72"^{2}, which is 20 mAs/X = 1,600/5,184, which is 1,600 X = 103,680, which is X = 65 mAs. **inverse square law [to maintain density], density maintenance law (Carlton, Bushong, Cullinan, Selman)**

506.   (B) Increases in exposure time cause mAs increases, which increase image density. **mAs, density (Cullinan, Carlton, Bushong)**

507.   (A) mAs and kVp are constantly changed during radiography. Distance is seldom used because for the majority of non-erect procedures, most radiographic equipment is incapable of distances greater than 40" to 45". **radiographic quality, prime factors, technical factors (Carlton, Cullinan)**

508.   (C) Central ray alignment primarily affects distortion. It has a minimal effect on recorded detail and little, if any, effect on density and contrast. **alignment, central ray, distortion, recorded detail, detail (Carlton, Bushong, Cullinan)**

509.   (A) High resolution films tend to be slow speed, high contrast, narrow latitude, and have high patient dose requirements. **film, sensitometry (Carlton, Cullinan, Bushong, Selman, Curry)**

510. (D) Radiographic density is increased by low, average atomic number tissues; thin anatomic parts; and disease processes that decrease tissue density. **attenuation, part thickness, anatomic part (Carlton, Curry, Cullinan, Bushong)**

511. (A) An automatic exposure device controls only the exposure time; therefore, an increase in mA will result in decreased exposure time. **automatic exposure control, phototiming (Carlton, Cullinan, Curry, Selman)**

512. (D) This is a definition of contrast. **contrast (Carlton, Cullinan, Bushong)**

513. (B) Magnification is calculated as FFD/FOD, so 180/169.6 = 1.06. Therefore, a 1.5 cm image is 1.06 times larger than the mass or 1.4 cm wide (1.5 cm/1.06 magnification factor). **magnification, size distortion, distortion (Cullinan, Curry, Carlton, Bushong, Selman)**

514. (C) The lumbar spine is normally imaged between 80 to 90 kVp. **kVp, contrast, technique factors, technical factors (Carlton, Cullinan)**

515. (A) Sodium sulfite serves as the preservative in both developer and fixer solutions. **processing, developer, fixer (Carlton, Bushong, Cullinan, Selman, Curry)**

516. (A) All of the examples given would increase recorded detail except decreased FFD, which will decrease it. **recorded detail, detail, distance, OFD (Carlton, Bushong, Selman, Cullinan)**

517. (D) In order of density, the tissues are: bone, muscle, water, and fat. **attenuation, tissue density (Carlton, Bushong, Curry)**

518. (A) Recorded detail and distortion are geometric properties that are not affected by the use of contrast media. Density and contrast are photographic properties that are affected by the primary beam absorbed by contrast media. **contrast media, density, contrast, recorded detail, detail, distortion (Carlton, Cullinan, Bushong)**

519. (A) The formula for converting from one grid ratio to another is mAs_1/mAs_2 = grid conversion factor$_1$/grid conversion factor$_2$. Therefore, 3 mAs/mAs$_2$ = 6.5/5.5, which is 6.5 mAs$_2$ = 16.5, which is mAs$_2$ = 2.5 mAs. **grids, grid conversion, bucky factor (Carlton, Cullinan, Bushong)**

520. (B) kVp is the primary controller of image contrast. **contrast, mAs (Cullinan, Carlton, Selman, Bushong, Carroll)**

521. (A) Decreasing OFD decreases image magnification and increases recorded detail. **recorded detail, detail, magnification (Carlton, Bushong, Cullinan, Selman, Carlton)**

522. (D) Decreasing the film/screen speed from 400 to 200 will decrease density to half. Only choice D provides a doubling of density to compensate, by increasing kVp by 15%. **density, film/screen combinations (Carlton, Bushong, Cullinan, Selman, Carlton)**

523. (B) Reducing beam size will decrease density because less scatter produces less overall image density. **beam restriction, density (Carlton, Bushong, Cullinan, Selman, Carlton)**

524. (D) Decreasing the grid ratio results in less primary beam being absorbed by the grid. This produces more density. Decreasing the grid ratio also results in less absorption of scattered radiation. This produces lower contrast. **grids, contrast (Carlton, Bushong, Cullinan, Selman, Carlton)**

525. (B) Only choice B maintains the density. When the kVp is reduced by 15% (from 75 to 64), the mAs level must be doubled. The original exposure used 32 mAs so the new mAs must be 64. 200 mA at 0.32 sec = 64 mAs. **15% rule, density, mAs (Carlton, Bushong, Carroll, Selman)**

526. (D) Magnification is calculated as FFD/FOD, so 100/95.6 = 1.05. **magnification, size distortion, distortion (Carlton, Cullinan, Curry, Bushong, Selman)**

527. (A) A fixed kVp system uses mAs as the primary variable and an optimal kVp which is fixed for a particular series of procedures. This reduces the number of variables and makes the system easier to remember. **exposure systems, fixed kVp (Carlton)**

528. (A) Recorded detail and distortion are geometric properties that are not affected by the use of a grid. Density and contrast are photographic properties that are affected by the scattered radiation absorbed by a grid. **grids, density, contrast, recorded detail, detail, distortion (Carlton, Cullinan, Bushong)**

529. (B) Average gradient is a measurement of the slope of the straight line portion of the D log E (H&D or characteristic) curve. High average gradient films typically exhibit high contrast, high speed, and narrow latitude. A typical high average gradient film is shown as film A in Figure 13. **D log E curves, sensitometry, characteristic curves, H&D curves (Cullinan, Bushong, Selman, Curry, Carlton)**

530. (B) This is a definition of a grid cassette. **grids, grid cassette, cassettes (Carlton, Bushong, Selman, Cullinan, Carlton, Curry)**

531. (C) A phototimer was an older type of automatic exposure control which is no longer in use. The term is often used to describe modern automatic exposure controls. **phototimer, automatic exposure control (Carlton, Bushong, Curry, Cullinan, Carroll, Selman)**

532. (C) A three-phase, 12-pulse generator will produce higher average photon energies, which will, in turn, produce more scatter and more image density. **density, generator phase (Carlton, Cullinan, Carroll, Bushong)**

533. (C) The reciprocity law states that as the mAs level increases, both x-ray exposure and radiographic density increase proportionally. **reciprocity law (Carlton, Carroll, Cullinan)**

534. (D) Grids, film processing, and anatomic part size all affect density. **density, distance, filtration, part size or thickness (Carlton, Cullinan, Carroll)**

535. (D) Decreasing the FFD will increase the magnification, decrease the recorded detail, and increase density. **recorded detail, magnification, contrast, air-gap (Cullinan, Carlton, Carroll, Bushong, Selman, Curry)**

536. (C) Increasing the kVp by 10 to 87 would constitute a 15% increase. The mAs value must be halved from 32 to 16 mAs to maintain the density. Changing from a 200 to a 100 relative speed film/screen combination requires a doubling of mAs to maintain the same density. Changing from 16 back to 32 mAs accomplishes this compensation, thus maintaining the density. **film/screen combinations (Cullinan, Carlton, Carroll)**

537. (B) Decreasing the size of the primary beam field will decrease the amount of scattered radiation produced, thus increasing contrast and decreasing density. In addition, it decreases the exposure dose to the patient. Choices 1 & 3 only are true, making B the correct answer. **beam restriction, collimation, contrast (Cullinan, Carlton, Carroll)**

538. (A) Increasing the distance will decrease the intensity of the primary beam, thus decreasing density. The increased distance will decrease magnification, thus increasing recorded detail. **grids, density, contrast (Cullinan, Carlton, Carroll)**

539. (D) If film/screen speed is halved (from 400 to 200), then mAs must be doubled to maintain the same density. **15% rule, film/screen combinations (Carlton, Bushong, Cullinan, Selman, Carlton, Carroll)**

540. (A) A fixed kVp system uses mAs as the primary variable and an optimal kVp which is normally higher than that possible with a variable kVp system under the same circumstances. The higher kVp permits lower mAs, thus reducing overall patient exposure dose. **exposure systems, fixed kVp (Carlton)**

541. (B) Magnification is calculated as FFD/FOD, so $100/89.2 = 1.12$. Therefore, a 3.4 cm image is 1.12 times larger than the mass, or 3.0 cm wide (3.4 cm/1.12 magnification factor). **magnification, size distortion, distortion (Cullinan, Curry, Carlton, Bushong, Selman)**

542. (A) The hand is normally imaged between 40 and 60 kVp. **kVp, contrast, technique factors, technical factors (Carlton, Cullinan)**

543. (B) Phenidone rapidly produces fine recorded detail shades of gray on the film while hydroquinone slowly produces heavy densities. **film processing, developer, reducing agents (Cullinan, Selman, Carlton, Bushong)**

544. (B) All of the examples given would decrease magnification or size distortion except increased film/screen speed, which would have no effect. **distortion, magnification, distance, OFD (Carlton, Bushong, Selman, Cullinan)**

545. (C) The anode heel theory demonstrates that radiation intensity is slightly greater at the cathode end of the x-ray tube. Therefore, the thickest body part should be positioned toward the cathode. Of the examples given, only the lateral lumbar spine with the cathode toward the pelvis fulfills these conditions. **anode heel effect (Cullinan, Selman, Carlton, Bushong)**

546. (D) Elongation and foreshortening are shape distortion. Magnification is size distortion. **distortion, magnification, foreshortening, elongation (Carlton, Bushong, Curry, Cullinan)**

547. (C) Aluminum and plastic fiber are the most common grid interspace materials. **grids (Carlton, Cullinan, Selman, Bushong, Curry)**

548. (D) Degenerative arthritis, fibrosarcoma, and osteoporosis all decrease beam attenuation, thus requiring decreased technical factors. **pathology, tissue density, density (Carlton, Cullinan, Bushong)**

549. (B) Depending on the author, the minimum mAs difference required to produce a visible density change is given as 25%, 30%, or 33%. In this example, both 8 and 16 mAs are more than 30% different from 12 mAs, while 14 mAs is significantly less than 25%. **density, mAs (Carlton, Carroll, Cullinan)**

550. (B) Compton effect interactions result in the production of much scattered radiation. This scatter provides inaccurate information to the image receptor that contributes to an overall gray density level that lengthens the scale of contrast, or makes it longer or lower. **contrast, photoelectric interaction (Carlton, Bushong, Cullinan, Selman)**

551. (A) An 8:1 grid requires approximately twice the mAs to maintain radiographic density achieved with a 6:1 grid. A 10:1 grid requires approximately 4X the mAs of a 6:1 grid; however, a kVp increase of 15% (from 80 to 92) reduces the required mAs increase to 2X. A 16:1 grid requires approximately 8X the mAs of a 6:1 grid, of which only 4X is compensated by the 15% kVp increase. **grids (Carlton, Cullinan, Selman)**

552. (C) The term D_{max} represents the maximum density value of which the film is capable. Therefore, continued exposure beyond this level begins the solarization or reversal process, thus decreasing the film density. **sensitometry (Carlton, Carroll, Cullinan, Selman)**

553. (C) Increased collimation reduces scatter, therefore increasing contrast and decreasing density. **contrast, density (Carlton, Carroll, Cullinan)**

554. (B) An automatic exposure device controls only the exposure time; therefore, a decrease in mA will result in increased exposure time. **automatic exposure control, phototiming (Carlton, Cullinan, Curry, Selman)**

555. (B) All of the examples given would increase magnification or size distortion, except decreased film/screen speed, which would have no effect. **distortion, magnification, distance, OFD (Carlton, Bushong, Selman, Cullinan)**

556. (C) An 8:1 grid requires approximately 25% of the density of a 12:1 grid. A 30% decrease in kVp (to 63 kVp) would be required. A 10:1 grid requires approximately half the density of a 12:1 grid. A 15% decrease in kVp would achieve this. A 16:1 grid requires approximately twice the density of a 12:1 grid. A 15% increase in kVp would achieve this. Because the kVp is slightly over 30% greater, a 15% decrease in kVp is needed. **grids (Carlton, Cullinan, Selman)**

557. (A) The basic variable kVp system is based on 2 kVp per cm plus a constant (usually 30, 40, or 50 kVp). **variable kVp, exposure systems (Carlton, Cullinan, Carroll)**

558. (C) The toe is the lowest portion of the curve. **D log E curves, sensitometry, characteristic curves, H&D curves (Carlton, Cullinan, Bushong, Selman, Curry)**

559. (B) The straight line portion of the curve is the center, which is nearly straight. **D log E curves, sensitometry, characteristic curves, H&D curves (Carlton, Cullinan, Bushong, Selman, Curry)**

560. (D) The shoulder is the higher part of the curve, where it begins to curve from the straight line portion. **D log E curves, sensitometry, characteristic curves, H&D curves (Carlton, Cullinan, Bushong, Selman, Curry)**

561. (A) D_{max} is the highest possible density that can be achieved by the film. **D log E curves, sensitometry, characteristic curves, H&D curves (Cullinan, Bushong, Selman, Curry, Carlton)**

562. (A) Film A is the fastest because it produces the greatest density for any given exposure point on the horizontal axis. **D log E curves, sensitometric curves, sensitometry, film speed (Carlton, Curry, Bushong, Carroll)**

563. (A) Film A is the fastest because it has the steepest straight line portion, thus producing the greatest difference between densities in the shortest range of exposures. **D log E curves, sensitometric curves, sensitometry, film contrast (Carlton, Curry, Bushong, Carroll)**

564. (C) Film C has the widest latitude because for any given range of densities it permits the widest range of exposures to be made without producing a density below or above the density range specified. **D log E curves, sensitometric curves, sensitometry, film contrast (Carlton, Curry, Bushong, Carroll)**

565. (B) Depending on the author, the minimum mAs difference required to produce a visible density change is given as 25%, 30%, or 33%. Choices 1 & 3 only change more than these percentages, while choice 2 does not. **density, mAs (Carlton, Carroll, Cullinan)**

566. (D) Beam restriction, film/screen combination, and filtration all affect density. **density, distance, filtration, part size or thickness (Carlton, Cullinan, Carroll)**

567. (B) Resolution is primarily determined by the screens, contrast by the film, and latitude by the film. **film/screen combinations, film, intensifying screens (Carlton, Bushong, Cullinan, Curry, Selman)**

568. (D) An off-level grid will absorb more radiation at one edge than the other. This results in normal density at one edge and decreased density at the other. **grids, off-level grid, grid errors (Cullinan, Carlton, Bushong, Selman)**

569. (C) Pneumothorax and emphysema decrease beam attenuation, thus requiring decreased technical factors. Pneumonia increases beam attenuation, thus requiring increased technical factors. **pathology, tissue density, density (Carlton, Cullinan, Bushong)**

570. (D) A compression band will decrease the thickness of the abdomen which decreases subject density, increases subject contrast, and increases radiographic density. **density, subject density, subject contrast, compression bands (Cullinan, Carlton, Carroll)**

571. (D) When no other factors are considered, the highest kVp always produces the lowest, or longest, scale of contrast. **contrast, kVp (Carlton, Bushong, Cullinan, Selman, Carlton)**

572. (A) The 15% rule accomplishes changes in contrast while maintaining density. A 15% increase in kVp while halving the mAs value or a 15% decrease in kVp while doubling the mAs value will maintain the density. **15% rule, contrast, density (Carlton, Cullinan, Carroll)**

573. (C) Recorded detail (definition) is controlled by geometric factors, especially the distances FFD and OFD. **detail, definition, recorded detail, geometric factors, distance (Carlton, Cullinan, Selman, Bushong, Carroll)**

574. (D) Small, effective focal spot size; long FFD, and short OFD all improve recorded detail. **recorded detail, penumbra (Carlton, Cullinan)**

575. (B) Because distance and film/screen combinations are identical they are not a factor. The mAs values are: A=4, B=8, C=8, D=8 so they must be considered. If the mAs value is adjusted to compensate for the kVp differences by using the 15% rule to use 85 kVp for all, the new mAs results are: A=8, B=8, C=8, D=8. The grid ratio is the only difference between the techniques, and the lowest ratio grid (8:1) would produce the darkest image. Thus, B is the correct answer. **density (Carlton, Cullinan)**

576. (D) Because distance, grid ratios, and film/screen combinations are identical they are not a factor. The mAs values are: A=80, B=40, C=20, D=20. If the mAs value is adjusted to compensate for the kVp differences by using the 15% rules to use 58 kVp for all, the new mAs results are A=40, B=40, C=40, D=80. Thus, D is the correct answer. **density (Carlton, Cullinan)**

577. (B) Because distance and grid ratios are identical, they are not a factor. The mAs values are: A=16, B=8, C=4, D=8 so they must be considered. If the mAs values are adjusted to compensate for the kVp differences by using the 15% rule to use 79 kVp for all, the new mAs results are: A=8, B=8, C=4, D=4. If mAs is adjusted to compensate for the film/screen combinations by using a 100 relative speed for all, the new mAs results are: A=16, B=32, C=16, D=4. Thus, B is the correct answer. **density (Carlton, Cullinan)**

578. (D) Because distances are identical they are not a factor. The mAs values are: A=60, B=60, C=40, D=60. If the mAs values are adjusted to compensate for the film/screen combinations by using a 100 relative speed for all, the new mAs results are: A=60, B=30, C=40, D=60. If the mAs values are adjusted to compensate for the kVp differences by using the 15% rule to use 90 kVp for all, the new mAs results are: A=60, B=60, C=40, D=120. Thus, the correct answer is D. **density (Carlton, Cullinan)**

579. (B) A variable kVp system uses kVp as the primary variable, thus permitting minute adjustments in image density. **exposure systems, fixed kVp (Carlton)**

580. (A) This is a definition of recorded detail. **recorded detail, detail (Carlton, Cullinan, Bushong)**

581. (A) Slow-speed film will provide the wide latitude desired. Increased patient exposure dose requirements are a result of slower speed and wider latitude film. High-contrast films tend to have faster speed and lower patient exposure dose requirements. **film/screen combinations, film, intensifying screens (Carlton, Bushong, Cullinan, Curry)**

582. (B) Low-resolution films tend to be high speed, low contrast, wide latitude, and have lower patient dose requirements. **film, sensitometry (Carlton, Cullinan, Bushong, Selman, Curry)**

583. (A) The formula for converting from one grid ratio to another is mAs_1/mAs_2 = grid conversion factor$_1$/grid conversion factor$_2$. Therefore, 12 mAs/mAs_2 = 5/3, which is 5 mAs_2 = 36, which is mAs_2 = 7 mAs. **grids, grid conversion, bucky factor (Carlton, Cullinan, Bushong)**

584. (B) Grid ratio is determined by lead strip height divided by interspace width, so: grid ratio = 1.5 mm/0.19 mm = 8:1 grids. **grid ratio (Cullinan, Curry, Selman, Carlton, Bushong)**

585. (A) A fixed kVp system uses mAs as the primary variable, thus permitting nearly equal contrast from projection to projection. **exposure systems, fixed kVp (Carlton)**

586. (C) The lateral L5-S1 lumbar spot is concave in relationship to the primary beam coming from the x-ray tube. This permits the diverging photons to pass through the joint spaces. The AP lumbar and PA thoracic spine have a convex relationship to the primary beam and superimpose the joint spaces. **alignment, distortion (Carlton, Cullinan)**

587. (B) Intensifying screen phosphor size and layer thickness effect density, contrast, and recorded detail. These factors have no effect on distortion. **intensifying screens, recorded detail, detail, density (Carlton, Bushong, Cullinan)**

588. (B) Average gradient is a measurement of the slope of the straight line portion of the D log E (H&D or characteristic) curve. High-contrast films typically exhibit high average gradients, high speed, and narrow latitude. A typical high average gradient film is shown as film A in Figure 13. **D log E curves, sensitometry, characteristic curves, H&D curves (Carlton, Cullinan, Bushong, Selman, Curry)**

589. (A) The anode heel effect is the absorption of the isotropically scattered radiation from the surface of the focal spot by the heel of the anode, thus reducing the total intensity of the x-ray beam exiting at the anode end of the tube. **anode heel effect (Carlton, Bushong, Curry, Cullinan, Selman)**

590. (C) An automatic exposure device controls only the exposure time; therefore, an increase in the density control will result in increased exposure time and image density. **automatic exposure control, phototiming (Carlton, Cullinan, Curry, Selman)**

591. (D) 68 kVp produces the maximum number of photons at the keV energy that is slightly higher than the binding energy of the inner shell electrons of barium. This increases the probability of photoelectric interactions, which increases the image contrast. **contrast media, iodine, photoelectric interactions (Carlton, Curry, Carroll, Cullinan)**

592. (C) Depending on the author, the minimum mAs difference required to produce a visible density change is given as 25%, 30%, or 33%. **density, mAs (Carlton, Carroll, Cullinan)**

593. (D) X-ray tube output, and, therefore, image density, is increased by a high vacuum inside the glass envelope, a smooth anode focal track, and decreased added filtration. **x-ray tubes (Cullinan, Carlton, Bushong, Selman, Carroll)**

594. (C) Primary beam field size and grid ratio produce changes in radiographic contrast. mAs does not. **contrast, collimation, grids (Cullinan, Carlton, Carroll)**

595. (A) old mAs/X = old distance^2/new distance^2, which is 18 mAs/X = 72"^{2}/40"^{2}, which is 18 mAs/X = 5,184/1,600, which is 5,184 X = 28,800, which is X = 6 mAs. **inverse square law [to maintain density], density maintenance law (Carlton, Bushong, Cullinan, Selman)**

596. (C) The prime factor that controls and regulates radiographic density is kVp. **density, prime factors (Carlton, Bushong, Cullinan, Selman, Carroll)**

597. (B) Compton effect interactions result in the production of much scattered radiation. This scatter provides inaccurate information to the image receptor that contributes to an overall gray density level that lengthens the scale of contrast, or makes it longer or lower. **contrast, photoelectric interaction (Carlton, Bushong, Cullinan, Selman)**

598. (B) The knee is normally imaged between 60 to 70 kVp. **kVp, contrast, technique factors, technical factors (Carlton, Cullinan)**

599. (D) A faster film/screen combination requires a decrease in primary beam quantity and/or quality. Decreasing mAs and kVp and increasing FFD all achieve this effect. **film/screen combinations (Cullinan, Carlton, Bushong, Selman, Curry)**

600. (A) Phenidone rapidly produces fine recorded detail shades of gray on the film, while hydroquinone slowly produces heavy densities. **film processing, developer, reducing agents (Cullinan, Selman, Carlton, Bushong)**

601. (A) All of the examples given would increase recorded detail except decreased FFD, which will decrease it. **recorded detail, detail, distance, OFD (Carlton, Bushong, Selman, Cullinan)**

602. (D) The anode heel theory demonstrates that radiation intensity is slightly greater at the cathode end of the x-ray tube. Therefore, the thickest body part should be positioned toward the cathode. All of the examples given fulfill these conditions. **anode heel effect (Cullinan, Selman, Carlton, Bushong)**

603. (A) In order of density, the tissues are: bone, muscle, water, and fat. **attenuation, tissue density (Carlton, Bushong, Curry)**

604. (D) Rare earth intensifying screens contribute to reduced patient exposure dose, permit the use of lower power generators, and increase tube life. **intensifying screens, rare earth (Carlton, Bushong, Curry, Cullinan)**

605. (A) Long FFD makes best use of a parallel grid. Anode angle and focal spot size have a minimal effect on grid effectiveness. **grids, parallel grids (Carlton, Bushong, Selman, Cullinan, Curry)**

606. (B) Ascites and cirrhosis increase beam attenuation, thus requiring increased technical factors. Bowel obstruction decreases beam attenuation, thus requiring decreased technical factors. **pathology, tissue density, density (Carlton, Cullinan, Bushong)**

607. (B) The 15% rule functions best between 50 and 80 kVp. **15% rule (Carlton, Carroll, Cullinan)**

608. (D) kVp, primary beam field size, and grid ratio all produce changes in radiographic contrast. **contrast, kVp, collimation, grids (Cullinan, Carlton, Carroll)**

609.   (C) If film/screen speed is halved (from 400 to 200), then the mAs value must be doubled to maintain the same density. The 15% rule states that an increase of 15% of the kVp will result in doubling of density. **15% rule, film/screen combinations (Carlton, Bushong, Cullinan, Selman, Carroll)**

610.   (D) When no other factors are considered, the lowest kVp always produces the highest, or shortest, scale of contrast. **contrast, kVp (Carlton, Bushong, Cullinan, Selman)**

611.   (B) Patient motion is decreased with increased mA, increased kVp, increased film/screen speed, and decreased FFD. **motion, recorded detail, detail (Carlton, Cullinan)**

612.   (A) Poor film-screen contact decreases resolution and increases density. **film-screen contact, recorded detail, detail, density (Cullinan, Carlton, Selman)**

613.   (D) Decreasing part thickness increases density and decreases contrast. It has no effect on recorded detail or distortion. **anatomic part, part thickness, contrast, density, recorded detail, detail, distortion (Carlton, Cullinan)**

614.   (D) Increasing the x-ray tube angle will decrease the density on one side of the central ray because the distance will become greater. It will also increase the density on the other side of the central ray because the distance will become less. Contrast will change because of the density changes. Distortion will increase because of the elongation and foreshortening of the object due to the geometry of the tube angle. **distortion, density, contrast, (Carlton, Cullinan, Selman, Bushong)**

615.   (D) Sodium sulfite is used as the preservative in both developer and fixer solutions. In the developer, it controls oxidation and serves as a buffer. In the fixer, it maintains the solution pH. **film processing, developer, fixer, preservative (Carlton, Cullinan, Selman, Bushong)**

616.   (C) Decreased OFD will minimize its magnification, or size distortion. Film/screen speed would have no effect. Both decreased FFD and increased focal spot size would increase magnification. **distortion, magnification, distance, OFD (Carlton, Bushong, Selman, Cullinan)**

617.   (B) The anode heel theory demonstrates that radiation intensity is slightly greater at the cathode end of the x-ray tube. Therefore, the thickest body part should be positioned toward the cathode. Of the examples given, only the AP thoracic spine with the cathode toward the neck does not fulfill these conditions. **anode heel effect (Cullinan, Selman, Carlton, Bushong)**

618.   (A) Elongation and foreshortening are shape distortion. Magnification is size distortion. **distortion, magnification, foreshortening, elongation (Carlton, Bushong, Curry, Cullinan)**

619.   (B) Resolution is primarily determined by the screens, contrast by the film, and latitude by the film. **film/screen combinations, film, intensifying screens (Carlton, Bushong, Cullinan, Curry, Selman)**

620. (C) Average gradient is a measurement of the slope of the straight line portion of the D log E (H&D or characteristic) curve. High-speed films typically exhibit high contrast, high average gradients, and narrow latitude. A typical high-speed film is shown as film A in Figure 13. **D log E curves, sensitometry, characteristic curves, H&D curves (Carlton, Cullinan, Bushong, Selman, Curry)**

621. (D) The convergence line is the point in space above the grid where the focused grid lines would meet if they were projected over the grid. The x-ray tube focal spot must be placed on the convergence line to avoid grid cut-off. **grids, focused grids (Carlton, Bushong, Selman, Curry, Cullinan)**

622. (A) Conditions that have decreased tissue attenuation require less quantity or quality of the incident x-ray beam. Decreased mAs, decreased kVp, and increased distance all achieve this effect. **pathology, tissue density, density (Carlton, Cullinan, Bushong)**

623. (C) Calipers permit the choice of exact technical factors for various patient part sizes. **calipers, measurement, part size (Carlton, Carroll, Cullinan)**

624. (C) Depending on the author, the minimum mAs difference required to produce a visible density change is given as 25%, 30%, or 33%. Choice 1 changes at least these percentages, while choices 2 & 3 do not. **density, mAs (Carlton, Carroll, Cullinan)**

625. (A) Depending on the author, the minimum mAs difference required to produce a visible density change is given as 25%, 30%, or 33%. In this example, both 30 and 40 mAs are less than 30% different from 35 mAs, while 47 mAs is enough to produce a visible density change. **density, mAs (Carlton, Carroll, Cullinan)**

626. (D) Distance, grids, and anatomic part size all affect density. **density, distance, filtration, part size or thickness (Carlton, Cullinan, Carroll)**

627. (A) Focal spot size has its major effect on recorded detail. **detail, recorded detail, focal spot size (Cullinan, Carlton, Carroll, Bushong, Selman)**

628. (C) Decreasing the focal spot size will increase the recorded detail. Focal spot size has a minimal and usually unobservable effect on magnification and density. **recorded detail, magnification, contrast, air-gap (Carlton, Cullinan, Carroll, Bushong, Selman, Curry)**

629. (B) Decreasing the kVp by 10 to 55 would constitute a 15% decrease. The mAs must be doubled from 6 to 12 mAs to maintain the density. Changing from a 200 to a 100 relative speed film/screen combination requires a doubling of the mAs value to maintain the same density. Increasing the size of the primary beam field will increase the amount of scattered radiation produced, thus decreasing contrast and increasing density. In addition, it increases the exposure dose to the patient. Choices 1 & 3 only are true, making B the correct answer. **beam restriction, collimation, contrast (Carlton, Cullinan, Carroll)**

630. (B) Increasing the size of the primary beam field will increase the amount of scattered radiation produced, thus decreasing contrast and increasing density. In addition, it increases the exposure dose to the patient. Choices 1 & 3 only are true, making B the correct answer. **beam restriction, collimation, contrast (Cullinan, Carlton, Carroll)**

631. (A) Increasing the distance will decrease the intensity of the primary beam, thus decreasing density. Although the decreased density will affect the visibility of recorded detail, the geometric factors controlling recorded detail itself will not change. **grids, density, contrast (Cullinan, Carlton, Carroll)**

632. (C) This is a definition of elongation. **distortion, foreshortening (Carlton, Cullinan)**

633. (A) Photoelectric interactions result in complete absorption of the incident photon, thus preventing it from reaching the image receptor. This lack of information, when combined with nearby information from photons that did not undergo photoelectric interactions, results in contrast permitting the image to become visible. **contrast, photoelectric interaction (Carlton, Bushong, Cullinan, Selman)**

634. (D) When no other factors are considered, the highest kVp always produces the lowest, or longest, scale of contrast. **contrast, kVp (Carlton, Bushong, Cullinan, Selman)**

635. (B) Fixer replenishment must occur at a higher rate than developer in most automatic processors. **automatic film processors (Carlton, Gray)**

636. (D) kVp, mAs, and subject density have no effect on recorded detail. **definition, recorded detail, motion (Carlton, Cullinan, Carroll)**

637. (D) The 15% rule accomplishes changes in contrast while maintaining density. A 15% increase in kVp while halving the mAs value or a 15% decrease in kVp while doubling the mAs value will maintain the density. **15% rule, contrast, density (Cullinan, Carlton, Carroll)**

638. (C) Because kVp, grid, and film/screen combinations are identical, they are not a factor. The mAs values are: A=8, B=8, C=8, D=8. Because the mAs values are identical, they also are not a factor. Distance is the only variable and because only C is at 40", it will produce the greatest image density. **density (Carlton, Cullinan)**

639. (A) Because distance, grid ratios, and film/screen combinations are identical, they are not a factor. The mAs values are: A=160, B=80, C=40, D=40. If the mAs values are adjusted to compensate for the kVp differences by using the 15% rules to use 80 kVp for all, the new mAs results are A=160, B=80, C=20, D=10. Thus, A is the correct answer. **density (Carlton, Cullinan)**

640.	(B) Because distance and grid ratios are identical, they are not a factor. The mAs values are: A=16, B=16, C=8, D=16, so they must be considered. If the mAs values are adjusted to compensate for the kVp differences by using the 15% rule to use 79 kVp for all, the new mAs results are: A=8, B=16, C=8, D=8. Thus, B is the correct answer. **density (Carlton, Cullinan)**

641.	(D) Because distances are identical, they are not a factor. The mAs values are: A=30, B=30, C=20, D=120. If the mAs values are adjusted to compensate for the film/screen combinations by using a 100 relative speed for all, the new mAs results are: A=30, B=15, C=20, D=120. If the mAs values are adjusted to compensate for the kVp differences by using the 15% rule to use 90 kVp for all, the new mAs results are: A=30, B=30, C=20, D=240. Therefore, the correct answer is D. **density (Carlton, Cullinan)**

642.	(A) old mAs/X = old distance^2/new distance^2, which is 2.4 mAs/X = 40"^{2}/32"^{2}, which is 2.4 mAs/X = 1,600/1,024, which is 1,600 X = 2,458, which is X = 1.5 mAs. **inverse square law [to maintain density], density maintenance law (Carlton, Bushong, Cullinan, Selman)**

643.	(D) If film/screen speed is doubled (from 200 to 400), then the mAs value must be halved to maintain the same density. **15% rule, film/screen combinations (Carlton, Bushong, Cullinan, Selman, Carroll)**

644.	(C) Because the area of interest is positioned directly in the center of the exposure area, the best image will be obtained by activating only the center ion chamber. **phototiming, automatic exposure device (Carlton, Cullinan, Bushong)**

645.	(C) Decreasing the focal spot size increases recorded detail. **recorded detail, detail, focal spot size (Carlton, Bushong, Cullinan, Selman)**

646.	(C) Decreasing the mA station from 100 to 50 will decrease density by half. Only choice C provides a doubling of density to compensate, by increasing the time from 0.08 to 0.16. **density, mAs (Carlton, Bushong, Cullinan, Selman)**

647.	(B) Removing the grid will permit a much greater intensity of radiation to reach the image receptor, making the film much darker. Decreasing mAs will compensate as will increasing the FFD. **grids, density (Carlton, Bushong, Cullinan, Selman)**

648.	(A) Increasing the field size will increase scattered radiation, which will decrease contrast and increase density. Recorded detail would not be affected. **collimation, field size (Carlton, Cullinan, Selman, Carroll)**

649.	(B) A slight reduction in film/screen combination relative speed will decrease the density slightly. **film/screen combinations, contrast (Carlton, Bushong, Cullinan, Selman)**

650.	(C) Only choice C maintains the density. When the mA is doubled (from 100 to 200), time must be halved. 0.04 sec is half of 0.08 sec. **density, mAs (Carlton, Bushong, Carroll, Selman)**

651. (D) Film/screen combination resolution can be measured by modulation transfer function, line spread function, and by a line pair per millimeter resolution tool. **resolution, film/screen combinations, film, intensifying screens (Carlton, Cullinan, Bushong, Selman, Curry)**

652. (B) High resolution films tend to be low speed, high contrast, narrow latitude, and have higher patient dose requirements. **film, sensitometry (Carlton, Cullinan, Bushong, Selman, Curry)**

653. (B) Radiographic density would increase with increased developer temperature and high temperature in film storage area. Fixing time has minimal effect on radiographic density. **density, film processing, film storage (Carlton, Bushong, Selman, Cullinan)**

654. (A) The formula for converting from one grid ratio to another is mAs_1/mAs_2 = grid conversion factor$_1$/grid conversion factor$_2$. Therefore, 4 mAs/mAs$_2$ = 4/7, which is 4 mAs$_2$ = 28, which is mAs$_2$ = 7 mAs. **grids, grid conversion, bucky factor (Carlton, Cullinan, Bushong)**

655. (A) Chronic osteomyelitis and acromegaly increase beam attenuation, thus requiring increased technical factors. Aseptic necrosis decreases beam attenuation, thus requiring decreased technical factors. **pathology, tissue density, density (Carlton, Cullinan, Bushong)**

656. (B) Narrow latitude films have steep straight line portions. This produces a film that responds to the entire range of densities within a narrow range of exposures, thus producing the highest density for any given exposure. This is essentially the definition of a high-speed film. **D log E curves, sensitometric curves, sensitometry, film latitude (Cullinan, Carroll, Curry, Carlton, Bushong)**

657. (D) The reciprocity law states that as the mAs value increases, both x-ray exposure and radiographic density increase proportionally. Reciprocity law failure occurs at very short (less than 0.01 second) and long (more than 10 seconds) exposures. **reciprocity law (Carlton, Carroll, Cullinan)**

658. (C) Both recorded detail and distortion are controlled by geometric factors, especially the distances FFD and OFD. **detail, recorded detail, definition, geometric factors, distance (Carlton, Cullinan, Selman, Bushong, Carroll)**

IMAGE PRODUCTION AND EVALUATION
Film Processing and Quality Assurance
5% (70) 659-728

659. (A) Developer contamination is evidenced by increased base-plus-fog, decreased speed, and lower contrast index readings during processor quality control sensitometry. **quality control, processing (Gray, Carlton, Carroll, Bushong)**

660. (C) Bending the film during handling before processing will produce a black, crescent, half moon artifact. **film, artifacts (Carlton, Cullinan)**

661. (A) Typical fixer replenishment rates average 6 to 8 ml/in of film transported through the entrance rollers. **automatic processing, film processing, processing, replenishment (Carlton, Bushong)**

662. (A) The transport system of an automatic processor controls the film immersion time, agitates the solutions, and moves the films through the processor. **automatic processing, film processing, processing (Selman, Carlton, Bushong, Cullinan)**

663. (A) The film identification blocker area is reserved for the patient's medical record information. The patient's name and the procedure performed are appropriate. The physician's age is not. **film identification (Carlton, Cullinan)**

664. (C) Extremely low humidity during film handling will produce static discharge artifacts that appear as black tree branching or smudge marks. **film, film handling (Carlton, Cullinan, Carroll, Selman)**

665. (D) 14" x 17" and 35 cm x 43 cm are equivalent. **cassettes, film (Carlton, Cullinan)**

666. (D) High-speed rare earths are the highest speed listed and will produce the lowest patient exposure dose. **intensifying screens (Carlton, Bushong, Selman, Cullinan, Curry)**

667. (B) An improperly seated crossover network can scratch the soft emulsion from the film as it passes over. This produces white lines for the length of the radiograph. **crossover network, automatic processing, artifacts (Carlton, Bushong, Selman)**

668. (B) A 90 second processor immerses the film for approximately 20 to 25 seconds in the fixer solution. **automatic processing (Selman, Carlton, Bushong)**

669. (A) Weak developer solution resulting from insufficient replenishment and developer solution contamination with fixer both will result in overall light gray films that lack clear white or completely black densities. **quality control, automatic processing (Carlton, Bushong, Cullinan)**

670. (C) This is a definition of a radiographic artifact. **artifact (Carlton, Bushong, Cullinan, Selman)**

671. (D) An orange-brown filter will produce light that is outside the sensitivity range of blue-violet sensitive film. **darkroom, safelights (Carlton, Cullinan, Bushong, Selman)**

672. (B) Adding concentrated chemicals to water reduces the possibility of chemistry splashing back toward the person doing the mixing. **replenishment, film processing, processing (Carlton, Selman)**

673. (A) The transport system of an automatic processor includes crossover networks, transport racks, and the drive system. **automatic processing, film processing, processing (Carlton, Bushong, Selman, Cullinan)**

674. (A) The radiograph is a subpoenable legal medical record. Although the information on the radiograph is considered to belong to the patient, the radiograph itself, as part of the medical record, is considered the property of the entity that is required to maintain the medical record. In most cases this is the hospital, clinic, or physician office for which it was produced. **film, film identification (Carlton)**

675. (B) The text described is a safelight test to determine how long a film may remain on the darkroom work surface without excessive fogging. **darkroom, safelight test (Carroll, Carlton, Gray)**

676. (A) Dirt or other foreign objects in a cassette will produce a white artifact on the radiograph as the light from the intensifying screens is absorbed and prevented from reaching the film to produce a latent image. **artifacts (Selman, Carlton, Bushong)**

677. (A) Both the recirculation system and the developer heater contribute to the regulation of the solution temperatures. **automatic processing, film processing (Carlton, Bushong, Cullinan, Selman)**

678. (A) A penetrometer is a step wedge, usually of aluminum or plastic. **penetrometer, step wedge (Gray, Carlton, Cullinan, Selman)**

679. (D) Base-plus-fog, a contrast index, and speed should all be evaluated daily on all radiographic film processing systems. **quality control, sensitometry, processor evaluation (Gray, Carroll, Carlton, Cullinan, Bushong, Selman)**

680. (C) Chemical precipitation uses chemicals to break down the fixer and release the silver for recovery. The process produces several toxic and explosive gasses. **silver recovery (Carlton, Cullinan)**

681. (B) A 7-watt to 15-watt bulb is recommended for safelights directed at film working surfaces but located at least 4 feet away. **darkroom, safelights (Carlton, Cullinan, Selman)**

682. (B) Both fixer fumes and increased developer temperature will fog film. Rough handling of film may damage the surface but would not add density to the image. **darkroom, base-plus-fog levels, sensitometry (Cullinan, Carlton, Bushong, Selman)**

683. (C) Orthochromatic film is sensitive to all wavelengths, except red. **film, safelight, film-screen combinations (Carlton, Carroll, Bushong)**

684. (A) Detail screens will produce the highest resolution but the slowest speed and highest patient exposure dose. **intensifying screens (Carlton, Bushong, Selman, Cullinan, Curry)**

685. (C) A clogged developer replenishment filter will result in insufficient replenishment of the strength of the developer solution. This is evidenced by no change in base-plus-fog, decreased speed, and lower contrast index readings during processor quality control sensitometry. **quality control, processing (Gray, Carlton, Carroll, Bushong)**

686. (D) Improperly aligned guide shoe deflectors will scratch the soft emulsion from the film, leaving a clear white scratch the length of the radiograph. **film, artifacts (Carlton, Cullinan)**

687. (B) Electrolytic silver recovery units are most efficient for the regular routine load of an average hospital diagnostic radiology department. **silver recovery (Carlton, Cullinan)**

688. (B) Typical developer replenishment rates average 4 to 5 ml/in of film transported through the entrance rollers. **automatic processing, film processing, processing, replenishment (Carlton, Bushong)**

689. (C) A transport rack of an automatic processor includes planetary rollers and guide shoe deflectors. The recirculation pump is a part of the recirculation system. **automatic processing, film processing, processing (Selman, Carlton, Bushong, Cullinan)**

690. (C) The radiographer producing the film is responsible for properly recording the identification information on the radiograph. **film, film identification (Carlton)**

691. (B) 30 to 60% humidity is the ideal condition for film storage. **film, film storage (Carlton, Carroll)**

692. (A) 8" x 10" and 20 cm x 25 cm are equivalent. **cassettes, film (Carlton, Cullinan)**

693. (C) Automatic film processor dryers use hot air between 120 to 150°F. **automatic processing, film processing, processing (Carlton, Bushong, Selman, Cullinan)**

694. (A) The entrance rollers determine how much replenisher is pumped into the developer and fixer tanks as each film passes into the processor. Although some newer processors use infrared light to sense incoming film size, this function is still accomplished at the entrance roller. **automatic processing, replenishment system (Carlton, Carroll, Bushong, Selman)**

695. (A) Rapid temperature changes during processing can cause a network of fine cracks in the emulsion, which is referred to as reticulation marks. **artifacts, film handling (Selman, Carlton)**

696. (D) Although white is preferred because it enhances the light level in a darkroom, any color is acceptable. **darkroom, safelight (Selman, Carlton, Bushong)**

697. (B) Crossover networks are positioned half in solution and half out. This permits chemical deposits to accumulate readily. **automatic processing, crossover networks (Carlton, Bushong, Selman)**

698. (B) The replenishment system of an automatic processor replaces depleted developer and fixer. **automatic processing, film processing, processing (Selman, Carlton, Bushong, Cullinan)**

699. (B) A corner of the film must be protected from the primary beam to reserve an area for a light-exposed identification marker. **film, film identification (Carlton, Cullinan)**

700. (C) Radiographic film should be stored at temperatures below 68°F. **film, film storage (Selman, Cullinan, Carlton)**

701. (A) Unexposed boxes of radiographic film should be stored on end to avoid abrasion and static discharge artifacts. **film handling (Carlton, Carroll, Bushong)**

702. (A) Detail screens will produce the highest resolution but the slowest speed and highest patient exposure dose. **intensifying screens (Carlton, Bushong, Selman, Cullinan, Curry)**

703. (B) An increase in developer temperature will increase base-plus-fog, increase speed, and decrease contrast index readings during processor quality control sensitometry. **quality control, processing (Carlton, Carroll)**

704. (B) Dirt or other foreign substance on a processor transport roller will be repeated the length of the radiograph as the roller imprints the artifact every time it turns. **film, artifacts (Carlton, Cullinan)**

705. (A) Metallic replacement cartridges or buckets filter used fixer through steel wool. The acid of the fixer permits the silver to precipitate onto the steel wool. **silver recovery (Carlton, Cullinan)**

706. (A) The guide shoe deflectors are made of metal. Wet films will adhere to them unless they are ribbed to break the surface tension of the solutions. **automatic processing, film processing, processing (Carlton, Cullinan, Bushong, Selman)**

707. (C) Processed films should be stored at about 60% humidity and 70°F. **film storage, processing (Carlton, Carroll)**

708. (C) 11" x 14" and 28 cm x 35 cm are equivalent. **cassettes, film (Carlton, Cullinan)**

709. (D) The dryer system forces hot air through tubes that have a slit through which the air is forced over the surface of the passing film to dry it. **automatic processing, dryer system (Carlton, Carroll, Bushong, Selman)**

710. (D) Improperly seated crossover networks or transport racks will cause films to jam as they attempt to enter the improperly aligned rollers. Films that are fed into the processor without using the guides on the feed tray may not travel in a straight line through the rollers and may jam when one edge is caught by the roller drive gears. **automatic processing, film processing (Carlton, Carroll)**

711. (B) An improperly seated crossover network or an improperly adjusted guide shoe deflector can scratch the soft emulsion from the film as it passes over. This produces white lines for the length of the radiograph. **crossover network, automatic processing, artifacts (Carlton, Bushong, Selman)**

712. (C) Insufficient washing will leave fixer solution in the film emulsion. This results in a slimy, wet feel that is not always removed by drying. Insufficient drying will also leave films wet. **quality control, automatic processing (Carlton, Bushong, Cullinan)**

713. (A) The stain left when improperly removed chemistry runs up or down a film during processing is called a curtain effect. **artifacts (Carlton, Bushong, Cullinan)**

714. (C) Crossover networks turn the film at the top of each solution tank, while guide shoes turn the film at the bottom of each tank. **film processing, automatic film processors, processing (Carlton, Cullinan, Bushong, Selman)**

715. (D) The film identification blocker area is reserved for the patient's medical record information. The patient's age, physician's name, and hospital's name are all appropriate. **film identification (Carlton, Cullinan)**

716. (A) Static discharge artifacts may appear as either black tree branching or black smudge marks after the film is processed. **film, artifacts (Carlton, Cullinan)**

717. (A) Extremely high humidity during film handling may produce waterspot artifacts from condensation of atmospheric moisture on the film. **film, film handling (Carlton, Cullinan, Carroll, Selman)**

718. (D) Fully opening cassettes on the darkroom loading bench permits dust and moisture to accumulate on the screens which become artifacts on the image. Using lotion on hands will leave fingerprints on the film when it is developed. Wearing a ring with a large stone increases the probability of scratching the top intensifying screen when removing film from the cassette. **darkroom, cassettes (Carlton, Cullinan)**

719. (D) Panchromatic film is sensitive to all wavelengths. **film, safelight, film-screen combinations (Carlton, Carroll, Bushong)**

720. (A) Base-plus-fog levels should be maintained at <0.20. **sensitometry, base-plus-fog (Carroll, Carlton, Cullinan)**

721. (B) Accidental exposure of a film bin requires immediate notification and correction to prevent loading cassettes with fogged film for use with patient exposures. This would require repeated exposures, with increased exposure dose, to patients. **darkroom, film handling (Carlton, Bushong, Cullinan)**

722. (D) Lead markers absorb radiation and leave an image on the film. Light exposure through paper prints an image of the writing on the paper onto the film. Permanent felt tip markers may be used to add information to a processed radiograph. **film identification, markers (Carlton, Cullinan, Bushong, Selman)**

723. (B) Dirt or other foreign substances on a processor transport roller will be repeated over the length of the radiograph as the roller imprints the artifact every time it turns, which is an interval equal to the circumference of the roller (pi times the diameter). **film, artifacts (Carlton, Cullinan)**

724. (B) Electrolytic silver recovery uses a unit that passes a current from a cathode to an anode through the fixer. This permits the ionized silver in the used fixer to be attracted to the negatively charge cathode where it plates for removal. **silver recovery (Carlton, Cullinan)**

725. (C) The dryer system removes excess water and shrinks and seals the film emulsion. **automatic processing, film processing, processing (Selman, Carlton, Bushong, Cullinan)**

726. (C) Both litigation and pediatric films should be retained longer than routine cases. In many states, the statute of limitations for pediatric patients does not begin until legal age. Once litigation has begun, films may be required at later dates as the case proceeds through the judicial system. **film storage, processing, storage (Carlton, Cullinan)**

727. (C) Abrasion lines can be formed when an interleaf of paper or cardboard next to a film is quickly removed. The abrasion lines will appear black when the trauma to the film occurred prior to processing. **film, artifacts (Carlton, Cullinan)**

728. (A) Only freezing will arrest film aging. **film, film storage (Carlton, Carroll)**

IMAGE PRODUCTION AND EVALUATION
Evaluation of Radiographs
6% (84) 729-812

729. (D) The original radiograph used 200 mAs. 200 mAs/0.5 s = 400 mA. **mAs, density (Selman, Bushong, Cullinan, Carlton, Carroll)**

730. (C) Low contrast images lack a great difference between adjacent shades of gray. **contrast (Carlton, Cullinan, Carroll)**

731. (A) Increased FOD decreases distortion. Decreased OFD decreases distortion. Decreased grid ratio has no effect on distortion. **distortion (Carlton, Carroll, Cullinan, Bushong)**

732.   (A) kVp controls the energy of the primary beam photons, which is considered the quality factor. **kVp (Carlton, Bushong, Selman, Cullinan)**

733.   (C) Film latitude and contrast are inversely proportional, so that when latitude increases, contrast decreases, and vice versa. **latitude, contrast, film, sensitometry (Carlton, Cullinan)**

734.   (D) The highest kVp produces the highest contrast when the density remains the same, as it does in all four examples. **contrast (Cullinan, Carlton, Bushong, Selman, Carroll)**

735.   (D) The highest grid ratio produces the highest contrast when the density remains the same, as it does in all four examples. **contrast, grids (Cullinan, Carlton, Bushong, Selman, Carroll)**

736.   (C) A 15% change in kVp will produce a visible change in contrast. Changes in mAs, mA, or time do not affect contrast when made within the straight line portion of the D log E curve. **contrast (Carlton, Carroll, Cullinan, Selman)**

737.   (D) Contrast can be raised only by decreasing the kVp. Of the two choices at less than the original 68 kVp, only 57 kVp at 5 mAs will maintain density according to the 15% rule. **15% rule, contrast (Cullinan, Carlton, Carroll)**

738.   (C) The valence of an atom has no effect on its ability to absorb or interact with x-ray photons. **contrast (Cullinan, Carlton, Carroll)**

739.   (A) There is a directly proportional relationship between exposure latitude and kilovoltage. As kVp increases, so does latitude, and vice versa. **latitude, kVp, sensitometry, (Cullinan, Selman, Carlton, Bushong, Carroll)**

740.   (D) Without proper density, evaluation of the image cannot occur. **density (Cullinan, Carlton, Bushong)**

741.   (C) A small plastic ball would have a density very similar to water and soft tissue and therefore would be nearly impossible to visualize radiographically without contrast media. **contrast (Carlton, Carroll)**

742.   (A) A hypersthenic body habitus would attenuate the greatest quantity of radiation, thus producing the lightest image density. **part thickness, body habitus (Ballinger, Carroll, Carlton, Cullinan)**

743.   (D) Film speed, developer activity, and collimation all affect radiographic density. **density (Cullinan, Carroll, Carlton, Bushong)**

744.   (A) Of the factors given, only increased developer time would produce greater density. **density, developer time (Carroll, Selman, Bushong, Cullinan, Carlton)**

745. (B) An off-level focused grid will permit the diverging portion of the central ray on the angled-down side to transit the grid, producing a relatively normal density image on one side. However, the angled-up side will place the grid lines perpendicular to the beam, thus absorbing a greater portion and producing a light image on the other side. **grids (Carroll, Cullinan, Carlton, Bushong)**

746. (D) Of the four primary factors, only distance also affects recorded detail. **recorded detail, detail (Cullinan, Carlton, Bushong, Carroll)**

747. (D) This is a definition of umbra. **umbra, penumbra, recorded detail (Carlton, Carroll, Cullinan, Bushong, Selman)**

748. (C) Time controls the number and quantity of photons. Photon wavelength is controlled by kVp. **mAs, density (Carlton, Bushong, Carroll, Cullinan)**

749. (D) Decreased FOD increases density. Increased kVp increases density. Decreased OFD increases scatter reaching the image receptor, which increases density. **density (Carlton, Carroll, Cullinan, Bushong)**

750. (D) Because mAs is relatively proportional to image density, reduction of image density by half requires a reduction of mAs by half or 50%. **mAs, density (Cullinan, Carlton, Carroll)**

751. (B) Slower film/screen combinations are also higher resolution, which would improve the recorded detail of an extremity. **recorded detail, detail (Cullinan, Carlton, Bushong, Carroll, Selman)**

752. (A) The right lumbar abdominal region would be the location of a large, right renal staghorn calculus. This would produce the least density in that area because the calcium in the calculus would attenuate more of the primary beam. **part thickness, body regions (Ballinger, Carroll, Carlton, Cullinan)**

753. (C) A decrease of 50% in time will reduce mAs to one half. According to the 15% rule, a 15% increase in kVp will maintain image density. **15% rule, density (Carlton, Cullinan, Carroll, Bushong)**

754. (B) Decreased FFD decreases resolution. High kVp has no effect on resolution. Increased OFD decreases resolution. **resolution, recorded detail, detail (Carlton, Carroll, Cullinan, Bushong)**

755. (A) A is 76 kVp at 22 mAs. 76 kVp is 8% more than 70 kVp, which constitutes half of the 15% rule, or a 50% increase in density. **density, 15% rule (Cullinan, Carlton, Bushong, Selman, Carroll)**

756. (B) According to the 15% rule, a 15% decrease in kVp will reduce image density by approximately one half. **15% rule, density (Cullinan, Carlton, Carroll)**

757. (D) An asthenic body habitus would attenuate the smallest quantity of radiation, thus producing the darkest image density. **part thickness, body habitus (Ballinger, Carroll, Carlton, Cullinan)**

758. (D) Film latitude, developer activity, and collimation all affect radiographic contrast. **contrast (Cullinan, Carroll, Carlton, Bushong)**

759. (B) Most diagnostic radiographic acceptance ranges include images with densities approximately 50 to 60% below optimal. This is equivalent to two 30% visible densities. **film critique, density, optimal density (Carlton, Carroll)**

760. (D) Grid ratio, kVp, and film/screen combination speed all have an effect on image contrast. **contrast, grids, film/screen combinations, kVp (Carlton, Bushong, Carroll, Cullinan)**

761. (A) kVp controls the average photon wavelength and quantity of photons. The number of photons is controlled by mAs. **kVp (Carlton, Bushong, Carroll, Cullinan)**

762. (B) Decreased FOD increases distortion. Increased kVp has no effect on distortion. Increased OFD increases distortion. **distortion (Carlton, Carroll, Cullinan, Bushong)**

763. (D) The possibility of motion reducing recorded detail would be most likely if the patient were standing. The PA projection would place the area of interest furthest from the film, thus increasing magnification and further reducing recorded detail. **motion, recorded detail, detail (Ballinger, Carlton, Cullinan, Carroll)**

764. (B) B is 98 kVp at 12 mAs. 98 kVp is 15% more than 85 kVp, thus doubling density. 24 mAs is half of 48, which would maintain density. However, the 12 mAs that is used reduces the density to half. **density, 15% rule (Cullinan, Carlton, Bushong, Selman, Carroll)**

765. (A) The lowest kVp will produce the highest contrast if image density remains the same, as it does in the examples. **contrast, 15% rule (Cullinan, Carlton, Carroll)**

766. (C) The original radiograph used 12 mAs. 12 mAs/0.04 s = 300 mA. **mAs (Selman, Bushong, Cullinan, Carlton, Carroll)**

767. (D) This is a definition of distortion. **distortion (Cullinan, Carroll, Carlton, Bushong)**

768. (A) A hypersthenic body habitus has the greatest volume of tissue. This results in less subject contrast, which would produce the lowest image contrast. **part thickness, body habitus (Ballinger, Carroll, Carlton, Cullinan)**

769. (A) Long wavelengths are produced by higher kVps, which decrease contrast. **contrast, kVp (Cullinan, Carlton, Carroll)**

770. (A) Decreasing grid frequency will decrease contrast and increase density. It has no effect on recorded detail. **grids, contrast, density (Carlton, Cullinan, Carroll)**

771. (B) Speed is a factor used to describe image density. **speed, density (Carroll, Cullinan, Carlton, Bushong, Curry)**

772. (A) The radiograph in Figure 14 exhibits insufficient density but satisfactory contrast because bony structures are visible and of appropriate contrast in some areas where density is sufficient. An increase in mAs will increase density without affecting contrast. **density, film critique (Carlton, Cullinan, Carroll)**

773. (B) 60 to 70 kVp would produce relatively low contrast, as desired for an iodine based contrast medium for an intravenous pyelogram. **kVp, contrast (Carlton, Cullinan, Carroll)**

774. (C) Grid ratio and film/screen speed do not affect recorded detail. Increased OFD decreases recorded detail. **recorded detail, detail, penumbra (Carlton, Cullinan, Carroll)**

775. (D) High contrast images exhibit a great difference between adjacent shades of gray. **contrast (Carlton, Cullinan, Carroll)**

776. (C) Decreased FOD increases density. Increased grid ratio decreases density. Increased OFD decreases the scatter that reaches the image receptor, which decreases density. **density (Carlton, Carroll, Cullinan, Bushong)**

777. (D) Posterior oblique projections would place the posterior lumbar facets closest to the image receptor, thus producing the best possible recorded detail. **recorded detail, detail (Carlton, Cullinan, Ballinger)**

778. (D) Film latitude, OFD, and collimation all affect radiographic density. **density (Cullinan, Carroll, Carlton, Bushong)**

779. (A) Both tissue thickness and composition are part of subject contrast. Metabolic activity has no effect on subject contrast radiographically. **contrast, subject contrast, tissue (Carroll, Cullinan, Carlton)**

780. (B) Mismatched film and screens result in decreased density because the film is not sensitive to all of the light emitted by the intensifying screens. **screen/film combinations, intensifying screens, film (Carlton, Cullinan, Bushong, Carroll)**

781. (D) Size and shape are the two types of distortion. **distortion (Carlton, Cullinan, Carroll)**

782. (B) Anode heel effect and central ray alignment have little effect on image contrast. Film speed directly affects image contrast. **contrast, anode heel effect, film speed (Carlton, Bushong, Carroll, Cullinan)**

783. (A) A light film has few silver atoms deposited in the silver halides of the film. **density (Carlton, Cullinan, Carroll)**

784. (C) Milliamperage controls the number and quantity of photons. Photon wavelength is controlled by kVp. **mAs, density (Carlton, Bushong, Carroll, Cullinan)**

785. (C) High kVp reduces contrast. Reduced OFD increases scattered radiation to the image receptor, thus reducing contrast. Use of a grid increases contrast. **contrast (Carlton, Carroll, Cullinan, Bushong)**

786. (D) D is 58 kVp at 2 mAs. 58 kVp is 15% more than 50 kVp, which produces a doubling in density. This is compensated by reducing the mAs value by half, from 3 to 1.5. The addition of 33% more mAs from 1.5 to 2 produces an image that is 33% darker. **density, 15% rule (Cullinan, Carlton, Bushong, Selman, Carroll)**

787. (B) Diagnostic film/screen combinations are often capable of 1 to 10 lp/mm. **resolution, recorded detail, detail (Cullinan, Carlton, Bushong, Carroll)**

788. (D) Because mAs is relatively proportional to image density, doubling image density requires a doubling of mAs. **mAs, density (Cullinan, Carlton, Carroll)**

789. (A) Magnification decreases recorded detail. **magnification, recorded detail, detail, distortion, size distortion (Carlton, Cullinan, Bushong, Selman, Carroll)**

790. (D) An asthenic body habitus has the smallest volume of tissue. This results in more subject contrast which would produce the highest image contrast. **part thickness, body habitus (Ballinger, Carroll, Carlton, Cullinan)**

791. (A) An increase of 100% in mA will double mAs. According to the 15% rule, a 15% decrease in kVp will maintain image density. **15% rule, density (Carlton, Cullinan, Carroll, Bushong)**

792. (C) An upside-down focused grid will permit the nearly perpendicular portion of the center of the diverging beam to reach the image receptor but will absorb a much greater percentage of the divergent outside edges of the beam, resulting in an image that has nearly sufficient density at the center but is light at both sides. **grids (Carlton, Carroll, Cullinan, Bushong)**

793. (A) The possibility of motion reducing recorded detail would be most decreased if the patient were in a comfortable supine position. **motion, recorded detail, detail (Ballinger, Carlton, Cullinan, Carroll)**

794. (A) Increased OFD and decreased FFD both decrease recorded detail. Contrast has no effect on recorded detail. **recorded detail, detail, penumbra (Carlton, Cullinan, Carroll)**

795. (C) This is a definition of penumbra. **penumbra, recorded detail (Carlton, Carroll, Cullinan, Bushong, Selman)**

796. (B) Increased FOD increases resolution. High kVp has no effect on resolution. Reduced OFD increases resolution. **resolution, recorded detail, detail (Carlton, Carroll, Cullinan, Bushong)**

797. (C) C is 120 kVp at 4 mAs. Reducing mAs from 8 to 4 reduces density by half. **density, mAs (Cullinan, Carlton, Bushong, Selman, Carroll)**

798. (C) Anterior oblique projections would place the sacroiliac joints farthest to the image receptor, thus producing the poorest recorded detail. **recorded detail, detail (Carlton, Cullinan, Ballinger)**

799. (B) Increasing kVp (by 15%) and decreasing mAs (by half) produces less contrast according to the 15% rule. **15% rule, density, contrast (Cullinan, Carlton, Bushong, Selman)**

800. (B) The original radiograph used 30 mAs. 30 mAs/0.15 s = 200 mA. **mAs (Selman, Bushong, Cullinan, Carlton, Carroll)**

801. (B) Film speed and base-plus-fog effect radiographic contrast. FFD has no effect on contrast. **contrast (Cullinan, Carroll, Carlton, Bushong)**

802. (B) Most diagnostic radiographic acceptance ranges include images with densities up to 90 to 100% above optimal. This is equivalent to three 30% visible densities. **film critique, density, optimal density (Carlton, Carroll)**

803. (C) Slower speed, low contrast films have wider latitude, which permits the recording of a wider range of exposures values. **latitude, sensitometry (Carlton, Cullinan, Carroll)**

804. (B) Both decreased kVp and increased grid frequency will reduce scattered radiation reaching the image receptor. FFD has little effect on scatter production. **scatter (Carlton, Bushong, Selman, Cullinan, Carroll)**

805. (C) Changes in distance also change recorded detail. **distance, recorded detail, detail (Cullinan, Carroll, Carlton)**

806. (C) According to the magnification formula FFD/FOD, 40/20 = 2.00. **magnification factor, distortion (Carlton, Cullinan, Carroll, Bushong)**

807. (C) Anode heel effect and intensifying screen speed affect image density. Central ray alignment has little noticeable effect on image density. **density, anode heel effect, intensifying screen speed (Carlton, Bushong, Carroll, Cullinan)**

808. (B) A dark film has experienced a great amount of reduction during development. **density, processing, development, reduction, film processing (Carlton, Cullinan, Carroll)**

809. (B) kVp controls the average photon wavelength and penetrating ability of photons. The number of photons is controlled by mAs. **kVp (Carlton, Bushong, Carroll, Cullinan)**

810. (A) Use of a grid and low kVp increase contrast. Reduced OFD increases scattered radiation to the image receptor, thus reducing contrast. **contrast (Carlton, Carroll, Cullinan, Bushong)**

811. (C) C is 60 kVp at 8 mAs. 8 mAs is nearly half of 14, thus reducing density to half. **density, 15% rule (Cullinan, Carlton, Bushong, Selman, Carroll)**

812. (D) The highest kVp will produce the longest scale of contrast, if image density remains the same, as it does in the examples. **contrast, 15% rule (Cullinan, Carlton, Carroll)**

RADIOGRAPHIC PROCEDURES
General Procedural Considerations
2% (28) 813-840

813. (A) Upper ribs should be examined on inspiration to push the diaphragm down. **ribs (Ballinger, Bontrager, Eisenberg POSITIONING)**

814. (C) This is a definition of pelvimetry. **pelvimetry (Ballinger, Bontrager, Eisenberg POSITIONING)**

815. (A) This is a definition of the anatomic position. **anatomic position (Ballinger, Bontrager, Eisenberg POSITIONING)**

816. (B) This is a definition of distal. **distal (Ballinger, Bontrager, Eisenberg POSITIONING)**

817. (D) A patient is lying on his or her left side when he or she is in a left decubitus position. This places the left side of the body on the x-ray table, closest to the image receptor. **decubitus position (Ballinger, Bontrager, Eisenberg POSITIONING)**

818. (C) The lateral cervicothoracic region should be examined with suspended breathing. The position of the diaphragm is not critical. **cervicothoracic region, cervical spine, thoracic spine (Ballinger, Bontrager, Eisenberg POSITIONING)**

819. (D) This is a definition of pronation. **pronation (Ballinger, Bontrager, Eisenberg POSITIONING)**

820. (D) This is a definition of an oblique position. **oblique (Ballinger, Bontrager, Eisenberg POSITIONING)**

821. (B) An AP projection would increase the probability of a pediatric patient holding still because the patient is easier to restrain and is more likely to cooperate when he or she can see what is happening. **skull, pediatric patients (Ballinger, Bontrager, Eisenberg POSITIONING)**

822.   (C) Underwear with wide elastic banding may change tissue density sufficiently to produce an image artifact in the form of a band of lesser density across the abdomen.   Pants with metallic or plastic fasteners will produce image artifacts of the fasteners.   Dentures are not within the area of interest for a stomach examination.   **stomach (Ballinger, Bontrager, Eisenberg POSITIONING)**

823.   (D) This is a definition of extension.   **extension (Ballinger, Bontrager, Eisenberg POSITIONING)**

824.   (A) A transverse plane divides the body into superior and inferior divisions. **transverse plane (Ballinger, Bontrager, Eisenberg POSITIONING)**

825.   (A) This is a definition of projection.   **projection (Ballinger, Bontrager, Eisenberg POSITIONING)**

826.   (B) Lower ribs should be examined on expiration to push the diaphragm up. **ribs (Ballinger, Bontrager, Eisenberg POSITIONING)**

827.   (D) This is a definition of a lateral projection. **lateral (Ballinger, Bontrager, Eisenberg POSITIONING)**

828.   (B) This is a definition of adduction.   **adduction (Ballinger, Bontrager, Eisenberg POSITIONING)**

829.   (B) This is a definition of the coronal plane.   **coronal plane (Ballinger, Bontrager, Eisenberg POSITIONING)**

830.   (D) Continued breathing during a lateral projection of the thoracic spine will produce a blurring of the ribs.   This permits better visualization of the underlying thoracic vertebra. **thoracic spine (Ballinger, Bontrager, Eisenberg POSITIONING)**

831.   (D) This is a definition of caudal. **caudal (Ballinger, Bontrager, Eisenberg POSITIONING)**

832.   (A) This is a definition of dorsal. **dorsal (Ballinger, Bontrager, Eisenberg POSITIONING)**

833.   (D) The sagittal plane divides the body into right and left sections. **sagittal plane (Ballinger, Bontrager, Eisenberg POSITIONING)**

834.   (B) The abdomen should be examined on expiration to push the diaphragm up and reduce tissue thickness. **abdomen (Ballinger, Bontrager, Eisenberg POSITIONING)**

835.   (D) This is a definition of proximal.   **proximal (Ballinger, Bontrager, Eisenberg POSITIONING)**

836.   (C) This is a definition of flexion. **flexion (Ballinger, Bontrager, Eisenberg POSITIONING)**

837. (B) This is a definition of abduction. **abduction (Ballinger, Bontrager, Eisenberg POSITIONING)**

838. (A) The chest should be examined on inspiration to push the diaphragm down. **chest (Ballinger, Bontrager, Eisenberg POSITIONING)**

839. (C) The right iliac abdominal region is located immediately inferior to the right lumbar region. **abdominal regions (Ballinger, Bontrager, Eisenberg POSITIONING)**

840. (A) This is a definition of the sagittal plane. **sagittal plane (Ballinger, Bontrager, Eisenberg POSITIONING)**

RADIOGRAPHIC PROCEDURES
Specific Imaging Procedures
26% (364) 841-1204

841. (C) The AP internal rotation shoulder demonstrates the humerus in the true lateral position. **shoulder (Ballinger, Bontrager, Eisenberg)**

842. (D) The ulnar styloid process is located immediately distal to the head of the ulna. **elbow, ulna (Ballinger, Bontrager, Eisenberg)**

843. (A) This is a definition of the hyoid bone. **hyoid (Ballinger, Bontrager, Eisenberg)**

844. (C) The esophagus, thyroid, and thymus gland all are found in the mediastinum. **mediastinum (Ballinger, Bontrager, Eisenberg)**

845. (A) This is a definition of an enzyme. **digestion (Anthony, Hole)**

846. (C) This is a definition of chyme. **digestion (Anthony, Hole)**

847. (B) To include both the stomach and duodenal loop, the centering point should be the duodenal bulb. **stomach (Ballinger, Bontrager, Eisenberg)**

848. (C) This is a definition of a nephrotomy. A nephrectomy is the surgical removal of a kidney. **nephrotomy (Ballinger)**

849. (C) The removal of nitrogenous waste, regulation of water levels, and the regulations of the acid-base balance and electrolyte levels are normal functions of the renal system. The presence of RBCs in urine is a pathologic condition. **urinary system, kidney (Hole, Anthony)**

850. (A) The acromion process is most lateral. The coracoid process is most superior. **scapula (Ballinger, Anthony, Hole)**

851. (B) Os magnum, capitate, and capitatum all are names for the same wrist bone. **wrist (Ballinger, Anthony, Hole)**

852. (A) The hand should rest on the lateral surface for a lateral projection of the 2nd digit. The hand must be rotated medially from a PA position to place the lateral surface on the image receptor. **hand (Ballinger, Bontrager)**

853. (A) The lateromedial position with the central ray entering laterally and exiting medially provides a profile view of the olecranon process of the ulna free from superimposition. **elbow (Ballinger, Bontrager)**

854. (C) The base of the 3rd metatarsal is the centering point for the AP foot. **foot (Ballinger, Bontrager, Eisenberg)**

855. (A) The radial notch is the depression on the lateral side of the ulnar coronoid process with which the radial head articulates. **ulna (Ballinger, Anthony, Hole)**

856. (D) The central ray should be angled 40° cephalad for the axial plantodorsal projection of the os calcis or calcaneus. **calcaneus, os calcis (Ballinger, Bontrager, Eisenberg)**

857. (D) The pisiform and greater multangular (trapezium) are most anterior as seen on a lateral wrist radiograph. **wrist (Ballinger, Bontrager, Eisenberg)**

858. (C) The lateral (external) oblique projection of the elbow demonstrates the radial head especially well. **elbow (Ballinger, Bontrager, Eisenberg)**

859. (C) The cervical region (labeled 1) is lordotic. The regions of the spinal (vertebral) column that are convex anteriorly are called lordotic. **lordosis, vertebra, spine (Ballinger, Bontrager, Eisenberg, Hole, Anthony)**

860. (C) The lumbar region (labeled 3) is lordotic. The regions of the spinal (vertebral) column that are convex anteriorly are called lordotic. **lordosis, vertebra, spine (Ballinger, Bontrager, Eisenberg, Hole, Anthony)**

861. (C) The term venography is used to indicate imaging of the venous system. **venography (Snopek, Tortorici, Ballinger)**

862. (B) In both the LPO and RAO positions, the hepatic flexure is projected in a more open position. **colon, digestive system (Ballinger, Bontrager, Eisenberg)**

863. (B) This is a definition of edema. **edema (Eisenberg PATHOLOGY)**

864. (B) Inversion of the feet causes the lesser trochanter to be rotated to a more medial projection where it can be seen on an AP projection. **hip (Ballinger, Bontrager, Eisenberg)**

865. (C) For the majority of patients, the umbilicus is approximately level with L3-L4. **umbilicus (Ballinger)**

866.   (D) Because the foot assumes a nearly true lateral position with the medial side down toward the image receptor, the lateromedial projection is preferred. However, if a structure of interest is lateral, a mediolateral projection can, and should be, used. **foot (Ballinger, Bontrager, Eisenberg)**

867.   (B) The left petrous portion of the temporal bone exhibits more recorded detail when closest to the image receptor. **temporal bone, petrous portion (Ballinger, Bontrager, Eisenberg)**

868.   (B) This is a definition of an aneurysm. **aneurysm (Eisenberg PATHOLOGY)**

869.   (A) The sphenoidal sinus appears between the foramen magnum and the maxillary sinuses on a submentovertical projection of the skull. **sphenoidal sinuses, submentovertical (Ballinger, Bontrager, Eisenberg)**

870.   (C) The pisiform is the only carpal bone that has a single name. **wrist (Ballinger, Bontrager, Eisenberg)**

871.   (B) Demonstrating the maximum amount of posterior breast tissue is the primary consideration when compressing for mammography. **mammography (Ballinger, Bontrager, Eisenberg)**

872.   (A) The orbitomeatal base line runs from the external auditory meatus to the outer canthus of the eye. **skull topography (Ballinger, Bontrager, Eisenberg)**

873.   (B) The surgical neck of the femur is illustrated by #2 in Figure 16. **hip, pelvis, femur (Ballinger, Hole, Anthony, Eisenberg, Bontrager)**

874.   (C) The lesser trochanter of the femur is illustrated by #3 in Figure 16. **hip, pelvis, femur (Ballinger, Hole, Anthony, Eisenberg, Bontrager)**

875.   (A) The acetabulum is illustrated by #1 in Figure 16. **hip, pelvis, femur (Ballinger, Hole, Anthony, Eisenberg, Bontrager)**

876.   (C) The central ray for a routine PA chest should be directed at the level of T6-T7. **chest (Ballinger, Bontrager, Eisenberg)**

877.   (C) The ureters are illustrated by #3 and #5 in Figure 17. **urinary system, kidney (Hole, Anthony, Ballinger, Eisenberg, Bontrager)**

878.   (D) The renal pelvis is illustrated by #6 in Figure 17. **urinary system, kidney (Hole, Anthony, Eisenberg, Bontrager)**

879.   (B) The lower pole of the left kidney is illustrated by #2 in Figure 17. **urinary system, kidney (Hole, Anthony, Eisenberg, Bontrager)**

880.   (D) An angle of 15° cephalad will project the central ray perpendicular to the anterior and posterior surfaces of the sacrum. **sacrum (Ballinger, Bontrager, Eisenberg)**

881.   (D) The parotid glands are salivary glands. The term sialography is used to describe the examination of these glands. **parotid gland, salivary glands, sialography (Ballinger, Bontrager, Eisenberg, Snopek)**

882.   (D) The articular facets of the lumbar spine are about 45° from the transverse process, so an oblique projection demonstrates them best. **spine, lumbar oblique, facets (Ballinger, Bontrager, Eisenberg)**

883.   (A) Supination of the hand opens the ulnar-radial spaces, while pronation causes superimposition of the ulna and radius. **forearm (Ballinger, Bontrager, Eisenberg)**

884.   (B) The apophyseal articulations of the thoracic spine are best visualized with a 20° oblique position. **thoracic spine, thoracic vertebrae (Ballinger, Bontrager, Eisenberg)**

885.   (D) A moveable core guide wire has a variable inside portion. **guide wire (Snopek, Tortorici)**

886.   (A) The PA skull position by the Caldwell method requires that the orbitomeatal line be perpendicular to the image receptor. The midsagittal plane is parallel to the central ray. The central ray is angled 15° caudad, not cephalad. **skull (Ballinger, Bontrager, Eisenberg)**

887.   (D) The urinary system consists of the kidneys, ureters, bladder, and urethra. **urinary system (Anthony, Hole, Ballinger, Bontrager, Eisenberg)**

888.   (B) The common bile duct is formed by the union of the common hepatic duct and the cystic duct. **digestive system, gallbladder, liver (Anthony, Hole, Ballinger, Bontrager, Eisenberg)**

889.   (D) A lateral chest radiography should visualize the heart and diaphragm, costophrenic angles and apices of the lungs, and the ribs posterior to the vertebral column should be superimposed. **thoracic viscera, chest (Ballinger, Eisenberg)**

890.   (C) The zygomatic process of the temporal bone (#6) and the zygomatic process of the zygomatic (malar) bone (#7) combine to form the zygomatic arch in Figure 18. **skull, zygomatic arch (Hole, Anthony, Ballinger, Eisenberg, Bontrager)**

891.   (C) The sagittal suture forms the articulation of the parietal bones and is illustrated by #10 in Figure 18. **skull, sagittal suture (Hole, Anthony, Eisenberg, Bontrager)**

892.   (C) The maxillary bones are the largest bones of the face and are illustrated by #5 in Figure 18. **skull, maxillary bone (Hole, Anthony, Eisenberg, Bontrager)**

893.   (A) The lesser tuberosity is visualized between the humeral head and greater tuberosity on a true AP position of the humerus. **humerus (Ballinger, Bontrager, Eisenberg)**

894.	(A) A PA projection of the sinuses is achieved if the patient is positioned so the midsagittal plane and orbitomeatal line are perpendicular to the image receptor and the central ray is perpendicular, exiting at the nasion. **paranasal sinuses, sinuses (Ballinger, Bontrager, Eisenberg)**

895.	(C) The proper centering point for a lateral position of the sella turcica is 3/4" anterior and 3/4" superior to the external auditory meatus. **skull (Ballinger, Bontrager, Eisenberg)**

896.	(A) The lateral skull position requires that the interpupillary line be perpendicular and the midsagittal plane be parallel to the image receptor. The infraorbitomeatal line is perpendicular to the central ray. **skull (Ballinger, Bontrager, Eisenberg)**

897.	(A) Hypersthenic patients tend to exhibit an angle between the midsagittal plane and the tabletop when the skull is positioned for a lateral projection. Placement of a properly adjusted support device, such as a sponge or pillow, under the parietal bone will bring the midsagittal plane parallel with the tabletop. **skull (Ballinger, Bontrager, Eisenberg)**

898.	(A) The zygomatic arch is composed of the temporal and zygomatic bones. **skull (Anthony, Hole, Ballinger, Bontrager, Eisenberg)**

899.	(A) The pyloric orifice is the opening between the duodenum and the stomach. It is controlled by the pyloric sphincter. **digestive system, gastrointestinal, stomach (Anthony, Hole, Ballinger, Bontrager, Eisenberg)**

900.	(C) The submandibular gland is also known as the submaxillary gland. **salivary glands (Anthony, Hole, Ballinger, Bontrager, Eisenberg)**

901.	(C) The esophagus is posterior to the trachea, anterior to the vertebral column, and medial to the heart. **mediastinum, thoracic viscera, esophagus, digestive system (Anthony, Hole, Ballinger, Bontrager, Eisenberg)**

902.	(A) The body of the sternum is also known as the gladiolus. **bony thorax, sternum (Hole, Anthony, Ballinger, Bontrager, Eisenberg)**

903.	(A) The pedicle forms the eye of the apophyseal joint "scotty dog" that can be demonstrated on oblique projections of the lumbar spine. **vertebral column, lumbar spine (Ballinger, Bontrager, Eisenberg)**

904.	(D) A 10° to 15° LPO positions the patient semi-supine and permits visualization of the hip joint and proximal left femur. **femur (Ballinger, Bontrager, Eisenberg)**

905.	(B) The brachycephalic skull is broad from side to side and has an angle of 54° between the internal structures and the midsagittal plane. However, it is short from front to back. The dolichocephalic skull is long from front to back. **skull (Ballinger, Bontrager, Eisenberg)**

906. (A) The average normal transit time for the stomach to empty is 2 to 3 hours. **digestive system, gastrointestinal (Ballinger, Hole, Anthony, Eisenberg)**

907. (D) Postoperative cholangiography is capable of detecting the status of the sphincter of the hepatopancreatic ampulla, the presence of previously undetected stones, and the patency and size of the biliary ducts. **digestive system, cholangiography (Ballinger, Bontrager, Eisenberg)**

908. (D) Full exhalation for an AP abdomen raises the diaphragm and demonstrates a greater portion of the abdomen. **digestive system, abdomen (Ballinger, Bontrager, Eisenberg)**

909. (A) The nucleus pulposus is the central mass of semigelatinous material inside an intervertebral disk. The annulus fibrosus is the tough cartilaginous material surrounding the nucleus pulposus. The pedicles are part of the bony vertebrae, not the intervertebral disk. **vertebral column, intervertebral disk (Ballinger, Bontrager, Eisenberg, Anthony, Hole)**

910. (D) L4 is at the level of the iliac crest. **surface landmarks (Ballinger, Bontrager, Eisenberg)**

911. (B) There are 7 tarsals: calcaneus, talus, scaphoid, cuboid, and 3 cuneiforms. **foot (Ballinger, Bontrager, Eisenberg)**

912. (C) This is a definition of pneumothorax. **pneumothorax (Eisenberg PATHOLOGY)**

913. (A) The normal position of the humeral head in a scapular Y position is superimposed over the junction of the Y. When it appears beneath the coracoid process, there is an anterior dislocation. When it appears beneath the acromion process, there is a posterior dislocation. **shoulder (Ballinger, Eisenberg PATHOLOGY)**

914. (C) The trapezium is immediately proximal to the carpometacarpal joint of the thumb. **hand (Ballinger, Bontrager, Eisenberg)**

915. (C) The placement of the two leads at the ends of the wire is at the apex and left ventricle of the heart shadow, thus proving them to be electrocardiographic leads. **electrocardiography, ECG (Torres, Ehrlich)**

916. (C) The patient in Figure 19 was erect when the exposure was made because there is free air under the right diaphragm. Free air rises only when the patient is erect. **abdomen, chest (Ballinger, Eisenberg PATHOLOGY)**

917. (B) The medial (internal) oblique elbow projects the ulnar coronoid process free of superimposition. **elbow (Ballinger, Bontrager, Eisenberg)**

918. (C) There are 7° between the orbitomeatal and infraorbitomeatal skull base lines. There are 8° between the orbitomeatal and glabellomeatal lines. **skull (Ballinger, Bontrager, Eisenberg)**

919. (C) Urography includes retrograde pyelography. Cystography refers to examinations of the urinary bladder, while nephrotomography refers to tomographic examination of the kidneys. **urinary system (Anthony, Hole, Ballinger, Bontrager, Eisenberg)**

920. (B) The presence of barium in the cecum signals its transit through the ileocecal valve. This completes a small bowel study. **small bowel, small intestine (Ballinger, Bontrager, Eisenberg)**

921. (C) The LAO or RPO position will project the ribs that normally overshadow the heart free of superimposition. **bony thorax, ribs (Ballinger, Bontrager, Eisenberg)**

922. (C) Phonation of "ah" during exposure of the atlas and axis in the AP open mouth position affixes the tongue to the floor of the mouth, thus avoiding superimposing its soft tissue over the odontoid process. **vertebral column, atlas and axis, cervical (Ballinger, Bontrager, Eisenberg)**

923. (A) The femoral head articulates with the hip bone at the acetabulum. **pelvis, hip, femur (Ballinger, Bontrager, Eisenberg)**

924. (C) This is a definition of a lipoma. **lipoma (Eisenberg PATHOLOGY)**

925. (B) The lamina is illustrated by #7 in Figure 20. **vertebral column, spine (Ballinger, Bontrager, Eisenberg, Anthony, Hole)**

926. (B) The vertebral foramen is illustrated by #3 in Figure 20. **vertebral column, spine (Ballinger, Bontrager, Eisenberg, Anthony, Hole)**

927. (C) The superior facet of an apophyseal joint (also known as the superior articular process) is illustrated by #6 in Figure 20. **vertebral column, spine (Ballinger, Bontrager, Eisenberg, Anthony, Hole)**

928. (D) A rib is illustrated by #2 in Figure 20. **vertebral column, spine (Ballinger, Bontrager, Eisenberg, Anthony, Hole)**

929. (C) The midsagittal plane and orbitomeatal line should be perpendicular to the image receptor for a PA axial position (Caldwell method) of the sinuses. **paranasal sinuses, sinuses (Ballinger, Bontrager, Eisenberg)**

930. (D) The zygoma, sphenoid, and ethmoid bones form part of the orbit. It is completed by the lacrimal, frontal, maxilla, and palatine bones. **skull (Ballinger, Bontrager, Eisenberg)**

931. (D) The midsagittal plane intersects the glabella, nasion, acanthion, and mental point of the skull. **skull (Ballinger, Bontrager, Eisenberg)**

932. (D) The LAO best demonstrates the splenic flexure of the colon. **colon (Ballinger, Bontrager, Eisenberg)**

933. (D) The 11th to 12th pairs of ribs do not have anterior cartilage and are therefore known as floating ribs. **bony thorax, ribs (Hole, Anthony, Ballinger, Bontrager, Eisenberg)**

934. (A) An amphiarthrotic joint, which permits only a slight movement between the individual vertebrae but considerable movement of the entire column, is formed between two vertebral bodies. **vertebral column (Ballinger, Bontrager, Eisenberg)**

935. (B) The navicular (scaphoid) articulates with the proximal end of all three cuneiforms. **foot (Ballinger, Bontrager, Eisenberg, Anthony, Hole)**

936. (D) A Grashey method position for the glenoid fossa is obtained when the patient is rotated approximately 35° to 45° toward the affected side and the central ray is directed at the shoulder joint. **shoulder (Ballinger, Bontrager, Eisenberg)**

937. (D) The acetabulum is formed by the junction of the ilium, ischium, and pubis. **acetabulum, hip, pelvis (Ballinger, Bontrager, Eisenberg, Anthony, Hole)**

938. (D) The posterior profile position (Stenvers method) and anterior profile position (Arcelen method) are complimentary positions. **temporal bone, petrous portions (Ballinger, Bontrager, Eisenberg)**

939. (A) The inion, or external occipital protuberance, is located on the exterior surface of the occipital bone. **skull (Anthony, Hole, Ballinger, Bontrager, Eisenberg)**

940. (C) The suprarenal, or adrenal, glands are part of the endocrine system. **adrenal, suprarenal, endocrine (Hole, Anthony, Ballinger, Bontrager, Eisenberg)**

941. (B) Bile is secreted by the liver and stored in the gallbladder. **digestive system, bile, liver (Anthony, Hole, Ballinger, Bontrager, Eisenberg)**

942. (C) The carina is the bifurcation of the trachea. **thoracic viscera, chest, trachea, respiratory system (Ballinger, Bontrager, Eisenberg, Anthony, Hole)**

943. (B) The trachea forms a junction with the larynx at the level of the 6th cervical vertebra. **thoracic viscera, trachea, respiratory system (Anthony, Hole, Ballinger, Bontrager, Eisenberg)**

944. (B) The approximate superior angle of the neck of the femur is 120° to 130°, although it varies with age, sex, and body type. **pelvis, femur, hip (Ballinger, Bontrager, Eisenberg, Hole, Anthony)**

945. (B) The image in Figure 21 is a carotid angiogram subtraction film. **subtraction (Ballinger, Snopek, Tortorici, Carlton)**

946. (B) The carotid siphon is illustrated by #5 in Figure 21. **cerebral angiography (Ballinger, Bontrager, Eisenberg, Tortorici, Snopek)**

947. (C) The internal carotid artery is illustrated by #3 in Figure 21. **cerebral angiography (Ballinger, Bontrager, Eisenberg, Tortorici, Snopek)**

948. (D) The gonion is the angle of the mandible. **mandible, skull (Anthony, Hole, Ballinger, Bontrager, Eisenberg)**

949. (C) The fontanels are areas of incomplete ossification that are present in newborn infants. **skull (Anthony, Hole, Ballinger, Bontrager, Eisenberg)**

950. (C) The stomach moves superiorly when a patient changes from an upright to recumbent position. **stomach, digestive system, gastrointestinal (Ballinger, Bontrager, Eisenberg)**

951. (B) Endoscopic retrograde cholangiopancreatography (ERCP) uses a fiberoptic endoscope to place a cannula into the hepatopancreatic ampulla and into the common bile duct. **digestive system, biliary system, pancreas (Ballinger, Snopek, Tortorici)**

952. (D) The psoas muscles, liver, and kidneys can all be demonstrated on an AP abdomen projection. **digestive system, abdomen (Ballinger, Bontrager, Eisenberg)**

953. (D) The sternal angle is formed by the gladiolus and xiphoid process. **bony thorax, sternum (Hole, Anthony, Ballinger, Bontrager, Eisenberg)**

954. (C) The coccyx is demonstrated on a PA projection (in a prone position) by a central ray angle of 10° cephalad. **vertebral column, coccyx (Ballinger, Bontrager, Eisenberg)**

955. (A) The urinary bladder and rectum are within the pelvic cavity. The kidneys are in the abdominal cavity. **body cavities (Ballinger, Bontrager, Eisenberg, Anthony, Hole)**

956. (C) T10 is at the level of the xiphoid tip. **surface landmarks (Ballinger, Bontrager, Eisenberg)**

957. (B) The obturator foramen of the pelvis is the largest foramina in the body. **pelvis (Ballinger, Bontrager, Eisenberg)**

958. (A) The tibia includes the medial malleolus. The fibula includes the lateral malleolus. **foot (Ballinger, Bontrager, Eisenberg, Hole, Anthony)**

959. (C) An embolism is a clot that has detached from a thrombosis and is moving freely in the circulatory system. **thrombosis, embolism (Eisenberg PATHOLOGY)**

960. (C) External rotation of the arm during an inferosuperior axial shoulder joint projection brings the lesser tubercle into profile and superimposes the greater tubercle onto the head of the humerus, thus minimizing superimposition onto the glenohumeral joint space. **shoulder (Ballinger, Bontrager, Eisenberg)**

961. (B) Supination of the hand avoids superimposition of the radius and ulna. **elbow, forearm (Ballinger, Bontrager, Eisenberg)**

962. (A) The left lung has 2 lobes, the right lung has 3. **lung (Hole, Anthony, Ballinger, Eisenberg, Bontrager)**

963. (C) The duodenum is illustrated by #13 in Figure 22. **small bowel, digestive system (Ballinger, Bontrager, Eisenberg, Anthony, Hole)**

964. (B) The pancreas is illustrated by #3 in Figure 22. **pancreas (Ballinger, Bontrager, Eisenberg, Anthony, Hole)**

965. (A) The descending colon is illustrated by #5 in Figure 22. **colon, digestive system (Ballinger, Bontrager, Eisenberg, Anthony, Hole)**

966. (B) The cecum is illustrated by #9 in Figure 22. **colon, digestive system (Ballinger, Bontrager, Eisenberg, Anthony, Hole)**

967. (D) The rugae are the folds of the gastric lining. **digestive system, gastrointestinal, stomach (Anthony, Hole, Ballinger, Bontrager, Eisenberg)**

968. (A) Sialography is the examination of the salivary glands and ducts. **salivary glands (Ballinger, Bontrager, Eisenberg)**

969. (D) The thymus gland is located directly posterior to the manubrium so it is anterior to the trachea, superior to the heart, and medial to the sternoclavicular joints. **mediastinum, thoracic viscera, thymus (Anthony, Hole, Ballinger, Bontrager, Eisenberg)**

970. (B) The PA abdomen projection significantly reduces gonadal dose, especially in males. **digestive system, abdomen (Ballinger)**

971. (B) Fluid in the pleural cavity is best demonstrated by a lateral decubitus chest radiograph with the patient lying on the affected side, in this case the right side. **thoracic viscera, chest (Ballinger, Bontrager, Eisenberg)**

972. (A) An AP projection of the cervical spine with a 15° to 20° cephalad angulation will open the intervertebral disk spaces. **vertebral column, cervical (Ballinger, Bontrager, Eisenberg)**

973. (C) The patient should be in a 40° LPO position to demonstrate the left ilium in an AP projection. **pelvis (Ballinger, Bontrager, Eisenberg)**

974. (C) This is a definition of a ureterocele. **ureterocele (Eisenberg PATHOLOGY)**

975. (B) The body of the pubis is illustrated by #7 in Figure 24. **pelvis (Ballinger, Bontrager, Eisenberg, Anthony, Hole)**

976. (B) The anterior superior spine of the ilium (ASIS) is illustrated by #7 in Figure 24. **pelvis (Ballinger, Bontrager, Eisenberg, Anthony, Hole)**

977. (C) The sacrum is illustrated by #15 in Figure 24. **sacrum, pelvis (Ballinger, Bontrager, Eisenberg, Anthony, Hole)**

978. (B) The anterior inferior iliac spine is illustrated by #3 in Figure 24. **pelvis (Ballinger, Bontrager, Eisenberg, Anthony, Hole)**

979. (C) The lesser sciatic notch is illustrated by #12 in Figure 24. **pelvis (Ballinger, Bontrager, Eisenberg, Anthony, Hole)**

980. (C) The third cuneiform is most lateral, the first is most medial. There is no fourth cuneiform. **foot (Ballinger, Bontrager, Eisenberg, Hole, Anthony)**

981. (C) This is a definition of an infarct. **infarct (Eisenberg PATHOLOGY)**

982. (A) Both the transverse plane, which is controlled by the interpupillary baseline, and the midsagittal plane must be corrected to achieve a properly positioned lateral skull image. **cranium, skull, lateral (Eisenberg, Ballinger, Bontrager)**

983. (A) Both the Stenvers (posterior profile position) and Arcelin (anterior profile position) demonstrate the petrous portions of the temporal bone. **temporal bone, petrous portion (Ballinger, Bontrager, Eisenberg)**

984. (C) The hyoid serves as an attachment for the muscles of the throat and tongue but does not articulate with any other bone. **hyoid (Anthony, Hole, Ballinger, Bontrager, Eisenberg)**

985. (A) The clinoid processes, both anterior and posterior, are part of the sphenoid. The crista galli is part of the ethmoid. **skull (Anthony, Hole, Ballinger, Bontrager, Eisenberg)**

986. (C) The respiratory excursion of the kidneys is approximately 2.5 cm (1"). **urinary system (Ballinger, Bontrager, Eisenberg)**

987. (C) The duct of Wirsung, also called the pancreatic duct, is located in the center of the pancreas. **digestive system, pancreas (Hole, Anthony, Ballinger, Bontrager, Eisenberg)**

988. (C) There are normally four parathyroid glands. They are located on the posterior aspect of the thyroid gland, one above the other on each side. **parathyroid, neck (Anthony, Hole, Ballinger, Bontrager, Eisenberg)**

989. (C) The 7th rib is the longest rib. **bony thorax, ribs (Ballinger, Bontrager)**

990. (B) This is a definition of a sarcoma. **sarcoma (Eisenberg PATHOLOGY)**

991. (C) The centering point for an AP scapula is 2" inferior to the coracoid process. **scapula (Ballinger, Bontrager, Eisenberg)**

992. (B) The carpal bridge tangential position demonstrates the posterior bridge of the wrist. **wrist (Ballinger, Bontrager, Eisenberg)**

993. (B) The AP axial Towne method produces an image of the elongated occipital bone as shown in Figure 26. **skull, cranium, Towne method (Ballinger, Eisenberg, Bontrager)**

994. (D) A central ray angle of 40° was used in Figure 26a because the foramen magnum is completely above the petrous portions of the temporal bone. **skull, cranium, Towne method (Ballinger, Eisenberg, Bontrager)**

995. (C) The lambdoidal suture is illustrated by #1 in Figure 26b. **skull, cranium, Towne method (Ballinger, Bontrager, Eisenberg)**

996. (B) The inion and external occipital protuberance is illustrated by #2 in Figure 26b. **skull, cranium, Towne method (Ballinger, Bontrager, Eisenberg)**

997. (C) The posterior clinoid process is illustrated by #5 in Figure 26b. **skull, cranium, Towne method (Ballinger, Bontrager, Eisenberg)**

998. (A) A central ray angle of 30° was used in Figure 26b because the foramen magnum is completely within the petrous portions of the temporal bone. **skull, cranium, Towne method (Ballinger, Eisenberg, Bontrager)**

999. (C) The orbitomeatal line must be positioned 37° to the image receptor for a parietoacanthial projection (Waters method) of the paranasal sinuses. **paranasal sinuses, sinuses (Ballinger, Bontrager, Eisenberg)**

1000. (D) The midsagittal plane should be positioned 53° from the surface of the image receptor for a parieto-orbital oblique position (Rhese method) of the optic foramen. **skull (Ballinger, Bontrager, Eisenberg)**

1001. (D) The general survey AP axial position by the Towne method requires that the orbitomeatal line be perpendicular and the midsagittal plane be parallel to the image receptor. The central ray is directed 30° caudally. **skull (Ballinger, Bontrager, Eisenberg)**

1002. (C) There are 14 bones in the facial bones; 2 nasal, 2 lacrimal, 2 maxillary, 2 zygomatic, 2 palatine, 2 inferior nasal conchae, 1 vomer, 1 mandible. **skull (Anthony, Hole, Ballinger, Bontrager, Eisenberg)**

1003. (C) Placing the Colcher-Sussman method pelvimeter ruler 10 cm below the level of the symphysis pubis places it at the level of the ischial tuberosities. This permits the radiologist to perform magnification measurements more accurately. **female reproductive system, pelvimetry (Ballinger, Bontrager, Eisenberg)**

1004. (C) It takes about 15 to 20 minutes for intravenously injected contrast medium to achieve its greatest concentration in the renal collecting system during urography. **urinary system (Ballinger, Bontrager, Eisenberg)**

1005. (A) The prostate gland is located anterior to the rectum, surrounding the proximal part of the male urethra. **urinary system, reproductive system (Anthony, Hole, Ballinger, Bontrager, Eisenberg)**

1006. (B) The lateral best demonstrates the rectum. **colon (Ballinger, Bontrager, Eisenberg)**

1007. (C) The central ray should be directed 30° to 40° caudad for a PA axial position of the colon. **colon (Ballinger, Bontrager, Eisenberg)**

1008. (C) The average normal transit time for food from the mouth through the rectum is 24 hours. **digestive system, gastrointestinal (Ballinger, Hole, Anthony, Eisenberg)**

1009. (B) The mediastinum contains all of the thoracic organs except the lungs. **thoracic viscera, mediastinum (Anthony, Hole, Ballinger, Bontrager, Eisenberg)**

1010. (D) The femoral head is the most medial of the structures at the proximal end of the femur. **pelvis, hip, femur (Ballinger, Bontrager, Eisenberg, Hole, Anthony)**

1011. (D) The Beclere, Camp-Coventry, and Holmblad methods all demonstrate the intercondyloid fossa of the femur. **intercondyloid fossa (Ballinger, Bontrager, Eisenberg)**

1012. (C) The AP internal rotation shoulder demonstrates the lesser tubercle of the humerus medially and in profile. **shoulder (Ballinger, Bontrager, Eisenberg)**

1013. (A) The primary advantage of the ulnar flexion wrist is to obtain a better image of the navicular (scaphoid) free from foreshortening that occurs during a PA projection. **wrist (Ballinger, Bontrager, Eisenberg)**

1014. (B) The duodenal bulb is most often located at the level of L2 in an average-sized patient. **stomach (Ballinger, Bontrager, Eisenberg)**

1015. (C) Only the intravenous urogram, also known as an intravenous pyelogram, demonstrates renal function. Cystourethrography and retrograde pyelography demonstrate anatomy only. **urinary system (Anthony, Hole, Ballinger, Bontrager, Eisenberg)**

1016. (C) The epiglottis is the thin flap that covers the laryngeal entrance during swallowing. **digestive system, chest, epiglottis (Hole, Anthony, Ballinger, Bontrager, Eisenberg)**

1017. (A) Foreign bodies tend to enter the right bronchus more than the left because the right bronchus lies in a more vertical position and is larger. **thoracic viscera, lungs, respiratory system (Ballinger, Bontrager, Eisenberg)**

1018. (B) The symphysis pubis is the joint where the two pubic bones articulate. **pelvis (Ballinger, Bontrager, Eisenberg, Anthony, Hole)**

1019. (A) An erect position avoids engorgement of the pulmonary vessels. A 72" FFD will reduce magnification of the heart size shadow when compared to a 40" FFD. Image contrast is not increased by either the erect position or the larger FFD. **thoracic viscera, chest (Ballinger, Bontrager, Eisenberg)**

1020. (B) The central ray should be angled 15° to 20° cephalad for an AP projection of the cervical vertebrae. **vertebral column, cervical (Ballinger, Bontrager, Eisenberg)**

1021. (B) The liver is illustrated by #7 in Figure 28. **sectional anatomy, abdomen (Ballinger, Bontrager, Eisenberg, Anthony, Hole)**

1022. (A) The stomach is illustrated by #1 in Figure 28. **sectional anatomy, abdomen (Ballinger, Bontrager, Eisenberg, Anthony, Hole)**

1023. (C) The aorta is illustrated by #4 in Figure 28. **sectional anatomy, abdomen (Ballinger, Bontrager, Eisenberg, Anthony, Hole)**

1024. (A) The lungs and heart are within the abdominal cavity. The stomach is in the abdominal cavity. **body cavities (Ballinger, Bontrager, Eisenberg, Anthony, Hole)**

1025. (B) The talus articulates with the superior facet of the calcaneus (navicular). **foot (Ballinger, Bontrager, Eisenberg)**

1026. (B) The trochlea articulates with the coronoid epicondyle of the ulna. **elbow, humerus, forearm, ulna (Anthony, Hole, Ballinger, Bontrager, Eisenberg)**

1027. (A) In both the RPO and LAO positions the splenic flexure is projected in a more open position. **colon, digestive system (Ballinger, Bontrager, Eisenberg)**

1028. (A) A posterior profile position (Stenvers method) of the petrous portion of the temporal bone requires a 12° cephalad central ray angulation. **temporal bone, petrous portion (Ballinger, Bontrager, Eisenberg)**

1029. (A) The parieto-orbital oblique position (Rhese method) for the optic foramen has the central ray and acanthiomeatal line perpendicular to the image receptor. The midsagittal plane forms an angle of 53° with the image receptor. **skull (Ballinger, Bontrager, Eisenberg)**

1030. (A) The antrum of Highmore is the maxillary sinus which is located in the maxilla. **skull (Anthony, Hole, Ballinger, Bontrager, Eisenberg)**

1031. (A) The sagittal and lambdoidal sutures meet at the bregma. **skull (Anthony, Hole, Ballinger, Bontrager, Eisenberg)**

1032. (C) The small bowel is approximately 22 feet in length, the entire gastrointestinal tract is 29 to 30 feet in length. **digestive system, gastrointestinal (Ballinger, Anthony, Hole)**

1033. (C) The LAO position projects the gallbladder free from superimposition of the vertebral column. **digestive system, gallbladder (Ballinger, Bontrager, Eisenberg)**

1034. (A) The salivary glands are the sublingual, submandibular, and parotid. **salivary glands (Hole, Anthony, Ballinger, Bontrager, Eisenberg)**

1035.   (B) The cervical intervertebral foramina are directed 45° anterior and 15° inferior. **vertebral column, cervical spine (Ballinger, Bontrager, Eisenberg)**

1036.   (C) T4 is at the level of the sternal angle. **surface landmarks (Ballinger, Bontrager, Eisenberg)**

1037.   (B) The transthoracic lateral Lawrence method is designed to obtain a projection of the proximal 2/3 of the humerus without moving the arm. **shoulder (Ballinger, Bontrager, Eisenberg)**

1038.   (D) The elbow is comprised of the humerus, radius, and ulna. **elbow (Ballinger, Bontrager, Eisenberg, Anthony, Hole)**

1039.   (C) The PA radial flexion position opens the interspaces between the medial carpals. **wrist (Ballinger, Bontrager, Eisenberg)**

1040.   (C) For an RAO projection, the thorax should be obliqued an average of 15° to 20° to project the sternum free from vertebral superimposition. **bony thorax, sternum (Ballinger, Bontrager, Eisenberg)**

1041.   (C) The knee joint is best located by palpating the femoral and tibial condyles at the medial aspect of the knee. **knee (Ballinger, Bontrager, Eisenberg)**

1042.   (B) This is a definition of emphysema. **emphysema (Eisenberg PATHOLOGY)**

1043.   (C) The glenoid fossa of the scapula articulates with the head of the humerus. **shoulder girdle, scapula, humerus (Ballinger, Bontrager, Eisenberg)**

1044.   (B) The sigmoid colon is illustrated by #3 in Figure 29. **colon, digestive system (Ballinger, Bontrager, Eisenberg)**

1045.   (C) The gall bladder is illustrated by #6 in Figure 29. **biliary tract, gall bladder (Ballinger, Bontrager, Eisenberg)**

1046.   (A) The cecum is illustrated by #4 in Figure 29. **colon, digestive system (Ballinger, Bontrager, Eisenberg)**

1047.   (C) The descending colon (#2) is gas filled in Figure 29. **colon, digestive system (Ballinger, Bontrager, Eisenberg)**

1048.   (A) Operative cholangiography requires a short exposure time because the anesthetist must temporarily arrest respiration. Because the biliary tract is located in the upper right quadrant of the abdomen, the film must be centered to this area. A pressure injector is never used in cholangiography. **digestive system, cholangiography (Ballinger, Bontrager, Eisenberg)**

1049.   (A) A PA projection of the sinuses should be centered so the central ray exits at the nasion. **paranasal sinuses, sinuses (Ballinger, Bontrager, Eisenberg)**

1050. (B) The nose, zygoma, and chin should rest on the image receptor surface for a PA oblique axial position (Law method) of the facial bones. **facial bones (Ballinger, Bontrager, Eisenberg)**

1051. (C) The orbitomeatal line should be positioned 37° to the image receptor on a parietoacanthial position (Waters method). **facial bones (Ballinger, Bontrager, Eisenberg)**

1052. (D) The PA axial projection of the skull by the Haas method should demonstrate the petrous pyramids of the temporal bone symmetrically and the dorsum sellae within the shadow of the foramen magnum. It is essentially a reversed AP axial Townes method position. **skull (Ballinger, Bontrager, Eisenberg)**

1053. (C) The efferent arteriole leaves the renal glomerulus and communicates with the renal vein. **urinary system (Anthony, Hole, Ballinger, Bontrager, Eisenberg)**

1054. (A) The arms should be placed over the head for a dorsal decubitus abdomen position to remove them from the area of interest. **digestive system, abdomen (Ballinger, Bontrager, Eisenberg)**

1055. (D) The portal circulation connects the liver with the pancreas, spleen, stomach, gallbladder, and most of the intestinal tract. **digestive system, portal circulation (Anthony, Hole, Ballinger, Bontrager, Eisenberg)**

1056. (C) The Valsalva maneuver distends the subglottic larynx and trachea with air. **larynx, trachea (Ballinger)**

1057. (A) The scapulae are rotated laterally by rotating the palms of the hands upward when positioning for a PA chest. **thoracic viscera, chest (Ballinger, Bontrager, Eisenberg)**

1058. (B) The top of the cassette should be placed 1" to 1.5" above the iliac crest for an AP pelvis position. **pelvis (Ballinger, Bontrager, Eisenberg)**

1059. (B) The tibia is anterior and medial to the fibula. **leg, lower leg (Ballinger, Bontrager, Eisenberg, Anthony, Hole)**

1060. (D) Abduction of the arm to a right angle with the hand by the head when the patient is supine will pull the axillary border of the scapula lateral from the ribs. **scapula (Ballinger, Bontrager, Eisenberg)**

1061. (A) The thumb is the first digit. **digit, hand (Ballinger, Bontrager, Eisenberg, Hole, Anthony)**

1062. (C) The neck of the femur is illustrated by #10 in Figure 30. **lower extremity, femur, pelvis (Ballinger, Bontrager, Eisenberg, Anthony, Hole)**

1063. (C) The intertrochanteric crest (or line) is illustrated by #8 in Figure 30. **lower extremity, femur, pelvis (Ballinger, Bontrager, Eisenberg, Anthony, Hole)**

1064. (A) The lateral condyle is illustrated by #5 in Figure 30. **lower extremity, femur, knee (Ballinger, Bontrager, Eisenberg, Anthony, Hole)**

1065. (B) The proper centering point for the cassette for an AP projection of the abdomen when the patient is supine is at the iliac crests. **digestive system, abdomen (Ballinger, Bontrager, Eisenberg)**

1066. (B) The spleen is part of the lymphatic system. The liver, pancreas, and gallbladder are parts of the digestive system. **spleen, digestive system, lymphatic system (Hole, Anthony, Ballinger)**

1067. (A) Free air in the pleural cavity is best demonstrated by a lateral decubitus chest radiograph with the patient lying on the unaffected side, in this case, the left side. **thoracic viscera, chest (Ballinger, Bontrager, Eisenberg)**

1068. (A) The trachea is best demonstrated by having the patient slowly inhale during the exposure. **thoracic viscera, trachea, respiratory system, chest (Ballinger, Bontrager, Eisenberg)**

1069. (C) The normal sacrum is composed of 5 fused segments. **vertebral column, spine (Ballinger, Bontrager, Eisenberg)**

1070. (C) The Gaynor-Hart method for the carpal canal requires hyperextension of the wrist with the central ray directed 25° to 30° toward the base of the third metacarpal. **wrist (Ballinger, Bontrager, Eisenberg)**

1071. (C) The lacrimal bones are located at the anterior medial wall of the orbits. **skull (Anthony, Hole, Ballinger, Bontrager, Eisenberg)**

1072. (B) The cardiac orifice is the opening between the esophagus and the stomach. It is controlled by the cardiac sphincter. **digestive system, gastrointestinal, stomach (Anthony, Hole, Ballinger, Bontrager, Eisenberg)**

1073. (D) The trachea is anterior to both the esophagus and vertebral column and is superior to the heart. **thoracic viscera, trachea chest, respiratory system (Ballinger, Bontrager, Eisenberg, Anthony, Hole)**

1074. (D) The last intervertebral foramina (L5-S1) is demonstrated only through the specialized Kovacs method PA oblique axial position. **vertebral column, lumbosacral junction (Ballinger, Bontrager, Eisenberg)**

1075. (A) The central ray should be directed at the level of the superior portion of the greater trochanter for an AP projection of the hip. **pelvis, hip (Ballinger, Bontrager, Eisenberg)**

1076. (C) Sarcomas and adenocarcinomas are malignant. Adenomas are benign. **sarcoma, adenocarcinoma, adenoma (Eisenberg PATHOLOGY)**

1077. (C) External rotation of the humerus and arm during an AP projection of the shoulder will demonstrate the head of the humerus in profile. **shoulder (Ballinger, Bontrager, Eisenberg)**

1078. (B) The sphenoid sinuses are visualized through the open mouth on an open mouth modification of a parietoacanthial projection (Waters method). **paranasal sinuses, sinuses (Ballinger, Bontrager, Eisenberg)**

1079. (B) The radial styloid process is illustrated by #5 in Figure 31. **wrist (Ballinger, Bontrager, Eisenberg, Anthony, Hole)**

1080. (C) The lunate is illustrated by #3 in Figure 31. **wrist (Ballinger, Bontrager, Eisenberg, Anthony, Hole)**

1081. (C) The navicular is illustrated by #6 in Figure 31. **wrist (Ballinger, Bontrager, Eisenberg, Anthony, Hole)**

1082. (C) To demonstrate air-fluid levels, all paranasal sinuses should be radiographed with the patient in an erect position. **paranasal sinuses, sinuses (Ballinger, Bontrager, Eisenberg)**

1083. (D) The central ray should be directed to a point 3" above the nasion for an AP axial position for temporomandibular joints. **temporomandibular articulations, temporomandibular joints (Ballinger, Bontrager, Eisenberg)**

1084. (A) The mandibular rami and orbital roofs should be superimposed on a lateral position of the facial bones. **facial bones (Ballinger, Bontrager, Eisenberg)**

1085. (A) The lambdoidal suture is, for the most part, formed by the articulation of the occipital and parietal bones. **skull (Anthony, Hole, Ballinger, Bontrager, Eisenberg)**

1086. (A) The duodenum and jejunum are joined at the angle of Treitz. **digestive system, gastrointestinal, duodenum, jejunum, Treitz (Ballinger, Hole, Anthony)**

1087. (B) The knee should be flexed approximately 20° to 30° for the lateral projection. **knee (Ballinger)**

1088. (B) The Lilienfeld and Lorenz methods demonstrate the scapula in a PA oblique position. The Lawrence method demonstrates the proximal humerus in a transthoracic lateral projection. **scapula (Ballinger, Bontrager, Eisenberg)**

1089. (B) The hand consists of 27 bones. **hand (Anthony, Hole, Ballinger, Bontrager, Eisenberg)**

1090. (D) The basilar artery is illustrated by #8 in Figure 32. **circulatory system, circle of Willis (Ballinger, Snopek, Tortorici, Anthony, Hole)**

1091. (A) The anterior communicating artery is illustrated by #2 in Figure 32. **circulatory system, circle of Willis (Ballinger, Snopek, Tortorici, Anthony, Hole)**

1092. (B) The posterior communicating artery is illustrated by #5 in Figure 32. **circulatory system, circle of Willis (Ballinger, Snopek, Tortorici, Anthony, Hole)**

1093. (B) The mastoid process is the structure of primary interest on an AP tangential position (modified Hickey method). **temporal bone, mastoid process (Ballinger, Bontrager, Eisenberg)**

1094. (B) The parietoacanthial position (Waters method) demonstrates the maxillary and frontal sinuses. It does not demonstrate the sphenoid sinus. **facial bones (Ballinger)**

1095. (D) The incus (anvil), stapes (stirrup), and malleus (hammer) are the 3 auditory ossicles located in the inner ear. **skull (Anthony, Hole, Ballinger, Bontrager, Eisenberg)**

1096. (B) It takes about 2 to 8 minutes for intravenously injected contrast media to appear in the pelvicalyceal system during urography. **urinary system (Ballinger, Bontrager, Eisenberg)**

1097. (B) The ensiform process is also known as the xiphoid process. **bony thorax, sternum (Hole, Anthony, Ballinger, Bontrager, Eisenberg)**

1098. (A) The foot must be internally rotated 15° to avoid foreshortening of the femoral neck and projecting the lesser trochanter beyond the medial edge of the femoral shaft on an AP hip. **pelvis, hip (Ballinger, Bontrager, Eisenberg)**

1099. (A) The coracoid process of the scapula is the centering point for an AP shoulder projection. **shoulder (Ballinger, Bontrager, Eisenberg)**

1100. (D) Triquetrum, cuneiform, and triangular (and triquetral) are all the same carpal. **wrist (Ballinger, Bontrager, Eisenberg, Hole, Anthony)**

1101. (D) A properly performed submentovertical (full basal) projection of the skull should demonstrate the petrous pyramids of the temporal bone symmetrically, the odontoid process of the axis, and the sphenoid sinuses. **skull (Ballinger, Bontrager, Eisenberg)**

1102. (B) The glabella is the smooth area between the superciliary ridges of the frontal bone. **skull (Anthony, Hole, Ballinger, Bontrager, Eisenberg)**

1103. (A) The ureters enter the bladder at the lateral superior margin. **urinary system (Anthony, Hole, Ballinger, Bontrager, Eisenberg)**

1104. (B) The divisions of the stomach are the cardia, fundus, body, and pyloric portion. The duodenum is the first portion of the small bowel. **digestive system, gastrointestinal, stomach (Ballinger, Bontrager, Eisenberg, Anthony, Hole)**

1105. (A) The liver is located in the upper right quadrant of the abdomen. **digestive system, liver (Anthony, Hole, Ballinger, Bontrager, Eisenberg)**

1106.   (C) Ten posterior ribs should be visualized above the diaphragm on a routine PA chest radiograph.   **thoracic viscera, chest (Ballinger, Bontrager, Eisenberg)**

1107.   (B) The central ray should be directed 5° to 7° cephalad for an AP projection of the knee.   **knee (Ballinger, Bontrager, Eisenberg)**

1108.   (D) The 4th metatarsal is illustrated by #5 in Figure 33.   **foot (Ballinger, Bontrager, Eisenberg, Anthony, Hole)**

1109.   (C) The cuboid is illustrated by #7 in Figure 33.   **foot (Ballinger, Bontrager, Eisenberg, Anthony, Hole)**

1110.   (B) The talus is illustrated by #9 in Figure 33.   **foot (Ballinger, Bontrager, Eisenberg, Anthony, Hole)**

1111.   (D) The navicular is illustrated by #1 in Figure 33.   **foot (Ballinger, Bontrager, Eisenberg, Anthony, Hole)**

1112.   (B) The orthoroentgenologic leg length measurement procedure involves three exposures with central ray positioning at the hip, knee, and ankle joints. It requires a neutral position of the lower leg.   **long bone measurement (Ballinger)**

1113.   (D) The wing-like lateral mass of the sacral body is termed the ala.   **vertebral column, spine (Ballinger, Bontrager, Eisenberg)**

1114.   (C) The dens or odontoid process is the superior process of the axis that fits into the anterior portion of the atlantal ring of the atlas to act as a pivot for the head.   **vertebral column, atlas (Ballinger, Bontrager, Eisenberg, Anthony, Hole)**

1115.   (A) The region below the pelvic brim is known as the lesser, or true, pelvis. The region above the pelvis brim is known as the greater, or false, pelvis.   **pelvis (Ballinger, Bontrager, Eisenberg)**

1116.   (A) LeFort I, II, and III fractures are severe injuries to the maxillae which result in instability of the facial bones.   **LeFort (Eisenberg PATHOLOGY)**

1117.   (B) An AP humerus position requires that the central ray be directed to the long axis of the part, midway between the elbow and shoulder joints.   **humerus (Ballinger, Bontrager, Eisenberg)**

1118.   (C) The RAO best demonstrates the hepatic flexure of the colon.   **colon (Ballinger, Bontrager, Eisenberg)**

1119.   (A) Positioning a patient in the left lateral position permits gas to rise to the right hemidiaphragm, where it is visualized more easily on a left lateral decubitus radiograph.   **digestive system, abdomen (Ballinger)**

1120.   (B) The most accurate verification of rotation on a PA chest radiograph is symmetrical distance of the sternoclavicular joints from the midline of the body. **chest, thoracic viscera (Ballinger, Bontrager, Eisenberg)**

1121.   (D) The bony thorax is composed of the ribs, sternum, and thoracic vertebrae. **bony thorax (Hole, Anthony, Ballinger, Bontrager, Eisenberg)**

1122.   (A) The first cervical vertebra is also called the atlas. **vertebral column, atlas (Ballinger, Bontrager, Eisenberg, Hole, Anthony)**

1123.   (D) The liver, kidneys, and stomach are all within the abdominal cavity. **body cavities (Ballinger, Bontrager, Eisenberg, Anthony, Hole)**

1124.   (D) The patellar base is superior to the apex. It is the largest sesamoid bone, and it lies slightly above the knee joint. **knee (Ballinger, Bontrager, Eisenberg, Anthony, Hole)**

1125.   (A) Osteitis deformans is more commonly known as Paget's disease. **Paget's disease (Eisenberg PATHOLOGY)**

1126.   (D) The sternoclavicular joint forms the medial end of the clavicle. **shoulder girdle, clavicle, sternum (Ballinger, Bontrager, Eisenberg)**

1127.   (C) The wrist should be obliqued 45° for the oblique position. **wrist (Ballinger, Bontrager, Eisenberg)**

1128.   (D) The coccyx is demonstrated on an AP projection by a central ray angle of 10° caudad. **vertebral column, coccyx (Ballinger, Bontrager, Eisenberg)**

1129.   (C) The pylorus is illustrated by #4 in Figure 34. **digestive system, stomach (Ballinger, Bontrager, Eisenberg, Anthony, Hole)**

1130.   (B) The lesser curvature is illustrated by #2 in Figure 34. **digestive system, stomach (Ballinger, Bontrager, Eisenberg, Anthony, Hole)**

1131.   (D) The duodenum is illustrated by #5 in Figure 34. **digestive system, stomach (Ballinger, Bontrager, Eisenberg, Anthony, Hole)**

1132.   (B) Alignment of the inferior tip of the mastoid process and the occlusal surface of the upper incisors so that a line between them is perpendicular to the image receptor properly positions the head for an AP, open mouth projection. **vertebral column, atlas and axis, cervical (Ballinger, Bontrager, Eisenberg)**

1133.   (B) Most patients experience at least partial ileus post-operatively. **ileus (Eisenberg PATHOLOGY)**

1134.   (D) This is a definition of hemorrhage. **hemorrhage (Eisenberg PATHOLOGY)**

1135.   (A) The transthoracic lateral Lawrence method demonstrates only the proximal 2/3 of the humerus. **humerus (Ballinger, Bontrager, Eisenberg)**

1136. (C) The central ray should be centered to exit at the nasion for a PA axial position (Caldwell method) of the sinuses. **paranasal sinuses, sinuses (Ballinger, Bontrager, Eisenberg)**

1137. (B) The tangential position (May method) of the facial bones is for the demonstration of the zygomatic arch. **facial bones (Ballinger, Bontrager, Eisenberg)**

1138. (B) There are 8 bones in the cranium: the frontal, ethmoid, 2 parietal, sphenoid, 2 temporal, and occipital. **skull (Anthony, Hole, Ballinger, Bontrager, Eisenberg)**

1139. (D) The central ray should be directed 30° to 40° cephalad for an AP axial position of the colon. **colon (Ballinger, Bontrager, Eisenberg)**

1140. (D) The RAO produces the best image of the duodenal bulb and pyloric canal during a stomach examination. **stomach, digestive system, gastrointestinal (Ballinger, Bontrager, Eisenberg)**

1141. (A) The appendix (or veriform process) is attached to the cecum. **digestive system, gastrointestinal, colon, appendix (Ballinger, Hole, Anthony)**

1142. (A) Both the dorsal and lateral decubitus abdomen position are useful in demonstrating air-fluid levels in the abdomen. The supine AP position is not. **digestive system, abdomen (Ballinger, Bontrager, Eisenberg)**

1143. (C) The lungs introduce oxygen into and remove carbon dioxide from the blood. **thoracic viscera, chest, lungs, respiratory system (Anthony, Hole, Ballinger, Bontrager, Eisenberg)**

1144. (A) On deep exhalation the ribs move inferiorly, posteriorly, and medially. **bony thorax, ribs (Ballinger, Bontrager, Eisenberg)**

1145. (D) The hip bone (innominatum or os coxae) is made up of the ilium, pubis, and ischium. **pelvis, hip (Ballinger, Bontrager, Eisenberg, Anthony, Hole)**

1146. (B) The left petrous portion of the temporal bone exhibits more recorded detail when closest to the image receptor. **temporal bone, petrous portion (Ballinger, Bontrager, Eisenberg)**

1147. (A) The lumbar bodies are deeper anteriorly than posteriorly and are slightly concave on their superior and inferior surfaces. They are connected to the vertebral spines by the pedicles, not by the lamina. **vertebral column, lumbar spine (Ballinger, Bontrager, Eisenberg)**

1148. (C) A lateral scapula is shown in Figure 35. **scapula (Ballinger, Bontrager, Eisenberg)**

1149. (A) The acromion process is illustrated by #1 in Figure 35. **scapula (Ballinger, Bontrager, Eisenberg)**

1150. (C) The head of the humerus is illustrated by #2 in Figure 35. **scapula (Ballinger, Bontrager, Eisenberg)**

1151. (D) Malignant neoplasms metastasize by seeding within body cavities, lymphatic spread, and embolistic spread. **metastasis (Eisenberg PATHOLOGY)**

1152. (A) When a patient cannot extend the elbow for an AP projection, two AP projections, one of the distal humerus, the other of the proximal forearm, must be obtained. **elbow (Ballinger, Bontrager, Eisenberg)**

1153. (A) The average normal transit time for food to travel from the mouth to the ileocecal valve is 2 to 3 hours. **digestive system, gastrointestinal (Ballinger, Hole, Anthony, Eisenberg)**

1154. (A) Endoscopic retrograde cholangiopancreatography (ERCP) is the examination of the pancreatic and biliary duct. **endoscopic retrograde cholangiopancreatography, ERCP (Ballinger, Eisenberg, Tortorici, Snopek)**

1155. (A) Lateral stressing of the lower leg will delineate the medial side of the knee during vertical ray contrast arthrography. **contrast arthrography (Ballinger)**

1156. (C) The central ray for a lateral chest should be directed to the level of the 6th to 7th thoracic vertebra. **chest (Ballinger, Bontrager, Eisenberg)**

1157. (A) The left, upper lobe of the lung is superior and anterior to the lower lobe. Both lobes extend medially to laterally so that neither is completely medial or lateral of the other. **thoracic viscera, chest, lung, respiratory system (Anthony, Hole, Ballinger, Bontrager, Eisenberg)**

1158. (D) The seventh cervical vertebra is also called the vertebra prominens because of its long, prominent spinous process. **vertebral column, vertebra prominens (Ballinger, Bontrager, Eisenberg, Hole, Anthony)**

1159. (B) The axiolateral (Danelius-Miller modification of the Lorenz method) is performed with the patient supine with the unaffected leg lifted, the film positioned with one end above the iliac crest, and the central ray directed at the neck of the femur entering medially and exiting laterally. **pelvis, hip (Ballinger, Bontrager, Eisenberg)**

1160. (B) There are two menisci in the knee joint, a lateral and a medial. **knee (Ballinger, Bontrager, Eisenberg, Hole)**

1161. (D) Only the lateral position clearly demonstrates all four paranasal sinuses. **paranasal sinuses, sinuses (Ballinger, Bontrager, Eisenberg)**

1162. (B) The proper central ray angulation for an axiolateral oblique position of the mandible is 25° cephalad. **mandible (Ballinger, Bontrager, Eisenberg)**

1163. (C) For a lateral position of the facial bones, the central ray should be centered to the malar surface of the zygomatic bone. **facial bones (Ballinger, Bontrager, Eisenberg)**

1164. (A) A fistula is an abnormal passage, usually between two organs. A sinus is similar except it leads to an abscess. **digestive system, abdomen (Ballinger, Eisenberg PATHOLOGY)**

1165. (C) The thymus gland reaches its maximum size at puberty. **thoracic viscera, thymus, mediastinum (Anthony, Hole, Ballinger, Bontrager, Eisenberg)**

1166. (C) The first 4 intervertebral foramina are best demonstrated on a lateral projection of the lumbar spine. The apophysial joints are best demonstrated on the oblique projections. **vertebral column, lumbar spine (Ballinger, Bontrager, Eisenberg)**

1167. (D) S1 is at the level of the anterior superior iliac spine. **surface landmarks (Ballinger, Bontrager, Eisenberg)**

1168. (D) The ilium includes the greater sciatic notch, posterior inferior spine, and anterior superior spine. **pelvis (Ballinger, Bontrager, Eisenberg)**

1169. (C) The medial (lateral) oblique of the lower leg will best demonstrate the tibiofibular articulations. **leg (Ballinger, Bontrager, Eisenberg)**

1170. (A) The os magnum is also known as the capitatim or capitate. **wrist (Ballinger, Bontrager, Eisenberg, Anthony, Hole)**

1171. (B) A central ray angulation of 15° to the orbitomeatal line is equivalent to 23° to the glabellomeatal line because the two baselines are 8° different from one another. **paranasal sinuses, sinuses (Ballinger, Bontrager, Eisenberg)**

1172. (D) All four sinuses, sphenoid, ethmoid, maxillary, and frontal, are located anterior to the external auditory meatus. **paranasal sinuses, sinuses (Ballinger, Bontrager, Eisenberg)**

1173. (A) The knee is in the AP position in Figure 36. **knee (Ballinger, Bontrager, Eisenberg)**

1174. (A) The lateral epicondyle is illustrated by #5 in Figure 36. **knee (Ballinger, Bontrager, Eisenberg)**

1175. (D) The intercondyloid fossa is illustrated by #1 in Figure 36. **knee (Ballinger, Bontrager, Eisenberg)**

1176. (C) The head of the fibula is illustrated by #3 in Figure 36. **knee (Ballinger, Bontrager, Eisenberg)**

1177. (B) The body of the mandible should be positioned parallel to the image receptor for an axiolateral oblique position of the mandible. **mandible (Ballinger, Bontrager, Eisenberg)**

1178. (C) The optic foramen should appear in the inferior lateral quadrant of the orbit on a properly positioned parieto-orbital oblique position (Rhese method). **optic foramen, skull (Ballinger, Bontrager, Eisenberg)**

1179. (C) For a submentovertical (full basal) projection of the skull, the infraorbitomeatal line should be parallel to the image receptor. **skull (Ballinger, Bontrager, Eisenberg)**

1180. (B) The glomerular capsule is connected to the proximal convoluted tubule. **urinary system (Anthony, Hole, Ballinger, Bontrager, Eisenberg)**

1181. (C) The haustra are the sacculations of the colon that are formed by the teniae coli of the wall. **digestive system, gastrointestinal, colon (Ballinger, Bontrager, Eisenberg)**

1182. (B) A second breath, or double-breathing technique, inflates the lungs more without strain. It has no effect on heart size or the position of large, pendulous breasts. **thoracic viscera, chest (Ballinger, Bontrager, Eisenberg)**

1183. (B) The apophyseal joints closest to the image receptor are demonstrated on AP oblique positions (RPO and LPO), while the apophyseal joints farthest from the image receptor are demonstrated on PA oblique positions (RAO and LAO). Therefore, the right apophyseal joints will be demonstrated by the LAO and RPO positions. **vertebral column, lumbar spine (Ballinger, Bontrager, Eisenberg)**

1184. (B) The approximate anterior angle of the neck of the femur is 15° to 20°, although it varies with age, sex, and body type. **pelvis, femur, hip (Ballinger, Bontrager, Eisenberg, Hole, Anthony)**

1185. (C) The joint spaces are opened when an AP foot is performed with a 15° posterior central ray angulation. **foot (Ballinger, Bontrager, Eisenberg)**

1186. (B) The central ray should be directed 30° to 35° caudad for an axiolateral position by the Lysholm method. **skull (Ballinger, Bontrager, Eisenberg)**

1187. (D) The ethmoid includes the perpendicular plate, crista galli, and cribriform plate. **skull (Anthony, Hole, Ballinger, Bontrager, Eisenberg)**

1188. (B) The body should be obliqued 35° to 45° for an RAO position of the colon. **colon (Ballinger, Bontrager, Eisenberg)**

1189. (A) A recumbent position must be used to increase venous pressure during an esophagram to demonstrate esophageal varices. Full exhalation or the Valsalva maneuver will assist in increasing venous pressure in a recumbent position, but they are not effective when the patient is erect. **digestive system, esophagus (Ballinger, Bontrager, Eisenberg)**

1190. (C) The human gastrointestinal tract is approximately 29 to 30 feet in length. **digestive system, gastrointestinal tract (Ballinger, Anthony, Hole)**

1191.   (A) The proper centering point for the cassette for an AP projection of the abdomen when the patient is erect is 2" to 3" above the iliac crests. **digestive system, abdomen (Ballinger, Bontrager, Eisenberg)**

1192.   (B) The lower ribs are best demonstrated by full exhalation, which raises the diaphragm to reveal the greatest number of lower ribs. **bony thorax, ribs (Ballinger, Bontrager, Eisenberg)**

1193.   (A) The manubrial (or jugular) notch is the deep depression in the superior aspect of the sternum. **bony thorax, sternum (Ballinger, Bontrager, Eisenberg)**

1194.   (B) A mediolateral lateral ankle position should have the central ray directed to the medial malleolus. **ankle (Ballinger, Bontrager, Eisenberg)**

1195.   (C) Osteochondroma (exostosis) is a benign projection of normal bone. Ewing's sarcoma and chondrosarcoma are malignant bone tumors. **osteochondroma, Ewing's sarcoma, chondrosarcoma (Eisenberg PATHOLOGY)**

1196.   (D) The semilunar (lunate), scaphoid (navicular), and pisiform, along with the triquetrum (triquetral, cuneiform, or triangular), make up the distal row of carpals. **wrist (Ballinger, Bontrager, Eisenberg)**

1197.   (C) This is a definition of interstitial pneumonia. **pneumonia (Eisenberg PATHOLOGY)**

1198.   (B) The right subclavian artery is illustrated by #7 in Figure 37. **circulatory system, arteries (Ballinger, Anthony, Hole)**

1199.   (B) The left common carotid artery is illustrated by #2 in Figure 37. **circulatory system, arteries (Ballinger, Anthony, Hole)**

1200.   (B) The aorta is illustrated by #5 in Figure 37. **circulatory system, arteries (Ballinger, Anthony, Hole)**

1201.   (D) The right vertebral artery is illustrated by #8 in Figure 37. **circulatory system, arteries (Ballinger, Anthony, Hole)**

1202.   (A) The renal artery is illustrated by #1 in Figure 38. **urinary system, kidney (Ballinger, Snopek, Tortorici, Anthony, Hole)**

1203.   (A) The renal cortex is illustrated by #5 in Figure 38. **urinary system, kidney (Ballinger, Snopek, Tortorici, Anthony, Hole)**

1204.   (C) A major calyx is illustrated by #7 in Figure 38. **urinary system, kidney (Ballinger, Bontrager, Eisenberg, Anthony, Hole)**

PATIENT CARE AND MANAGEMENT
Record Maintenance and Administrative Procedures
1% (14) 1205-1218

1205. (B) According to the *Principles of Professional Conduct* of the American Registry of Radiologic Technologists, radiologic technologists shall not diagnose. **code of ethics, ethics (Ehrlich, Torres, Gurley)**

1206. (D) The patient's medical record includes all documents regarding the patient that are collected. This includes records of medications given, consent forms, and radiographs. **medical record (Ehrlich, Torres)**

1207. (D) Although no method should be used by itself, questioning the patient, reading the wrist identification band, and checking the bed nameplate are all valid cross-checks of patient identification. **patient identification (Ehrlich, Torres, Gurley)**

1208. (A) The abbreviation c indicates "with." **abbreviations (Ehrlich, Torres, Gurley)**

1209. (D) Failure to carry out professional duties, performing, and threatening to perform, a procedure that a patient has refused are all grounds for legal action which could result in requirements to pay damages. **malpractice (Ehrlich, Tortorici)**

1210. (D) A radiographer is responsible to provide the physician with all information relative to radiologic diagnosis according to the *Principles of Professional Conduct* of the American Registry of Radiologic Technologists. This case clearly involves providing additional information from the patient history (pain in the opposite wrist but no pain on the side to be radiographed) to the physician before proceeding with the examination. **code of ethics, ethics (Ehrlich, Torres, Gurley)**

1211. (B) All states require persons prescribing the use of radiation to have a license to practice medicine. **code of ethics, ethics (Ehrlich, Torres, Gurley)**

1212. (B) Internal rotation of the leg will rotate the head of the femur into the acetabulum. Pain in the groin associated with this movement could indicate hip pathology. **professional ethics (Tortorici, Ehrlich)**

1213. (D) The abbreviation prn indicates "as needed." **abbreviations (Ehrlich, Torres, Gurley)**

1214. (A) As compared to a PA erect chest at 72", a supine AP chest at 40" would produce a magnified heart while not demonstrating air-fluid levels in the lungs. **chest (Ballinger, Bontrager, Eisenberg)**

1215. (A) Discussing patient information with a friend outside the medical setting is an invasion of the patient's privacy. **malpractice (Tortorici, Ehrlich)**

1216. (A) The abbreviation LLQ indicates "lower left quadrant." **abbreviations (Ehrlich, Torres, Gurley)**

1217. (C) Respondeat superior ("let the master answer") holds that the employer is responsible for the acts of the radiographer. **malpractice (Tortorici, Ehrlich)**

1218. (B) Minors and persons who have had their civil rights removed (such as prisoners) may undergo procedures upon the consent of their guardian. In the case of a prisoner, this is often the officer in charge of the prisoner. Beyond being a minor, the age of a patient is not a determinant in consent. **informed consent (Ehrlich, Torres, Gurley)**

PATIENT CARE AND MANAGEMENT
Patient Safety and Comfort
1% (14) 1219-1232

1219. (D) The center of gravity for a standing patient is in the pelvis, usually near the symphysis pubis. **body mechanics (Torres, Ehrlich)**

1220. (C) Pediatric patients respond and cooperate best if they can be examined without restraints and with parental involvement. However, many factors are involved in these decisions, and the preferred method is often not possible. **pediatric patients (Ehrlich, Torres)**

1221. (C) The knees should be bent, feet slightly apart, and the back as straight as possible to minimize spinal injury to the radiographer when moving patients. **body mechanics (Ehrlich, Torres)**

1222. (A) Fowler's position places the patient semi-sitting with the head raised from 45° to 60°. **Fowler's position (Ehrlich, Torres)**

1223. (A) When carrying a baby, his back and head must be supported at all times. **pediatric patient (Ehrlich, Torres)**

1224. (A) Both skin color and respiratory rate can provide a quick general assessment of a patient's overall condition. **physical signs (Ehrlich, Torres)**

1225. (C) A sheet restraint (i.e., mummy-style wrappings) is the most effective restraint for a small child. **pediatric patient (Torres, Ehrlich)**

1226. (B) A proper wheelchair to x-ray table transfer of a patient who can stand but cannot walk involves placing the wheelchair parallel to the x-ray table. Then, the radiographer stands facing the patient, places both hands on the patient's scapulae, and gently pulls the patient into an upright position. The patient then can be pivoted into the locked wheelchair. **transfer (Ehrlich, Torres)**

1227. (B) Lifting a large weight with the legs instead of the back will protect the spine. The other choices are reversed. Their correct order is: pull a weight instead of pushing it, keep the feet apart to develop a wide base, and use the patient's moving abilities as much as possible. **body mechanics (Ehrlich, Torres)**

1228. (C) A patient is supine when he or she is flat on his or her back. **supine position (Ehrlich, Torres)**

1229. (A) When transferring a patient from an x-ray table to a stretcher cart, the sheet should be rolled as close to the patient's body as possible. The persons transferring the patient should be positioned with half of the people on each side of the patient. **transfer (Ehrlich, Torres)**

1230. (A) Crying and kicking are normal responses to distress by a small child. **pediatric patient (Ehrlich, Torres)**

1231. (C) Very small children often respond best when the radiographer is at eye level and touching is avoided for a short time while attempts are made to gain the child's confidence. **pediatric patient (Torres, Ehrlich)**

1232. (D) Skin breakdown is known to be caused by immobility in a single position, prolong contact with wet surfaces, and tension to the skin surface during transfer procedures. **skin care (Ehrlich, Torres)**

PATIENT CARE AND MANAGEMENT
Disinfection and Sterile Technique
2.5% (35) 1233-1267

1233. (B) Medical asepsis is the process of reducing the probability of infectious organisms being transmitted to someone who is susceptible. **infection control (Torres, Ehrlich)**

1234. (C) When the sterilization of an object is in question, it must be discarded. **sterilization (Ehrlich, Torres)**

1235. (C) Infection proceeds from incubation to prodromal to full active to convalescent. **infection (Torres, Ehrlich)**

1236. (D) The trendelenburg position is with the patient's head slightly lower than the body. **trendelenburg position (Torres, Ehrlich)**

1237. (A) When returning a patient to his or her room, the bed should be lowered to the lowest position and the return of the patient should be reported to the appropriate nursing station. The patient's chart should not be taken from the nursing station unless by pre-arranged request of the radiologist or other authority. **transferring patients (Torres)**

1238. (C) Microorganisms that are capable of forming spores can survive high heat, chemicals, dry periods, etc., and remain viable when favorable conditions are available. **infection control (Torres, Ehrlich)**

1239. (B) Most patients feel more comfortable if the clothing to be removed is specified and the radiographic procedures are explained. Most patients do not feel comfortable if they must discover how to wear a patient gown. A short explanation usually alleviates this feeling. **patient care, care of valuables, communicating with patients (Ehrlich, Torres)**

1240. (A) A contaminated x-ray table should be cleaned by starting with the least contaminated area and working into the higher contamination areas. This avoids spreading contamination into previously uncontaminated areas. **infection control (Torres, Ehrlich)**

1241. (A) Disinfection involves the destruction of pathogens by using chemicals. **infection control (Ehrlich, Torres)**

1242. (B) Fungi are classified as either yeasts or molds. Protozoa are complex multi-celled microorganisms that are classified separately. **infection control (Torres, Ehrlich)**

1243. (D) A cap, face mask, and shoe covers are among the items usually required to be worn for entry into an operating room. **surgical asepsis (Torres, Ehrlich)**

1244. (B) Steam under pressure is the most effective and convenient method of sterilization for items that can withstand high temperatures. **sterilization (Ehrlich, Torres)**

1245. (C) The use of hand lotion prevents cracking of the skin surface, which would provide access to infectious materials. **infection control (Ehrlich, Torres)**

1246. (D) The four basic groups of microorganisms that can cause infections in humans include bacteria, viruses, and protozoa, as well as fungi. **infection control (Torres, Ehrlich)**

1247. (C) Mentally impaired patients usually respond best when they are treated as adults but with simple instructions. Talking loud serves no purpose for these patients and should be avoided. **communication (Ehrlich)**

1248. (D) A paraplegic patient has lost the use of the lower part of the body, including the legs. **mobility (Torres, Ehrlich)**

1249. (A) Failure to wear a face mask in a respiratory isolation unit and pricking of the skin by a used needle are serious violations of infectious control procedures and should be reported by filing an incident report. Failure to use hand lotion after hand washing is not a violation, although the use of hand lotion as often as possible is recommended. **infection control (Torres, Ehrlich)**

1250. (A) Disinfection is the process where as many microorganisms as possible are eliminated, although spores are seldom destroyed. **infection control (Torres, Ehrlich)**

1251. (A) Nosocomial infections are those that are acquired by a patient while in a health-care institution. **infection control (Torres, Ehrlich)**

1252. (B) It is recommended that needles not be recapped before discarding, and that all needles be considered contaminated. In addition, it is recommended that needles not be broken prior to being discarded as they may spray infectious material. **infection control (Torres, Ehrlich)**

1253. (B) A loud voice is required with geriatric patients only when indications of hearing difficulties are present. Simple instructions are recommended for all patients. Geriatric patients should be treated as adults. **communication (Ehrlich)**

1254. (A) Gas sterilization is the most effective and convenient method for items that cannot withstand high temperatures. **sterilization (Ehrlich, Torres)**

1255. (D) Infectious diseases can be transported from one person to another by insect vectors, airborne droplets, and by indirect contact through objects called fomites. **infection control (Torres, Ehrlich)**

1256. (B) If a sterile tray has been opened but the procedure is delayed for an hour, the tray should be covered and then watched to guarantee that no one contaminates it. **surgical asepsis, infection control (Torres, Ehrlich)**

1257. (C) Boiling (in water) will disinfect items but does not sterilize because many spores resist boiling for many hours. **disinfecting (Ehrlich, Torres)**

1258. (B) Because of the heat requirements for boiling and pressurized steam, gas sterilization usually is used to sterilize electronic equipment. However, especially sensitive equipment is sometimes sterilized by ionizing radiation in special laboratories equipped for the purpose. **sterilization (Ehrlich, Torres)**

1259. (B) The proper method of painting the skin with antiseptic as part of surgical skin preparation is to begin at the center of the area and move in a circular motion toward the outside. **surgical asepsis (Torres, Ehrlich)**

1260. (B) The hands of the person holding the sterile cassette bag are sterile as is the outside of the bag. The cassette, inside of the bag, and person holding the cassette are not sterile. **infection control, surgical asepsis (Torres, Ehrlich)**

1261. (B) Acquired immunodeficiency syndrome (AIDS) is not an airborne infection, although both measles and tuberculosis are. **infection control, isolation (Torres, Ehrlich)**

1262. (D) Dry heat, ionizing radiation, and gas are all effective methods of removing all microorganisms and their spores from an article, thus sterilizing it. **asepsis, sterilization (Ehrlich, Torres)**

1263. (D) Both blood and fecal contact along with breathing droplets from coughing can transmit infectious disease. Not all diseases are transmitted by all forms of contact. **infection control (Torres, Ehrlich)**

1264. (C) The gloves should be added last when dressing for a sterile operating room procedure. **surgical asepsis (Ehrlich, Torres)**

1265. (B) Infection proceeds from incubation to prodromal to full active to convalescent. The full active phase is when the person appears most sick. **infection (Torres, Ehrlich)**

1266.   (C) An autoclave is a device designed to sterilize items with steam under pressure. **sterilization (Ehrlich, Torres)**

1267.   (C) Urinary catherization requires the use of sterile technique. The cleaning of an ileus and the insertion of a naso-gastric tube do not. **infection control (Torres, Ehrlich)**

PATIENT CARE AND MANAGEMENT
Isolation Techniques
1% (14) 1268-1281

1268.   (D) Acquired immunodeficiency syndrome (AIDS), hepatitis B, and syphilis all require blood and body fluid precautions. **isolation (Torres, Ehrlich)**

1269.   (C) The gloves should be removed first, by grasping the inside. **isolation (Ehrlich, Torres)**

1270.   (D) During mobile radiography in a strict isolation unit, as long as the x-ray controls are not touched by contaminated items, they can be adjusted freely. Circumstances that would not involve touching the controls by contaminated items include before touching the patient or items in the room, by another radiographer who has not touched the patient or items in the room, and after touching the patient or items in the room as long as new gloves are put on first. **isolation, infection control (Torres, Ehrlich)**

1271.   (B) Respiratory isolation is designed to prevent airborne droplet contamination. **infection control (Torres, Ehrlich)**

1272.   (C) Enteric isolation is designed to avoid fecal material contamination. **infection control (Torres, Ehrlich)**

1273.   (D) Strict isolation requires the use of gown, mask, and gloves. **isolation (Torres, Ehrlich)**

1274.   (C) A patient with a communicable disease should be transferred by wrapping completely in a cotton sheet. **isolation (Torres, Ehrlich)**

1275.   (A) Touching by the hands is the most common method of spreading microorganisms. **infection control (Torres, Ehrlich)**

1276.   (B) Medically aseptic hand washing requires that the hands be kept lower than the elbows. **infection control (Torres, Ehrlich)**

1277.   (C) *Staphylococcus aureus* and herpes simplex require only contact isolation precautions. Acquired immunodeficiency syndrome (AIDS) requires blood and body fluid precautions. Other diseases requiring only contact isolation are respiratory infections, diphtheria, impetigo, streptococcal, rabies, and major skin wounds, burns, or drainages. **isolation (Torres, Ehrlich)**

1278. (D) Spattering of blood and body waste as well as rubbing the eyes with hands are primary concerns when avoiding contamination of the eyes when working with isolation patients. **isolation (Torres, Ehrlich)**

1279. (C) The only acceptable reason for not rinsing bedpans and urinals immediately after use by an isolation patient is when a specimen is required. **isolation (Torres, Ehrlich)**

1280. (D) The basic principles for dealing with patients who have a communicable disease include frequent hand washing; placement of needles in puncture-resistant receptacles; bagging and labeling contaminated materials for laundry and waste handling; and sterilization, disinfection, or disposal of all items. **isolation (Torres, Ehrlich)**

1281. (D) A second person should be available to assist during radiography of a patient with a communicable disease in order to handle items to and from contaminated area. **isolation (Torres, Ehrlich)**

PATIENT CARE AND MANAGEMENT
Monitoring Vital Signs
1% (14) 1282-1295

1282. (C) Normal adult respiration ranges between 10 to 20 breaths per minute. **vital signs (Torres, Ehrlich)**

1283. (A) The brachial artery, just above the elbow, is most commonly used to measure blood pressure. **vital signs (Torres, Ehrlich)**

1284. (A) An electrocardiogram (ECG or EKG) measures the electrical activity of the heart. **vital signs (Torres, Ehrlich)**

1285. (C) An apical pulse refers to the apex of the heart. **vital signs (Torres, Ehrlich)**

1286. (C) The normal adult oral temperature is 37° C, or 98.6° F. **vital signs (Torres, Ehrlich)**

1287. (B) The range of normal adult resting pulse rates is 60 to 90 beats per minute. **vital signs (Torres, Ehrlich)**

1288. (B) Rectal temperatures are the most accurate measure of body temperature. **vital signs (Torres, Ehrlich)**

1289. (B) Both mercury and aneroid sphygmomanometers, or blood pressure units, are available. The mercury units operate by measuring the pressure on a column of mercury, while the aneroid units, which are less accurate, operate by measuring the pressure of the air on a gauge. Ultrasonic (doppler) and other electronic blood pressure measurements also are available. There is no barometric type of sphygmomanometer. **vital signs (Torres, Ehrlich)**

1290. (A) Patients are considered hypertensive when the systolic pressure is consistently greater than 140 mm Hg, and the diastolic pressure is consistently greater than 90 mm Hg. **vital signs (Torres, Ehrlich)**

1291. (A) Systolic blood pressure is the top number in a blood pressure reading. It is measuring the pressure of the left ventricle's pumping ability. **vital signs (Torres, Ehrlich)**

1292. (D) The terms labored, shallow, and rapid often are used to describe variations in respiratory patterns. The terms noisy, regular, and irregular also are used. **vital signs (Torres, Ehrlich)**

1293. (D) Bradycardia describes a heart rate of less than 60 beats per minute. Tachycardia describes a heart rate of more than 100 beats per minute. **vital signs (Torres, Ehrlich)**

1294. (A) The radial pulse, over the radial artery at the base of the thumb, is the most common location for detecting the pulse. **vital signs (Torres, Ehrlich)**

1295. (B) Normal, adult diastolic blood pressure ranges from 60 to 80 mm Hg. **vital signs (Torres, Ehrlich)**

PATIENT CARE AND MANAGEMENT
Contrast Media
4% (56) 1296-1351

1296. (A) Contrast medium reactions are more severe during venous injection than during arterial injections because the kidneys remove some of the contrast medium before it reaches the heart during arterial injections. **contrast media, iodinated contrast agents (Snopek, Torres, Ehrlich)**

1297. (B) The absorption of primary photons causes positive contrast material to produce an area of reduced image density. **contrast material (Snopek, Tortorici, Torres)**

1298. (A) Sodium is the more toxic cation in organic iodide contrast media. Meglumine is less toxic. **contrast media, iodinated contrast agents (Snopek, Torres, Ehrlich)**

1299. (B) Viscosity describes the resistance of a contrast medium to free flow. **contrast media, iodinated contrast agents (Snopek, Torres, Ehrlich)**

1300. (A) Both electromechanical and compressed air angiographic pressure injectors have proven feasible in clinical use. **contrast media, iodinated contrast agents (Snopek, Torres, Ehrlich)**

1301. (A) Most radiologic contrast media are administered intravenously. **contrast media, iodinated contrast agents (Snopek, Torres, Ehrlich)**

1302. (D) Headaches, aphasia, and unconsciousness are all possible adverse effects of the use of contrast material. **adverse effects, contrast material (Torres, Tortorici, Ehrlich)**

1303. (A) An intravenous line is often connected to the vessel being used for injection during an angiogram to provide an open line for medications and for additional contrast material. It is not used to remove blood samples for arterial gasses. **patient care (Torres, Snopek, Tortorici)**

1304. (C) A vasodilator will relax vascular walls to permit greater blood flow. **drugs (Torres, Tortorici)**

1305. (D) The normal injection time for ethiodolized oil into the lymph vessels is usually 45 to 90 minutes. **lymphangiography, lymphography (Tortorici, Snopek)**

1306. (B) An anaphylactic reaction is characterized by an exaggerated response to a substance which had previously sensitized the organism. **shock (Torres, Ehrlich)**

1307. (B) Warming contrast material decreases its viscosity. **contrast material, injectors (Tortorici, Torres, Snopek)**

1308. (C) Nitroglycerin is a vasodilator. **drugs (Torres, Ehrlich)**

1309. (A) Anaphylactic shock is the type of shock seen most often during angiography because it is caused by the use of iodinated contrast materials. **medical emergencies (Torres, Ehrlich)**

1310. (A) Iodinated contrast media studies should be performed first, with all examinations performed in the following order of sequence: urinary, biliary, lower gastrointestinal, upper gastrointestinal. **contrast media, scheduling (Ehrlich, Torres)**

1311. (B) An intravenous set should be raised 18" to 24" above the vein. **patient care (Torres, Ehrlich)**

1312. (B) An enema tip should be inserted approximately 3" to 4", or until it passes the anal sphincter. **enema (Torres, Ehrlich)**

1313. (A) Anticoagulants should be withheld at least 4 hours prior to angiography. **preangiographic care (Tortorici)**

1314. (C) Neurogenic shock is caused by the pooling of blood due to the failure of arterial resistance. **shock (Torres, Ehrlich)**

1315. (A) An antihistamine, which is used to relieve symptoms caused by nasal, drug, food, and skin allergies. It should be considered for a patient who complains of having "tongue thickness." **adverse reactions (Ehrlich, Torres)**

1316. (B) Barium sulfate is used for visualization of the gastrointestinal tract. Barium sulfite is extremely toxic and is never used for radiologic imaging. **barium, contrast media (Torres, Ehrlich)**

1317. (B) When resistance is encountered when inserting an enema tip for a barium enema, assistance should be requested from a physician. Under no circumstances should the tip be forced into the rectum. **barium enema, enema (Torres, Ehrlich)**

1318. (B) A bismuth laxative is partially radiopaque and will produce artifacts after it coats the intestine. Castor oil, saline enemas, and soap suds enemas are all acceptable cleansing methods. **cathartics, laxatives, barium enema (Ehrlich, Torres)**

1319. (D) The gallbladder, kidneys, and adrenal glands can all be examined with iodinated contrast media. **iodinated contrast media, contrast media (Torres, Ehrlich, Ballinger)**

1320. (B) Allowing fluid to flow to the enema tip prior to inserting it in the rectum avoids instilling air into the colon. **enema, gastrointestinal tract (Ballinger, Ehrlich, Torres)**

1321. (A) A urinary catheter is used to administer contrast media for a cystogram. **cystography (Ballinger, Ehrlich)**

1322. (A) Barium has hygroscopic properties and will absorb fluid from the bowel. It also solidifies if it remains static without fluid suspension and may form a barium impaction. Both of these problems are more likely in geriatric patients, especially if they are inactive. **barium (Ehrlich, Torres)**

1323. (D) The use of iodinated contrast material causes all of the hemodynamic consequences listed: vasodilation, increased cardiac output, and increased heart rate. **contrast material (Snopek, Tortoricci)**

1324. (B) A hypertonic saline enema solution removes interstitial fluid from the bowel, thus promoting peristalsis. Only a small amount of fluid (120 to 180 ml) is needed for this type of enema. **enemas (Ehrlich, Torres)**

1325. (D) A tourniquet, alcohol wipes, and adhesive tape are all necessary to begin an intravenous infusion. **patient care (Torres, Ehrlich)**

1326. (A) Mixing barium with normal saline solution instead of tap water assists in minimizing electrolyte balance problems and cardiac insufficiency following increases in the amount of absorbed water following a barium enema. **barium enema (Ehrlich, Ballinger)**

1327. (D) The enema tip should be directed toward the umbilicus as it is inserted into the anus. **enema (Torres, Ehrlich)**

1328. (B) Nearly all reactions to iodinated contrast media occur within 2 to 10 minutes after injection. **iodinated contrast media, contrast media reactions (Torres, Ehrlich)**

1329. (D) Because the NPO fasting order may cause other problems with pediatric, diabetic, and geriatric patients, they should have priority over other patients for gastrointestinal examinations. **gastrointestinal tract, gastrointestinal (Ehrlich, Torres, Ballinger)**

1330. (B) Laxatives are known as cathartics. **cathartics, laxatives, enema (Ehrlich, Torres)**

1331. (A) When the sigmoid colon is filled, usually with 200 to 400 ml of fluid, the colon will sometimes experience a spasm that will pass with a brief pause and change of position. **gastrointestinal tract, enema, barium (Torres, Ehrlich)**

1332. (D) Percutaneous transhepatic cholangiography uses a long, thin needle which is inserted through the liver (transhepatically) into the biliary ducts. Because the needle is withdrawn through the peritoneum, it is possible to produce peritonitis as a side effect. **cholangiography (Ballinger, Snopek, Torres, Tortorici, Ehrlich)**

1333. (A) The only purpose of an inflatable balloon cuff on an enema tip is the retention of barium. **enema, barium (Torres, Ehrlich)**

1334. (D) Air, iodine, and barium all can be used to visualize the colon. **contrast media (Torres, Ehrlich)**

1335. (A) Breaks in the gastrointestinal mucosa due to trauma or disease may permit barium to extravasate into the peritoneal cavity or bloodstream where peritonitis or venous embolism may cause serious complications. Fibrosis or barium granuloma also are known complications of this process. **barium, contrast media (Torres, Ehrlich)**

1336. (C) Hypovolemic shock is caused by an abnormally low volume of circulating blood. **shock (Ehrlich, Torres)**

1337. (B) Both gastric ulcers and abdominal trauma are potential causes of bowel perforation. Polyps in the colon are unlikely causes of perforation. **barium, ulcers, abdominal trauma (Torres, Eisenberg PATHOLOGY, Ehrlich)**

1338. (D) Sneezing and coughing; itching at the site of injection, eyes, and nose; and apprehensiveness are all typical signs of anaphylactic shock and should be reported and acted upon immediately. **anaphylactic shock, contrast media reactions (Torres, Ehrlich)**

1339. (A) Non-ionic iodinated contrast media are less likely to cause anaphylactic shock, although they are more expensive. There is no appreciable difference in image quality with non-ionic media. **contrast media, iodine (Ehrlich, Torres)**

1340. (C) Barium solution that is to be administered rectally should be at a temperature of 102° to 105° F. **barium, enema (Ehrlich, Torres)**

1341.   (C) The average, normal, adult, barium enema examination without air contrast techniques requires approximately 1,500 ml of barium solution. **enema, barium (Torres, Ehrlich)**

1342.   (B) Intravenous injection is the most efficient method for the injection of medications to counteract adverse reactions. **medication administration (Tortorici, Ehrlich, Torres, Snopek)**

1343.   (C) Contrast media examinations should be performed in the following order of sequence: urinary, biliary, lower gastrointestinal, upper gastrointestinal. **contrast media, scheduling (Ehrlich, Torres)**

1344.   (B) Iodine is the only acceptable contrast medium for the examination of the gastrointestinal tract when bowel perforation is possible. **contrast media, iodinated contrast media (Torres, Ehrlich, Ballinger)**

1345.   (C) Gastroscopy and thyroid iodine uptake procedures should be done prior to a barium examination of the colon to avoid interference with the results. An upper gastrointestinal examination with barium should follow a barium enema. **scheduling, gastrointestinal tract (Ehrlich, Torres)**

1346.   (A) The NPO order indicates nothing by mouth, or fasting. **diet, gastrointestinal tract, abbreviations, acronyms (Torres, Ballinger, Ehrlich)**

1347.   (B) Excessive height of the barium solution bag during a barium enema examination can cause severe abdominal cramping and rupture of diverticula in the colon due to the excessive fluid pressure. **gastrointestinal tract, gastrointestinal, barium enema (Ballinger, Ehrlich, Torres)**

1348.   (A) Black tarry blood in the stool is an indication of upper gastrointestinal bleeding. Fresh red blood indicates hemorrhoids or pathology in the distal colon. **upper gastrointestinal, gastrointestinal (Eisenberg PATHOLOGY, Ehrlich, Ballinger)**

1349.   (B) A urogram indicates an examination of the entire urinary system, while a pyelogram indicates examination of the pylorus of the kidney. KUB is used to designate a plain film examination of the kidneys, ureters, and bladder. A cystogram is an examination of the urinary bladder only. **urinary system (Ballinger, Ehrlich)**

1350.   (B) Barium should be administered orally with a straw to avoid coating the mouth with barium. **barium (Torres, Ehrlich)**

1351.   (B) Sims position, which is a LAO, is the best position for insertion of an enema tip. **enema (Torres, Ehrlich)**

1352.   (A) A clear liquid diet should be prescribed for 24 hours prior to a barium examination of the gastrointestinal tract. This diet includes carbonated beverages, clear gelatin, clear broth, and coffee and tea with sugar. It excludes whole grain cereals, bread, vegetables, fried foods, and milk. **barium, contrast media (Torres, Ehrlich)**

1353. (D) The first five seconds of rescue activity for an unwitnessed cardiac arrest should be used to establish unresponsiveness. **cardiopulmonary resuscitation (Torres, Ehrlich)**

1354. (D) The most common cause of airway obstruction after an unwitnessed collapse is the tongue. **medical emergencies, obstruction (Snopek, Torres, Ehrlich)**

1355. (B) Hypoglycemia results from an excess amount of insulin in the bloodstream of a patient with diabetes mellitus. It is treated by the administration of sugar. **medical emergencies (Torres, Ehrlich)**

1356. (B) The heart is squeezed between the sternum and spine to produce artificial circulation. **cardiopulmonary resuscitation (Torres, Ehrlich)**

1357. (B) The primary function of establishing an intravenous line during angiography is to establish a direct route for introducing medication and for the injection of additional contrast media if needed. **cardiopulmonary resuscitation (Torres, Ehrlich)**

1358. (D) Oxygen, lidocaine, and epinephrine are all considered essential for CPR, as are sodium bicarbonate, atropine, calcium chloride, and morphine sulfate. **cardiopulmonary resuscitation (Torres, Ehrlich)**

1359. (D) When high-priority, acute, emergency orders are received at once, the procedure that can be accomplished in the shortest length of time should be done first. **acute emergencies, medical emergencies (Ehrlich, Torres)**

1360. (A) A cerebral vascular accident is often characterized by one-sided muscle weakness and eye deviation accompanied by difficult speech and a sudden stiff neck. **medical emergencies (Torres, Ehrlich)**

1361. (B) Two ventilations and 15 cardiac compressions is the proper sequence for adult cardiopulmonary resuscitation. **cardiopulmonary resuscitation (Torres, Ehrlich)**

1362. (C) Cardiac compressions should not be interrupted by more than 7 seconds once cardiopulmonary resuscitation has begun. **cardiopulmonary resuscitation (Torres, Ehrlich)**

1363. (B) Noisy breathing, wheezing, and labored breathing are all symptoms of a partially obstructed airway. **medical emergencies (Torres, Ehrlich)**

1364. (A) A patient should be moved to a lateral recumbent or sitting position when vomiting to avoid aspiration of vomitus. **acute emergencies, medical emergencies (Ehrlich, Torres)**

1365. (B) Epinephrine will resolve an acute asthmatic episode. **acute emergencies, medical emergencies (Ehrlich, Torres)**

1366. (B) The sternum should be compressed 1.5" to 2" during cardiopulmonary resuscitation of an adult. **cardiopulmonary resuscitation (Torres, Ehrlich)**

1367. (A) The Heimlich maneuver involves a quick forceful pressure upward against the diaphragm. It does not involve clearing the mouth or mouth-to-mouth resuscitation. **medical emergencies (Torres, Ehrlich)**

1368. (D) Tracheal intubation, cricothyreotomy, and bag-valve-mask are all valid artificial ventilation methods. **cardiopulmonary resuscitation (Torres, Ehrlich)**

1369. (D) Dyspnea is labored or difficult breathing. **medical emergencies, acute emergencies (Torres, Ehrlich)**

1370. (C) Benadryl (diphenhydramine) will assist in resolving a mild reaction to iodinated contrast media. **acute emergencies, medical emergencies (Ehrlich, Torres)**

1371. (C) Fingers should never be inserted into the mouth of a patient experiencing a seizure as they may bite them and cause serious damage. A physician should be called to move the tongue into a safe location. The patient should be assisted into a supine position on the floor, and objects should be moved out of the patient's reach. **medical emergencies, acute emergencies (Torres, Ehrlich)**

1372. (B) Clamping the nose with the fingers effectively seals the airway during cardiopulmonary resuscitation. **cardiopulmonary resuscitation (Torres, Ehrlich)**

1373. (A) Hypoglycemia results from an excess amount of insulin in the bloodstream of a patient with diabetes mellitus. It is treated by the administration of sugar. **medical emergencies (Torres, Ehrlich)**

1374. (A) Sodium bicarbonate and morphine sulfate are considered essential drugs for CPR. Nitroglycerine is not, although oxygen, epinephrine, atropine, lidocaine, and calcium chloride also are considered essential. **drugs (Torres)**

1375. (B) Effective cardiac compression requires the patient be supine with a hard surface under him or her. A clear airway is not required for effective cardiac compression, although it is necessary to resuscitate the patient. **cardiopulmonary resuscitation (Torres, Ehrlich)**

1376. (C) Ventilations only should be initiated if a patient has stopped breathing but the carotid pulse can still be detected. **cardiopulmonary resuscitation (Torres, Ehrlich)**

1377. (C) Diabetic reactions and anaphylaxis are potentially life-threatening. Asthmatic attacks are seldom life-threatening. **medical emergencies, acute emergencies (Torres, Ehrlich)**

1378. (B) Diaphoresis is profuse sweating. **medical emergencies, acute emergencies (Torres, Ehrlich)**

1379. (C) Epistaxis is another term for a nosebleed. **medical emergencies, acute emergencies (Ehrlich, Torres)**

1380. (A) During cardiopulmonary resuscitation, the second hand is placed on top of the first hand, which is positioned with the palm over the midline of the sternum above the xiphoid process. **cardiopulmonary resuscitation (Torres, Ehrlich)**

1381. (C) The carotid pulse is recommended during resuscitation procedures. **cardiopulmonary resuscitation (Torres, Ehrlich)**

1382. (C) 80 external cardiac compressions are recommended for one-rescuer CPR of an adult. **cardiopulmonary resuscitation (Torres, Ehrlich)**

1383. (D) The elbows must be locked during cardiac compression, the carotid pulse checked every minute, and assistance must be requested during cardiopulmonary resuscitation. **cardiopulmonary resuscitation (Torres, Ehrlich)**

1384. (C) The heel of the hand should be placed on the sternum to initiate cardiac compression during cardiopulmonary resuscitation. **cardiopulmonary resuscitation (Torres, Ehrlich)**

1385. (C) A "stat" order receives highest priority. **medical emergencies, acute emergencies (Ehrlich, Torres)**

1386. (B) A triage procedure is used for efficient handling of large numbers of trauma patients at one time, as in a disaster. **medical emergencies, acute emergencies (Ehrlich, Torres)**

1387. (B) Cardiac compressions must begin immediately if the pulse ceases during the ventilation of a patient with an airway obstruction. **cardiopulmonary resuscitation (Torres, Ehrlich)**

1388. (D) Fifteen cardiac compressions followed by two ventilations is the proper sequence for adult cardiopulmonary resuscitation. **cardiopulmonary resuscitation (Torres, Ehrlich)**

1389. (B) Irreparable brain damage occurs within 3 to 5 minutes after cardiac arrest. **cardiopulmonary resuscitation (Torres, Ehrlich)**

1390. (B) 60 external cardiac compressions are recommended for two-rescuer CPR of an adult. **cardiopulmonary resuscitation (Torres, Ehrlich)**

1391. (A) Aspiration of food is the most common cause of respiratory arrest. **respiratory arrest (Torres, Ehrlich)**

1392. (B) Ataxia is defective muscle coordination. **medical emergencies, acute emergencies (Torres, Ehrlich)**

1393. (B) Ketoacidosis results when insufficient insulin is available to metabolize glucose, and mobilization of fatty acids begins. The condition may result if a patient misses an insulin injection due to a radiologic procedure or while waiting in a radiology department. **medical emergencies (Torres, Ehrlich)**

PATIENT CARE AND MANAGEMENT
Monitoring of Medical Equipment
0.5% (6) 1394-1400

1394. (C) A surgically implanted, biliary duct T-tube is designed to drain bile. **biliary system (Ballinger, Torres, Eisenberg, Ehrlich)**

1395. (C) In most institutions, it is permissible for radiographers to reconnect oxygen lines and urinary catheter lines because they require aseptic but not sterile procedures. A Swan-Ganz catheter is a direct line into the heart and requires strict surgical asepsis and precise positioning techniques. **drainage tubes, catheters, bedside radiography (Torres, Ehrlich, Snopek)**

1396. (A) A cystostomy tube drains fluid from the kidneys to outside the body. **drainage tubes, bedside radiography (Torres, Ehrlich)**

1397. (B) A closed chest drainage tube and a tracheostomy require surgical procedures during insertion. A nasogastric tube requires simply aseptic procedures only. **drainage tubes, bedside radiography (Torres, Ehrlich)**

1398. (C) Tissue drains includes the Penrose and Hemovac drains. The Cantor tube is a nasogastric tube. **drainage tubes, bedside radiography (Torres, Ehrlich)**

1399. (A) A nonrebreathing mask is capable of delivering up to 100% oxygen. A partial rebreathing mask may deliver 60 to 90% oxygen; a venturi mask 24 to 50%; and an aerosol mask 60 to 80%. **oxygen administration (Torres, Ehrlich)**

1400. (A) The Cantor and Levin tubes are gastric. A Penrose drain is used to drain tissues. **drainage tubes, bedside radiography (Torres, Ehrlich)**

Radiation Protection

B^5

A^6

D^7

A^8

B^9

Question # ┐
Answer ┐ |
↓ |
↓

Patient Protection 8% (16) 1-16

1. During which trimester of pregnancy does the maximum sensitivity of the fetus occur?
   1. first
   2. second
   3. third
      a. 1 only
      b. 2 only
      c. 3 only
      d. 1, 2, & 3

2. What is the threshold level for radiation injury to the central nervous system?
      a.   500 to 1,000 rad
      b. 2,000 to 4,000 rad
      c. 5,000 to 10,000 rad
      d. 20,000 to 100,000 rad

3. Which of the following errors would most likely cause the greatest excessive exposure to the patient?
      a. collimation 3 cm wider than necessary
      b. low kVp and high mAs
      c. poor positioning resulting in a repeated projection
      d. incoming line voltage fluxuation

4. Which type of gonad shield should be used during a sterile procedure?
   1. flat contact
   2. shaped contact
   3. shadow
      a. 1 only
      b. 2 only
      c. 3 only
      d. 1, 2, & 3

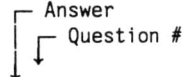

┌─ Answer
│ ┌─ Question #

5. Which of the following exposure factor systems contribute to a reduction of patient exposure dose?
   1. fixed kVp systems
   2. variable kVp systems
B¹⁵   3. automatic exposure controls
      a. 1 & 2 only
      b. 1 & 3 only
      c. 2 & 3 only
      d. 1, 2, & 3

6. Which of the interactions between ionizing radiation and matter cause more patient exposure dose?
      a. photoelectric effect
C¹⁶   b. coherent (classical) scatter
      c. Compton effect
      d. pair production

7. Which primary beam field size would produce the greatest scatter dose to the patient?
      a. 4" x 4"
      b. 6" x 6"
      c. 6" x 8"
      d. 8" x 8"

C¹⁷   8. Which skin surface receives the greatest exposure when the patient is positioned for an LPO abdomen?
      a. right anterior
      b. left anterior
      c. right posterior
      d. left posterior

9. Which of the following procedures should be rescheduled, if possible,
D¹⁸   for a pregnant patient?
      1. barium enema
      2. cervical spine
      3. abdomen and pelvis
      a. 1 & 2 only
      b. 1 & 3 only
      c. 2 & 3 only
B¹⁹   d. 1, 2, & 3

440

10. Which of the following technical factors would result in the greatest patient exposure dose?
    a. 70 kVp, 3 mAs, 200 relative film/screen speed
    b. 70 kVp, 1.5 mAs, 400 relative film/screen speed
    c. 60 kVp, 6 mAs, 200 relative film/screen speed
    d. 60 kVp, 3 mAs, 400 relative film/screen speed

11. Which of the following are removed from the primary beam by filtration?
    a. short wavelength, low-energy photons
    b. short wavelength, high-energy photons A^1
    c. long wavelength, low-energy photons
    d. long wavelength, high-energy photons

12. Which of the following technical factors would produce the greatest patient exposure dose?
    a. 70 kVp, 6 mAs, 72" FFD
    b. 70 kVp, 1.5 mAs, 40" FFD
    c. 80 kVp, 3 mAs, 72" FFD B^2
    d. 80 kVp, 1.5 mAs, 40" FFD

13. Which of the following beam restriction devices is adjustable?
    1. aperture diaphragms
    2. collimators
    3. cones and cylinders
       a. 1 only C^3
       b. 2 only
       c. 3 only
       d. 1, 2, & 3

14. Which of the following best defines a non-stochastic radiation effect?
    a. radiation damage that can be described by a non-threshold, non-linear, dose-response curve
    b. radiation damage that increases the probability of inducing a late effect but will not increase the severity of C^4
       the effect
    c. radiation damage that exhibits a threshold above which the severity of the effect is increased
    d. radiation damage that is exhibited after birth but is not congenital

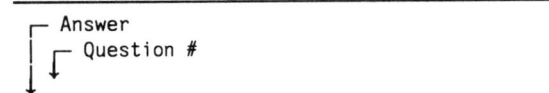

Answer
Question #

15. What is the primary concern regarding radiation exposure to the gonads?
    a. somatic effects
    b. genetic effects
    c. threshold effects
    d. non-threshold effects

A^{25}

16. Which of the following would reduce patient exposure during fluoroscopy?
    1. increase mA
    2. use intermittent fluoroscopy
    3. decrease primary beam field size
       a. 1 & 2 only
       b. 1 & 3 only
       c. 2 & 3 only
       d. 1, 2, & 3

A^{26}

Personnel Protection 4% (8) 17-24

17. What is the whole body, lifetime accumulated occupational maximum permissible dose?
    a. 0.5 rem
    b. 5 rem

B^{27}

    c. 5(N-18) rem, where N = age in years
    d. 5(18-N) rem, where N = age in years

18. What are the recognized basic methods of protection from radiation?
    1. time
    2. distance

B^{28}

    3. shielding
       a. 1 & 2 only
       b. 1 & 3 only
       c. 2 & 3 only
       d. 1, 2, & 3

C^{29}

19. How many scattering events should x-rays undergo before they reach a radiographer behind a shielded wall?
    a. 1
    b. 2
    c. 3
    d. 5

20. Which of the following are exempted from whole body, occupational effective dose equivalent limits?
    a. hands and feet
    b. liver and stomach
    c. cornea and brain
    d. gonads

C^{10}

21. Which of the following is within the normal, monthly, occupational exposure dose range for a radiographer working in diagnostic radiography?
    a. 20 mrem
    b. 500 mrem
    c. 20 rem
    d. 1,000 rem

C^{11}

22. What is the required lead equivalency for the drape used during fluoroscopy to intercept the scattered radiation produced in the patient?
    a. 0.25 mm Al
    b. 0.25 mm Pb
    c. 1.5 mm Al
    d. 1.5 mm Pb

D^{12}

23. Which of the following is the major source of the majority of scattered radiation received by the radiographer assisting with a fluoroscopic examination?
    a. fluoroscopic x-ray tube
    b. image intensifier
    c. patient
    d. fluoroscopist

B^{13}

24. Which of the following is a requirement for the exposure activation switch of a fluoroscopic unit?
    1. it cannot be located in the fluoroscopic room
    2. it must be a dead-man type
    3. it must produce an audible signal at all times when activated
    a. 1 only
    b. 2 only
    c. 3 only
    d. 1, 2, & 3

C^{14}

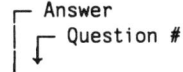

Radiation Exposure and Monitoring 4% (8) 25-32

B³³ 25. Which of the following is a monitoring device that records exposure to radiation by discharging a wire due to the ionization of the air within a chamber?
  a. pocket ionization chamber
  b. film badge
  c. cutie pie
  d. thermoluminescent dosimeter

D³⁴ 26. Which radiation unit/s is/are used to report personnel monitoring exposure of occupational workers?
  1. rem
  2. roentgens
  3. rad
  a. 1 only
  b. 2 only
  c. 3 only
  d. 1, 2, & 3

D³⁵ 27. If two personnel monitoring devices are worn, which would record t he thyroid dose?
  a. neck outside lead apron
  b. neck inside lead apron
  c. waist outside lead apron
  d. waist inside lead apron

B³⁶ 28. What is the SI unit of exposure in air?
  a. roentgen
  b. coulomb per kilogram
  c. gray
  d. sievert

B³⁷ 29. What is the mR/mAs if an exposure at 80 kVp and 12 mAs produces a dosimeter reading of 68.4 mR?
  a.   0.9 mR
  b.   1.2 mR
  c.   5.7 mR
  d. 960.0 mR

C³⁸

444

30. What is the recommended annual, whole body dose equivalent limit for students under 18 years of age?
    a. 0.1 mSv
    b. 0.5 mSv
    c. 1.0 mSv
    d. 5.0 mSv

A^{20}

31. What is the annual dose equivalent limit for a nurse?
    a.   0.1 rem
    b.   0.5 rem
    c.   5.0 rem
    d. 1,000 rem

A^{21}

mR/mAs CHART

source to receptor distance = 40" (100 cm)

kVp	mR/mAs
50	0.7
60	1.1
70	1.9
80	3.1
90	5.4
100	6.8
110	7.3
120	8.1

B^{22}

C^{23}

Figure 37

32. What is the approximate entrance exposure that would be measured at the tabletop for a single exposure of 100 kVp and 15 mAs according to Figure 37?
    a.   6.8 mR
    b. 14.7 mR
    c. 102.0 mR
    d. 680.0 mR

B^{24}

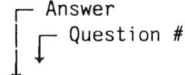

Answer

Question #

Radiographic Equipment 11% (22) 33-54

33. What term describes the positively charged electrode of a modern diagnostic x-ray tube?
    a. cathode
    b. anode
    c. input phosphor
    d. output phosphor

A⁴⁴

34. Upon striking the anode, approximately what percentage of the energy of the x-ray beam is converted to x-radiation?
    a. >99%
    b. 66%
    c. 50%
    d. <1%

A⁴⁵

35. Which of the following components normally are located in the high voltage branch of the x-ray circuit?
    a. timer circuit
    b. pre-reading kVp meter
    c. line voltage compensator
    d. rectifier

D⁴⁶

36. What is the principle function of the high-tension transformer?
    a. to produce high tube current mA
    b. to create a high potential difference
    c. to convert the AC to a DC waveform
    d. to produce a high filament temperature

C⁴⁷

37. A three-phase, twelve-pulse unit has a maximum anode heat storage capacity of 100,000 heat units. How many consecutive 800 mA, 0.12 s, and 80 kVp exposures may be made without exceeding the anode capacity?
    a. 7
    b. 9
    c. 13
    d. 26

D⁴⁸

38. What is the unit of electrical current?
    a. volt
    b. ohm
    c. ampere
    d. farad

39. What is the most common phosphor used for the input screen phosphor of a fluoroscopic image intensification tube?
    a. calcium tungstate
    b. gadolinium
    c. cesium iodide
    d. xenon

C^{30}

40. What constant factor is used to determine heat units for a three-phase, six-pulse generator?
    a. 1.00
    b. 1.35
    c. 1.41
    d. 1.50

B^{31}

41. What term describes the output voltage curve produced by the rotation of a generator armature?
    a. Fourier
    b. inverse
    c. inverse square
    d. sine

42. In the 80 to 100 kVp range, approximately what percentage of emitted x-ray photons are produced by bremstrahlung interactions?
    a. 1
    b. 10
    c. 50
    d. 90

43. What term is used to describe the fastest time in which an automatic exposure control can terminate an exposure?
    a. backup time
    b. minimum reaction time
    c. exposure time
    d. overload

C^{32}

44. Which of the following can be used to increase the voltage produced by an electrical generator?
    1. increasing the strength of the magnetic field
    2. increasing the speed with which magnetic lines of force cut through conductors
    3. decreasing the angle between the magnetic field and the conductors
    a. 1 & 2 only
    b. 1 & 3 only
    c. 2 & 3 only
    d. 1, 2, & 3

A^{55}

45. Which of the following factors will decrease effective focal spot size?
    1. smaller anode angle
    2. smaller actual focal spot size
    3. greater FFD
    a. 1 & 2 only
    b. 1 & 3 only
    c. 2 & 3 only
    d. 1, 2, & 3

D^{56}

46. What material is commonly used for x-ray tube cathode filaments?
    a. copper
    b. molybdenum
    c. rhenium
    d. tungsten

C^{57}

47. What is the power rating of a three-phase x-ray generator capable of 120 kVp at 800 mA?
    a.   6.6 kVp/mA
    b.   96 watts
    c.   96 kilowatts
    d. 200 watts

B^{58} 48. What is a diode?
    a. a capacitor adapted for high-voltage use
    b. a transistor
    c. a rheostat
    d. a rectifying semiconductor

B^{59}

Question #
Answer

49. How many lines comprise a standard video raster pattern?
    a. 60
    b. 120
    c. 525
    d. 1050

C^{39}

50. Which of the following components of a diagnostic x-ray tube have a positive charge during the production of x-rays?
    1. anode
    2. cathode
    3. focal track
        a. 1 & 2 only
        b. 1 & 3 only
        c. 2 & 3 only
        d. 1, 2, & 3

B^{40}

51. What is the approximate speed of a high speed rotating anode?
    a.   100 to 200 rpm
    b.   3,000 to 3,500 rpm
    c.   10,000 to 12,000 rpm
    d.   30,000 to 50,000 rpm

D^{41}

52. What term is used to describe the effect produced when a varying current is supplied to the primary side of a transformer and causes a current to flow in the secondary side of the transformer without electrical contact between the two?
    a. mutual induction
    b. self induction
    c. primary induction
    d. secondary induction

D^{42}

53. What is the speed of light?
    a. 3 x 10^8 meters/second
    b. 6.24 x 10^{18} meters/second
    c. 186,000 meters/second
    d. 2.14 x 10^{-14} meters/second

B^{43}

54. Which of the following best describes the electrical properties of plastic?
    a. conductor
    b. semiconductor
    c. superconductor
    d. insulator

Maintenance and Malfunctions of Radiographic Unit and Accessories
4% (8) 55-62

C^{64}

55. Which of the following grids could be used upside down without affecting the quality of the radiographic image?
    a. linear parallel
    b. focused parallel
    c. focused cross-hatch
    d. focused circular

B^{65}

56. Which of the following describe a phosphorescent effect in radiographic intensifying screens?
    1. screen lag
    2. luminescence
    3. afterglow
      a. 1 & 2 only
      b. 1 & 3 only
      c. 2 & 3 only
      d. 1, 2, & 3

A^{66}

57. If an exposure is made with a single-phase, full-wave rectified x-ray unit on 60 Hz current at 0.05 s, how many dots should be imaged with a spinning top test?
    a. 18
    b. 12

C^{67}

    c. 6
    d. 3

58. Which of the following are potential causes of anatomic motion appearing on a radiograph?
    1. vibration of the bucky tray by the reciprocating grid mechanism
    2. accidental bumping of the x-ray control console
    3. drifting of the overhead tube due to faulty locks and detentes

C^{68}

      a. 1 & 2 only
      b. 1 & 3 only
      c. 2 & 3 only
      d. 1, 2, & 3

59. Which of the following is a reasonable range of acceptable mA linearity error?
    a. 0.1%
    b. 10%
    c. 20%
    d. 30%

60. What is the most likely cause of black tree-like marks on a processed radiograph?
    a. bending of the film before processing
    b. oil or lotion on fingers that handled the film before processing
    c. a small piece of paper in the cassette during exposure
    d. static electricity discharge in the darkroom

C[49]

61. What quality control test is performed by blocking all automatic exposure control chambers, except one, with a lead block?
    a. backup timer verification
    b. minimum response time verification
    c. ion chamber sensitivity and accuracy
    d. system reproduceability

62. Which of the following require periodic fluoroscopy or filming to verify their protective ability?
    1. lead gloves
    2. lead walls
    3. lead aprons
    a. 1 & 2 only
    b. 1 & 3 only
    c. 2 & 3 only
    d. 1, 2, & 3

A[50]

C[51]

Selection of Technical Factors 16% (32) 63-94

63. Which of the following factors are considered to be prime factors that regulates radiographic density?
    1. mA
    2. time
    3. kVp
    a. 1 & 2 only
    b. 1 & 3 only
    c. 2 & 3 only
    d. 1, 2, & 3

A[52]

A[53]

D[54]

Answer
Question #

64. A film/screen combination is rated with an arbitrary number of 100. If another film/screen combination is rated at 200, what adjustment must be made to correctly compensate radiographic density?
    a. increase kVp by 7%
    b. increase kVp by 15%
    c. decrease kVp by 15%
    d. increase mAs by a factor of 2

A[74]

65. If a satisfactory radiograph is produced with 80 mAs at 40", what mAs change should be made to produce an identical radiograph at 55"?
    a. 100 mAs
    b. 151 mAs
    c. 156 mAs
    d. 160 mAs

66. Which of the following effective focal spots will produce the greatest recorded detail on any given radiograph?

A[75]
    a. 0.03 mm
    b. 1.2 mm
    c. 2.2 mm
    d. 3.0 mm

67. Which of the following conditions does not contribute to poor recorded detail?
    a. large effective focal spot size
    b. short FFD

B[76]
    c. short OFD
    d. large OFD

68. Which of the following optical density (OD) numbers demonstrate the approximate range of radiographic densities visible to the human eye?
    a. 0.00 to 1.00
    b. 0.00 to 10.00
    c. 0.25 to 2.50

B[77]
    d. 1.00 to 5.00

For items 69 to 72 use the following information: A satisfactory radiograph of a hip has been produced using the technical factors listed below. In each of the questions one factor has been changed. Indicate the result that will be seen on the radiograph as a result of each factor change if all other factors remain the same.

B[78]

300 mA
0.12 s
84 kVp
40" FFD
3" OFD
12:1 grid ratio
400 relative speed film/screens
2.5 mm focal spot
10" x 12" field size

D^{60}

69. Changing the OFD to 2.5" would result in:
    a. increased magnification
    b. decreased magnification
    c. decreased recorded detail C^{61}
    d. higher contrast

70. The use of a 200 relative speed film/screen combination and 72 mAs would result in:
    a. increased magnification
    b. increased density
    c. decreased density
    d. essentially no change

71. Collimating to an 11" x 14" primary beam field would result in: B^{62}
    a. higher contrast
    b. lower contrast
    c. increased recorded detail
    d. focal spot blooming

72. Changing the grid ratio to 16:1 would result in:
    a. decreased density and higher contrast
    b. decreased density and lower contrast
    c. increased density and higher contrast
    d. increased density and lower contrast

73. How is a grid ratio determined?
    a. lead strip height divided by interspace width A^{63}
    b. lead strip width divided by interspace width
    c. lead strip width divided by lead strip height
    d. interspace width divided by lead strip width

Equipment Operation and Maintenance

74. Which of the following have the ability to increase image density by increasing x-ray tube output?
    1. a high vacuum inside the glass envelope
    2. a smooth anode focal track
    3. increased added filtration
        a. 1 & 2 only
        b. 1 & 3 only

A⁸³
        c. 2 & 3 only
        d. 1, 2, & 3

75. Which of the following will reduce the production of scattered radiation?
    1. low kVp
    2. large part thickness
    3. high speed film
        a. 1 only
        b. 2 only

C⁸⁴
        c. 3 only
        d. 1, 2, & 3

76. Which of the following projections take advantage of the divergence of the primary beam to reduce distortion?
    1. PA lumbar spine
    2. PA thoracic spine

D⁸⁵
    3. lateral L5-S1 lumbar spot
        a. 1 & 2 only
        b. 1 & 3 only
        c. 2 & 3 only
        d. 1, 2, & 3

C⁸⁶
77. What is the actual size of a heart that casts a shadow 10.2 cm wide on a PA chest radiograph produced at 180 cm when the heart is located 4 cm from the film?
        a. 1.02 cm
        b. 10.0 cm
        c. 10.2 cm
        d. 10.4 cm

78. Which of the following kVp ranges are appropriate for imaging the cervical spine?

B⁸⁷
        a.   40 to 50
        b.   60 to 70
        c.   80 to 90
        d.   110 to 120

454

79. Which of the following is increased by increasing part thickness?
    a. recorded detail
    b. distortion
    c. contrast
    d. density

80. Which of the following are hardening agents used in automatic film processing solutions?
    1. hydroquinone
    2. glutaraldehyde
    3. potassium alum
    a. 1 & 2 only
    b. 1 & 3 only   B^{69}
    c. 2 & 3 only
    d. 1, 2, & 3

81. Which of the following characteristics are common for radiographic films with a high average gradient?
    1. high contrast   D^{70}
    2. low speed
    3. narrow latitude
    a. 1 & 2 only
    b. 1 & 3 only
    c. 2 & 3 only
    d. 1, 2, & 3

82. An 8:1 ratio grid has a non-grid conversion factor of 4 and a 12:1 B^{71} grid has a non-grid conversion factor of 5.5. What mAs should be used to produce a radiograph of similar density with the 12:1 grid when a satisfactory radiograph is produced using 76 kVp and 14 mAs with the 8:1 ratio grid?   A^{72}
    a. 2.5 mAs
    b. 3.5 mAs
    c. 10 mAs
    d. 19 mAs

A^{73}

B⁹³

83. Which of the following pathologic conditions would require decreased technical factors to maintain image density as compared to normal tissue?
    1. emaciation
    2. atrophy
    3. abscess
        a. 1 & 2 only
        b. 1 & 3 only
        c. 2 & 3 only
        d. 1, 2, & 3

A⁹⁴

84. Which of the following conditions contribute to decreased recorded detail?
    1. small effective focal spot size
    2. short FFD
    3. long OFD
        a. 1 & 2 only
        b. 1 & 3 only
        c. 2 & 3 only
        d. 1, 2, & 3

85. Which of the following technical factors would produce a radiograph with the lowest contrast?
    a. 200 mA, 0.12 s, 80 kVp
    b. 200 mA, 0.06 s, 92 kVp
    c. 400 mA, 0.03 s, 92 kVp
    d. 200 mA, 0.03 s, 106 kVp

A⁹⁵

86. Which of the following are decreased by increased film fog?
    a. distortion
    b. recorded detail
    c. contrast
    d. density

B⁹⁶

87. Which of the following can be used to compensate for a slower film/screen combination?
    1. decrease mAs
    2. increase kVp
    3. increase FFD
        a. 1 only
        b. 2 only
        c. 3 only
        d. 1, 2, & 3

88. Which of the following is most affected by involuntary motion?
    a. density
    b. contrast
    c. distortion
    d. recorded detail

    C^{79}

89. Which of the following are typical of low-resolution film?
    1. high speed
    2. high contrast
    3. wide latitude
        a. 1 & 2 only
        b. 1 & 3 only
        c. 2 & 3 only
        d. 1, 2, & 3

    C^{80}

90. Toward what structure are the grid lines directed in a focused grid?
    a. toward the x-ray tube focal spot
    b. toward the area of interest in the patient
    c. toward the x-ray tabletop
    d. toward the image receptor

91. Which of the following films would most likely produce the widest latitude?

    B^{81}

    1. low contrast
    2. fast
    3. low base-plus-fog
        a. 1 only
        b. 2 only
        c. 3 only
        d. 1, 2, & 3

92. Which of the following changes will occur with an increase in abdominal compression?

    D^{82}

    1. decreased density
    2. higher contrast
    3. increased recorded detail
        a. 1 only
        b. 2 only
        c. 3 only
        d. 1, 2, & 3

93. What is the actual size of a cyst in the proximal tibia that casts a shadow 2.1 cm wide on an AP knee radiograph produced at 100 cm when the mass is located 1.4 cm from the film?
    a. 1.01 cm
    b. 2.1 cm
    c. 2.2 cm
    d. 2.3 cm

B^{102} 94. Which of the following will increase the production of scattered radiation?
    1. high kVp
    2. large part thickness
    3. small OFD
    a. 1 & 2 only
C^{103} b. 1 & 3 only
    c. 2 & 3 only
    d. 1, 2, & 3

Film Processing and Quality Assurance 5% (10) 95-104

95. Which of the following could produce increased base-plus-fog levels during sensitometric evaluation of radiographic film?
C^{104} 1. excessive heat in storage area
    2. cracked safelight filter
    3. excessively warm processor wash water
    a. 1 & 2 only
    b. 1 & 3 only
    c. 2 & 3 only
    d. 1, 2, & 3

96. Which of the following are acceptable storage methods for radiographic cassettes?
    1. on end
    2. flat
A^{105} 3. at an angle
    a. 1 only
    b. 2 only
    c. 3 only
    d. 1, 2, & 3

97. Which of the following is a device used for producing a standard optical step wedge on a radiographic film?
    a. densitometer
    b. dosimeter
    c. sensitometer
    d. galvanometer

    D⁸⁸

98. Why must film be brought to room temperature before breaking the moisture-proof seal in the package?
    a. to avoid moisture from the air condensing on the film
    b. to prevent the emulsion from cracking with the rapid temperature change
    c. to bring the emulsion up to sensitivity gradually thus avoiding areas of low sensitivity
    d. to maintain the adhesion between the emulsion and base

    B⁸⁹

99. Which automatic processor system stabilizes solution temperatures, agitates solutions, and mixes replenishment chemistry into the tanks?
    1. replenishment system
    2. recirculation system
    3. temperature control system
    a. 1 only
    b. 2 only
    c. 3 only
    d. 1, 2, & 3

    A⁹⁰

100. What are the causes of age fog?
    1. background radiation
    2. heat
    3. primary beam radiation
    a. 1 & 2 only
    b. 1 & 3 only
    c. 2 & 3 only
    d. 1, 2, & 3

    A⁹¹

101. What is the approximate developer immersion time for a film in a 90 second processor?
    a. 1 to 5 seconds
    b. 20 to 25 seconds
    c. 45 to 60 seconds
    d. 90 seconds

    B⁹²

102. Why should an automatic film processor be allowed to run for 15 to 20 minutes prior to developing the first films?
    1. to bring the developer solution up to the appropriate temperature
    2. to permit proper replenishment of the developer to compensate for oxidation that has occurred while the unit was shut down
    3. to permit agitation and recirculation to mix the solutions well
        a. 1 & 2 only
        b. 1 & 3 only
        c. 2 & 3 only
        d. 1, 2, & 3

C^{111}

B^{112} 103. Which of the following color safelights would produce safe conditions for working with yellow-green sensitive film?
        a. blue-violet
        b. yellow-green
        c. dark red
        d. orange-brown

104. What procedure should be used to assure equal wear of automatic film processor rollers as well as straight transport through the system?
        a. feed films with alternate sides facing up
        b. feed all films from the right side of the feed tray
        c. alternately feed films from the right and left sides of the feed tray
        d. feed all films at the center of the feed tray

C^{113}

Evaluation of Radiographs 6% (12) 105-116

C^{114} 105. What are the effects of higher grid ratio on image quality?
    1. contrast increases
    2. density decreases
    3. distortion decreases
        a. 1 & 2 only
        b. 1 & 3 only
        c. 2 & 3 only
        d. 1, 2, & 3

B^{115}

106. Approximately what percentage change in kVp will double image density within the diagnostic range of kVp and within average patient part sizes?
    a. 5%
    b. 15%
    c. 25%
    d. 50%

C^{97}

107. Which portion of a chest image will be most affected by an increase in chemical fog?
    a. areas with low-density anatomic structures
    b. areas with high-contrast anatomic structures
    c. areas with medium-density anatomic structures
    d. areas with high-density anatomic structures

108. When used to control density, which of the following will change when kVp is increased?
    1. contrast decreases
    2. recorded detail increases
    3. scatter production increases
    a. 1 & 2 only
    b. 1 & 3 only
    c. 2 & 3 only
    d. 1, 2, & 3

A^{98}

109. Which of the following will increase recorded detail?
    1. increased FFD
    2. increased intensifying screen speed
    3. decreased focal spot size
    a. 1 & 2 only
    b. 1 & 3 only
    c. 2 & 3 only
    d. 1, 2, & 3

B^{99}

110. Which of the following describes a misrepresentation of the true size and shape of an object?
    a. density
    b. contrast
    c. recorded detail
    d. distortion

A^{100}

B^{101}

111. Which of the following projections would produce the best recorded detail of the orbits?
    a. AP
    b. PA
    c. RAO and LAO
    d. RPO and LPO

D[121]

112. If a satisfactory image is achieved using 68 kVp and 2.5 mAs, which of the following sets of technical factors would maintain the same image density while decreasing contrast?
    a. 79 kVp at 1.3 mAs
    b. 79 kVp at 0.7 mAs
    c. 68 kVp at 1.3 mAs
    d. 57 kVp at 5 mAs

B[122]

113. Which of the following will increase image contrast?
    1. decreased automatic exposure control density
    2. decreased primary beam field size
    3. decreased kVp
    a. 1 & 2 only
    b. 1 & 3 only
    c. 2 & 3 only
    d. 1, 2, & 3

D[123]

114. Which of the following will reduce scattered radiation?
    1. increased kVp
    2. increased OFD
    3. decreased primary beam field size
    a. 1 & 2 only
    b. 1 & 3 only
    c. 2 & 3 only
    d. 1, 2, & 3

B[124]

115. Which of the following exposure factors is most closely related to the quantity of photons in the x-ray beam?
    1. kVp
    2. mAs
    3. distance
    a. 1 only
    b. 2 only
    c. 3 only
    d. 1, 2, & 3

C[125]

462

Question # ⌐
Answer ⌐ |
         ↓ |
            ↓

116. Which abdominal region would produce an image with the greatest density if the stomach was retaining a large amount of gas and no technical factors compensation were made?
    a. right lumbar
    b. left iliac
    c. right hypochondriac   B[106]
    d. left hypochondriac

General Procedural Considerations 2% (4) 117-120

117. Into what divisions is the body divided by the coronal plane?
    a. superior and inferior   A[107]
    b. anterior and posterior
    c. medial and lateral
    d. right and left

118. Which term describes the direction toward the head of the body?
    a. dorsal
    b. ventral
    c. cephalad
    d. caudal

119. Which term describes the sole of the foot?   B[108]
    1. dorsal
    2. ventral
    3. plantar
    a. 1 only
    b. 2 only
    c. 3 only
    d. 1, 2, & 3

120. Which part of the patient's body is closest to the image receptor if   B[109]
the patient is supine?
    a. anterior
    b. posterior
    c. right side
    d. left side

                                                       D[110]

Specific Imaging Procedures 26% (52) 120-172

D¹³⁰

121. What projection of the chest will be obtained with the patient standing erect with the back against an upright bucky unit and the central ray directed to the second thoracic vertebra at an angle of 15° to 20° cephalad?
     a. AP
     b. lateral
     c. AP axial
     d. lordotic AP

122. What is the proper centering point for a posteroanterior projection of the second finger?
     a. distal interphalangeal joint
     b. proximal interphalangeal joint
     c. metacarpalphalangeal joint
     d. midway between the proximal interphalangeal joint and metacarpalphalangeal joint

123. How many degrees of obliquity properly position the cervical spine f or an oblique projection?
     a. 30°
     b. 35°
     c. 40°
     d. 45°

124. Which position best demonstrates the superior intervertebral foramina of the lumbar spine?

     a. AP
     b. lateral
     c. anterior oblique
     d. posterior oblique

C¹³¹

125. Which pairs of ribs are considered to be floating?
     1. 10th
     2. 11th
     3. 12th

A¹³²
     a. 1 & 2 only
     b. 1 & 3 only
     c. 2 & 3 only
     d. 1, 2, & 3

126. Which of the following will be demonstrated with a lateral cervical spine projection?
    1. vertebral interspaces
    2. inferior five articular facets
    3. spinous processes
        a. 1 & 2 only
        b. 1 & 3 only
        c. 2 & 3 only
        d. 1, 2, & 3

D^{116}

127. Which of the following bones have a styloid process at the distal end?
    1. radius
    2. humerus
    3. ulna
        a. 1 & 2 only
        b. 1 & 3 only
        c. 2 & 3 only
        d. 1, 2, & 3

B^{117}

128. Which position best demonstrates the axillary portions of the ribs?
        a. AP
        b. PA
        c. oblique
        d. lateral

C^{118}

129. Which of the following are avoided by extending the neck when radiographing the atlas and axis in a lateral position?
    1. base of the skull superimposed over the axis
    2. rami of the mandible superimposed over the axis
    3. rami of the mandible superimposed over the atlas
        a. 1 & 2 only
        b. 1 & 3 only
        c. 2 & 3 only
        d. 1, 2, & 3

C^{119}

B^{120}

465

Answer
Question #

130. Which of the following articulate with the radius?
1. navicular
2. lunate
3. scaphoid
   a. 1 & 2 only
   b. 1 & 3 only
   c. 2 & 3 only
   d. 1, 2, & 3

D 139

C 140

B 141

D 142

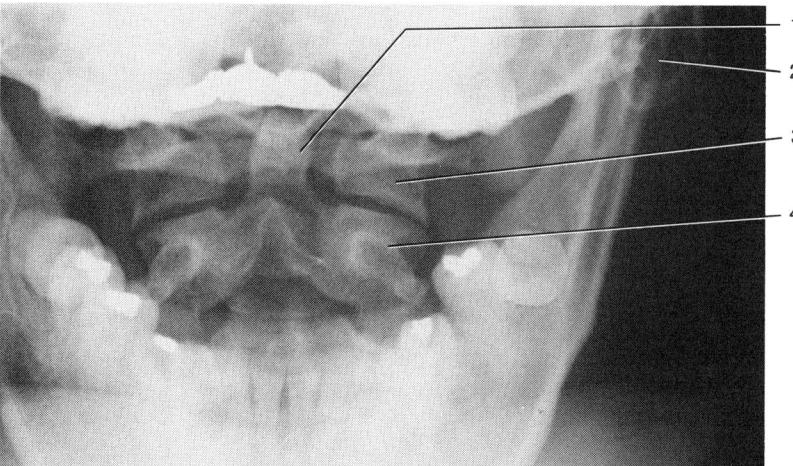

Figure 38

131. Which number in Figure 38 illustrates the atlas?
   a. 1
   b. 2
   c. 3
   d. 4

A 143

132. Which number in Figure 38 illustrates the dens?
   a. 1
   b. 2
   c. 3
   d. 4

A 144

466

133. Which number in Figure 38 illustrates the mastoid tip?
    a. 1
    b. 2
    c. 3
    d. 4

134. Which of the following axiolateral position methods for examining the temporal bone uses a 35° caudal central ray angle? D^{126}
    1. Henschen
    2. Lysholm
    3. Schuller
        a. 1 only
        b. 2 only
        c. 3 only
        d. 1, 2, & 3

135. What is the proper central ray angulation for an AP axial positi on for temporomandibular joints? B^{127}
        a. 25° caudal
        b. 25° cephalad
        c. 35° caudal
        d. 35° cephalad

136. What is the proper central ray angulation for a PA oblique axial position (Law method)? C^{128}
        a. 15° cephalad
        b. 25° to 30° cephalad
        c. 37° cephalad
        d. 53° cephalad

137. Where should the petrous ridges of the temporal bone appear on a parietoacanthial position (Waters method)?
        a. below the maxillae
        b. in the lower third of the orbits
        c. in the upper third of the orbits C^{129}
        d. above the orbits

138. Within which bone is the superior orbital fissure located?
        a. sphenoid
        b. ethmoid
        c. palatine
        d. maxilla

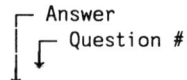

139. What joint is formed by the articulation of the condyloid process of one bone with the mandibular fossa of another?
    a. acromioclavicular
    b. knee
    c. wrist
    d. temporomandibular

B¹⁵⁰   140. What is the proper centering point for a PA chest?
    a. T2-T3
    b. T4-T5
    c. T6-T7
    d. T8-T9

C¹⁵¹   141. What result is desired when a patient is instructed to use shallow breathing during an RAO projection of the sternum?
    a. the heart shadow will be blurred
    b. the pulmonary markings will be blurred
    c. diaphragmatic motion will be blurred
    d. air in the lungs will produce an air-gap increase in contrast

B¹⁵²   142. What structure is located by drawing a line between the anterior superior iliac spine and the superior margin of the symphysis pubis, and then drawing a line from the center of that line to a point 1" distal to the lateral-most portion of the greater trochanter?
    a. intertrochanteric crest
    b. greater trochanter
    c. lesser trochanter
    d. femoral neck

A¹⁵³   143. Which of the following will demonstrate the patellofemoral joint?
    1. Merchant method
    2. Settegast method
    3. Holmblad method
    a. 1 & 2 only
    b. 1 & 3 only
    c. 2 & 3 only
    d. 1, 2, & 3

144. Which of the following refers to a posterior defect of the spinal canal due to lack of fusion of the elements of the vertebrae?
    a. spina bifida
    b. spondylolisthesis
    c. chondrosarcoma
    d. multiple myeloma

145. Which position for the clavicle will provide the best resolution?
    1. AP
    2. PA   B¹³³
    3. AP axial
        a. 1 only
        b. 2 only
        c. 3 only
        d. 1, 2, & 3

146. If the colon is demonstrated with an air-fluid level in which
    barium appears laterally and air medially within the ascending
    colon, which of the following positions was used to produce the
    image?   B¹³⁴
        a. right lateral decubitus
        b. left lateral decubitus
        c. AP erect
        d. PA prone

147. Which of the following are required for proper positioning of the
    elbow for a lateral projection?
        a. no flexion   C¹³⁵
        b. 45° flexion
        c. 90° flexion
        d. 180° flexion

148. Which position produces the best image of the gastric fundus
    during a barium stomach examination?
        a. erect PA   B¹³⁶
        b. supine PA
        c. prone PA
        d. semi-supine LPO

149. Which of the following describes a procedure for the visualization
    of the biliary tract, where a needle is inserted through the right
    lateral intercostal space and advanced toward the hilum of the   A¹³⁷
    liver, with contrast material then injected as the needle is
    withdrawn until the desired structures are visualized.
        a. percutaneous transhepatic cholangiography
        b. endoscopic retrograde cholangiopancreatography   A¹³⁸
        c. postoperative cholangiography
        d. operative cholangiography

150. In which directions do the ribs move on deep inhalation?
    1. anteriorly
    2. inferiorly
    3. laterally
        a. 1 & 2 only
        b. 1 & 3 only
        c. 2 & 3 only
        d. 1, 2, & 3

A^{158}

151. Which of the following are true of the male pelvis compared with the female?
    1. it is lighter
    2. it is narrower and deeper
    3. the sacrum is more narrow
        a. 1 & 2 only
        b. 1 & 3 only
        c. 2 & 3 only
        d. 1, 2, & 3

A^{159}

152. How many articulations are there between the radius and ulna?
        a. 1
        b. 2
        c. 3
        d. 4

153. What is the proper central ray angulation for an axiolateral position (Law method) of the mastoid process when the midsagittal plane is rotated 15° toward the image receptor from a true lateral position?
    1. 15° caudad
    2. 15° anterior
    3. 15° medial
        a. 1 only
        b. 2 only
        c. 3 only
        d. 1, 2, & 3

A^{160}

154. Which of the following describe the proper location of structures within the skull when an AP axial projection has been performed properly by the Townes method?
    1. the petrous pyramids of the temporal bone are projected symmetrically
    2. the dorsum sellae and posterior clinoid processes are projected within the shadow of the foramen magnum
    3. the inion is located near the center of the film
        a. 1 & 2 only
        b. 1 & 3 only
        c. 2 & 3 only
        d. 1, 2, & 3

B^{145}

155. Which of the following are part of the mandible?
    1. rami
    2. mental protuberance
    3. cornua
        a. 1 & 2 only
        b. 1 & 3 only
        c. 2 & 3 only
        d. 1, 2, & 3

A^{146}

156. Which of the following are true regarding the left kidney?
    1. it lies slightly more inferior than the right kidney
    2. it is slightly longer than the right kidney
    3. it is slightly narrower than the right kidney
        a. 1 & 2 only
        b. 1 & 3 only
        c. 2 & 3 only
        d. 1, 2, & 3

C^{147}

D^{148}

157. What is peristalsis?
    a. a pathologic condition of the colon resulting from diverticulosis
    b. a pathologic condition of the colon resulting from diverticulitis
    c. the normal contractive waves of the digestive system
    d. a narrowing of the colon

A^{149}

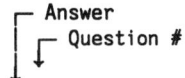

Answer
  Question #

158. Which of the following is best demonstrated on a LPO projection of the lumbar spine?
    a. left apophysial joints
    b. right apophysial joints
    c. 1st to 4th intervertebral foramina
    d. 5th intervertebral foramen

D^{167}

159. Which of the following are opposites of one another?
    1. osteopetrosis
    2. osteoporosis
    3. osteochondroma
      a. 1 & 2 only
      b. 1 & 3 only
      c. 2 & 3 only
      d. 1, 2, & 3

B^{168}

C^{169}

D^{170}

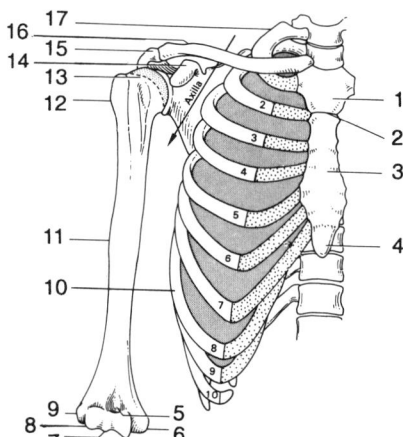

Figure 39 (from Akesson EJ, Loeb JA, Wilson-Pauwels L: Thompson's Core Textbook of Anatomy, 2nd ed. Philadelphia, JB Lippincott, 1990)

C^{171}

160. Which of the following is illustrated by #1 in Figure 39?
    a. manubrium
    b. sternal angle
    c. sternal body
    d. xiphoid process

472

161. Which number in Figure 39 illustrates the medial epicondyle?
      a. 6
      b. 7
      c. 8
      d. 9

162. Which number in Figure 39 illustrates the acromion process of
the scapula?
      a. 13
      b. 14
      c. 15 D^{154}
      d. 16

163. Which rib is illustrated by #10 in Figure 39?
      a. 7th
      b. 8th
      c. 9th
      d. 10th

164. Which portion of the colon is usually most superior? A^{155}
      a. hepatic flexure
      b. splenic flexure
      c. transverse
      d. sigmoid

165. Which is the largest salivary gland?
      a. suborbital
      b. parotid
      c. sublingual C^{156}
      d. submandibular

166. What type of respiration will best demonstrate the upper ribs?
      1. inhalation
      2. exhalation
      3. shallow breathing
         a. 1 only
         b. 2 only
         c. 3 only C^{157}
         d. 1, 2, & 3

167. What is the proper position of the hips for a localized lateral projection of the L5-S1 lumbosacral junction?
    a. affected side extended, unaffected side flexed
    b. affected side flexed, unaffected side extended
    c. both sides flexed
    d. both sides extended

A[176] 168. Which of the following are on the lateral side of the humerus?
    1. capitulum
    2. trochlea
    3. greater tubercle
    a. 1 & 2 only
    b. 1 & 3 only
    c. 2 & 3 only
    d. 1, 2, & 3

C[177] 169. Which of the following axiolateral position methods for examining the temporal bone uses a 25° caudal central ray angle?
    1. Henschen
    2. Lysholm
B[178]   3. Schuller
    a. 1 only
    b. 2 only
    c. 3 only
    d. 1, 2, & 3

170. What is the centering point for a parietoacanthial projection (Waters method) of the paranasal sinuses?
    a. glabella
    b. nasion
A[179]   c. inion
    d. acanthion

171. Which of the following are recommended in preparing a patient for urographic examination?
    1. reduced hydration for 24 hours
    2. non-gas-forming laxative
    3. NPO after midnight the day of the examination
    a. 1 & 2 only
    b. 1 & 3 only
    c. 2 & 3 only
D[180]   d. 1, 2, & 3

172. Which of the following positions is achieved by having the patient sit on the side of the x-ray table with legs hanging down and then grasp the ankles for support while the central ray is centered perpendicularly through the lumbosacral region at the level of the greater trochanters?
    A[161]
    - a. RAO
    - b. LAO
    - c. PA axial
    - d. axial (Chassard-Lapine method

Record Maintenance and Administrative Procedures 1% (2) 173-174 C[162]

173. What is the most appropriate action if a patient denies knowledge of the possible effects of the use of contrast media?
    - a. terminate the examination
    - b. explain the effects and request verification of understanding from the patient   B[163]
    - c. proceed with the examination
    - d. consult with legal counsel

174. Which of the following procedures normally would require a signed form to verify informed consent?   B[164]
    1. angiogram
    2. cardiac catherization
    3. lung tomograms
    - a. 1 & 2 only
    - b. 1 & 3 only   B[165]
    - c. 2 & 3 only
    - d. 1, 2, & 3

Patient Safety and Comfort 1% (2) 175-176

175. What position places the patient on one side, the top arm flexed and the bottom arm extended behind the body, and the body obliqued with the top knee flexed level with the pelvis?
    - a. Fowler's   A[166]
    - b. Sims'
    - c. supine
    - d. trendelenburg

176. Which of the following serve as barriers that can reduce communication between a radiographer and patient?
    1. increased physical distance
    2. crossing arms or legs
    3. using simple layman's terminology
        a. 1 & 2 only
        b. 1 & 3 only
        c. 2 & 3 only
        d. 1, 2, & 3

A^{185}

Disinfection and Sterile Technique 2.5% (5) 177-181

177. Which is acceptable when washing the hands as part of surgical scrub?
    a. touching the faucet handles
    b. picking up a hand brush if it is dropped into the sink
    c. permitting water to run from the elbows
    d. permitting water to run from the hands

A^{186}

178. Where should a lead apron be worn during surgery?
    a. over the surgical gown
    b. under the surgical gown but over the scrub suit
    c. under the scrub suit
    d. as a lead apron would contaminate the surgical apparel, it cannot be worn during surgery

C^{187}

179. Which of the following is bacterial in origin?
    1. tuberculosis
    2. herpes simplex
    3. acquired immunodeficiency syndrome (AIDS)
        a. 1 only
        b. 2 only
        c. 3 only
        d. 1, 2, & 3

C^{188}

180. Which of the following can contribute to making a radiographer a susceptible host to infection from a patient?
    1. fatigue
    2. stress
    3. low-grade fever
        a. 1 & 2 only
        b. 1 & 3 only
        c. 2 & 3 only
        d. 1, 2, & 3

A^{189}

181. Which of the following rules for sterile fields is not true?
1. a sterile field cannot be left unattended
2. a sterile drape that is below the tabletop is considered unsterile
3. sterile persons must pass front-to-front
    a. 1 only
    b. 2 only
    c. 3 only
    d. 1, 2, & 3

D 172

Isolation Techniques 1% (2) 182-183

182. What is the primary purpose of strict (reverse) isolation procedures if a patient does not have an infectious disease?
    a. to protect persons entering the isolation room
    b. to protect the patient from persons entering the isolation room
    c. to suppress insect vectors
    d. to counteract viral infections with bacteria

B 173

183. Which of the following require only simple respiratory isolation?
1. pertussis
2. influenzal meningitis
3. pneumonic plague
    a. 1 & 2 only
    b. 1 & 3 only
    c. 2 & 3 only
    d. 1, 2, & 3

A 174

Monitoring Vital Signs 1% (2) 184-185

184. What is the normal range of adult systolic blood pressure?
    a. 30 to 50 mm Hg
    b. 60 to 80 mm Hg
    c. 110 to 140 mm Hg
    d. 140 to 180 mm Hg

B 175

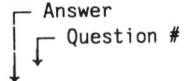

C[195]

185. Which of the following locations are good areas to check for signs of cyanosis as an indicator of respiratory distress?
     1. nail beds
     2. mouth and gums
     3. conjunctiva of the eyes
        a. 1 & 2 only
        b. 1 & 3 only
        c. 2 & 3 only
        d. 1, 2, & 3

C[196]

Contrast Media 4% (8) 186-193

186. Toxicity is most significant with contrast media components that interact at the level of which of the following?
     a. cells
     b. tissues
     c. organ
     d. system

A[197]

187. What is the primary difference between lymphangiographic and arteriographic injectors?
     a. arteriographic injectors warm the contrast media
     b. arteriographic injectors deliver a slower flow rate
     c. lymphangiographic injectors deliver a slower flow rate
     d. the two injectors are interchangeable

B[198]

188. What term describes a solution with an ionic concentration higher t han normal body fluids?
     a. isotonic
     b. hyperostotic
     c. hyperosmolar
     d. osmotic

B[199]

189. Which type of shock is most likely during iodinated contrast media studies?
     a. anaphylactic
     b. hypoglycemic
     c. hypovolemic
     d. septic

190. Which of the following are characteristics of non-ionic contrast material?
    1. cause fewer adverse reactions
    2. do not disrupt homeostasis
    3. do not disassociate in solution
        a. 1 & 2 only
        b. 1 & 3 only
        c. 2 & 3 only
        d. 1, 2, & 3

C[181]

191. What is a safe rate for intravenous infusion?
        a.   2 to 6 drops/min
        b. 15 to 20 drops/min
        c. 25 to 35 drops/min
        d. 40 to 50 drops/min

192. Which of the following are true of positive contrast material?
        a. image density is increased
        b. they are gaseous
        c. they are radiolucent
        d. they increase x-ray absorption

B[182]

193. Which type of cleansing enema is designed to cause mild irritation of the intestine in order to promote peristalsis and defecation?
        a. normal saline
        b. hypertonic saline
        c. oil retention
        d. soap suds

A[183]

Emergency Situations 3% (6) 194-199

194. Which of the following are common reactions to the symptoms of a heart attack?
    1. when the symptoms are mild, they may be ignored or attributed to some other cause
    2. occur suddenly without warning
    3. subside and return
        a. 1 & 2 only
        b. 1 & 3 only
        c. 2 & 3 only
        d. 1, 2, & 3

C[184]

195. What is the universal distress signal characterizing an apparent obstructed airway in the conscious adult?
    a. rapid heavy breathing
    b. violent choking
    c. one hand at the throat
    d. violent thrashing of the arms

196. What is the recommended rate of artificial ventilations for CPR of an adult?
    a. once every second
    b. once every 3 seconds
    c. once every 5 seconds
    d. once every 60 second

197. Which of the following medical emergencies is usually of slow onset?
    1. hyperglycemia
    2. hypoglycemia
    3. seizures
        a. 1 only
        b. 2 only
        c. 3 only
        d. 1, 2, & 3

198. Approximately what percentage of patients undergoing iodinated contrast media procedures can be expected to exhibit some type of reaction to the contrast media?
    a. 0.01%
    b. 3%
    c. 50%
    d. 95%

199. Which of the following is a mild form of neurogenic shock that is often referred to as fainting?
    a. anaphylaxis
    b. syncope
    c. epistaxis
    d. ataxia

Monitoring of Medical Equipment 0.5% (1) 200

200. For which of the following are nasogastric and nasointestinal tubes used?
    1. to maintain decompression
    2. feeding
    3. treating gastrointestinal disease
        a. 1 & 2 only
        b. 1 & 3 only
        c. 2 & 3 only
        d. 1, 2, & 3

D [190]

B [191]

D [192]

D [193]

D [194]

Patient Care and Management

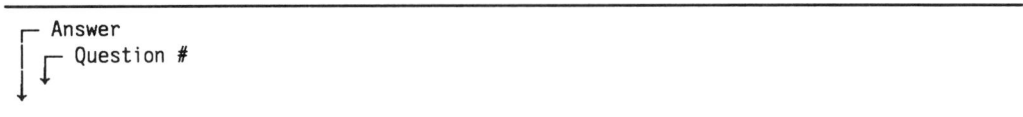

┌─ Answer
│ ┌─ Question #
↓ ↓

Question # ⌐
Answer ⌐ │
      ↓ │
        ↓

D^{200}

POST-TEST ANSWERS AND EXPLANATIONS

1. (A) The fetus is most sensitive during the organogenesis phase of development, which occurs during the first trimester. **pregnancy, trimester** (Bushong, Travis, Noz)

2. (B) The first central nervous system radiation injuries occur at 2,000 to 4,000 rad in humans. **central nervous syndrome, acute radiation syndrome** (Travis, Bushong)

3. (C) Repeating a projection approximately doubles the patient exposure for a single projection. **radiation protection (Carlton, Bushong)**

4. (C) Because a shadow shield is arranged so that it does not touch the patient, it is ideal for situations requiring sterile procedures. **gonad, radiation protection (Carlton, Bushong, Selman)**

5. (B) The higher average kVp settings used in fixed kVp technique systems permit lower average mAs levels which result in lower patient exposure dose. Automatic exposure controls eliminate the possibility of manual measurement and technique setting errors which can reduce patient exposure dose. The lower average kVp settings used in variable kVp technique systems usually require higher mAs levels which result in higher patient exposure dose. **fixed kVp, variable kVp, radiation protection (Carlton, Bushong)**

6. (A) Because a photoelectric effect interaction absorbs the entire energy of the incident photon, it is more likely to contribute to patient exposure dose. **interactions between x-rays and matter, filtration (Curry, Carlton, Bushong, Selman)**

7. (D) The largest field size produces the greatest amount of scatter. **beam restriction, collimation (Bushong, Curry, Carlton, Selman)**

8. (A) The right anterior skin surface is located closest to the tube and receives the maximum exposure dose. **left posterior oblique (Ballinger)**

9. (B) Both the barium enema and abdomen and pelvis procedures would require inclusion of the fetus in the primary beam. A cervical spine procedure would permit satisfactory shielding of the abdomen and fetus. **pregnancy (Bushong)**

10. (C) As all four sets of technical factors would produce similar image density, the higher kVp (70) permits less mAs to be used and, therefore, reduces patient exposure dose. Of the two 60 kVp techniques, the higher relative film/screen speed (400) permits a further reduction in mAs. Therefore, technique C, with the highest mAs, produces the greatest patient exposure dose. **intensifying screens, film/screen combinations (Carlton, Bushong, Cullinan, Curry)**

11. (C) Filtration removes low-energy, long-wavelength photons that would add patient dose without contributing to the image. **filtration (Carlton, Bushong, Selman, Cullinan, Curry)**

12. (D) A, B, and C all produce the same image density and approximately the same patient exposure dose. D produces twice the image density (the conversion from 72" to 40" should be 0.75 mAs to maintain the same image density). Therefore, D produces greater patient exposure dose. **inverse square law (Carlton, Bushong, Cullinan, Curry)**

13. (B) Collimators use adjustable lead shutters. Aperture diaphragms, cones, and cylinders are manufactured to an established size and must be changed to adjust the primary beam size. **beam restriction, collimators (Bushong, Selman, Carlton, Cullinan, Curry)**

14. (C) C is a definition of a non-stochastic (or non-random) effect. **stochastic, late effects, radiation effects (Travis)**

15. (B) The genetic effects of radiation damage that may be passed on to offspring are the primary concern when radiating the gonads, although somatic effects in the irradiated individual are also possible. **radiation effects, gonads, reproductive system (Bushong, Travis)**

16. (C) Intermittent fluoroscopy reduces patient exposure because many dynamic functions can be observed as well intermittently as by constant irradiation. Decreased primary beam field size reduces patient exposure because it decreases the amount of radiation exposing the body. An increase in mA would increase patient exposure because mA and exposure dose are directly related. **radiation protection, fluoroscopy (Carlton, Bushong, Selman)**

17. (C) NCRP Report No. 39. **maximum permissible dose (Bushong, Selman)**

18. (D) The three primary methods of protection again radiation are time, distance, and shielding. **radiation protection (Carlton, Bushong, Selman)**

19. (B) After a second interaction, most photons have lost sufficient energy to be safely reduced in penetrating power. **scatter, shielding (Noz, Bushong)**

20. (A) Because the extremities are not critical organs, they are permitted effective dose equivalency limits higher than the rest of the body. **effective dose limits, maximum permissible dose (Travis, Carlton, Bushong, Selman)**

21. (A) Normal monthly occupational exposure doses often range from 10 to 100 mrem. **dose equivalent limits, maximum permissible dose (Travis, Carlton, Bushong)**

22. (B) NCRP Report #102. **fluoroscopy, primary barrier (Travis, Bushong)**

23. (C) Because the vast majority of the primary beam is absorbed by the patient and image receptor, only those photons that scatter at the entrance skin surface or within the patient have the proper angle to present a radiation hazard to an assisting radiographer. **fluoroscopy, scattered radiation (Bushong, Noz, Selman, Carlton)**

24. (B) NCRP Report #102. **fluoroscopy, dead-man switch (Carlton, Bushong, Curry)**

25. (A) All ionization chambers function by discharging a wire to measure the ionization that has occurred after an exposure within a known volume of air. **personnel monitoring, ionization chambers (Bushong, Noz, Carlton)**

26. (A) The rem is an acronym representing "radiation equivalent in man" and is the best unit for reporting human exposure. **personnel monitoring, rem (Carlton, Bushong, Noz, Selman)**

27. (B) The monitor at the neck inside the apron is closest to the thyroid. **personnel monitoring (Carlton, Bushong)**

28. (B) The coulomb per kilogram is the SI unit of exposure that replaces the roentgen. **radiation units (Carlton, Bushong, Noz)**

29. (C) 68.4 mR/12 mAs = 5.7 mR/mAs. **radiation protection, mR/mAs (Carlton, Bushong)**

30. (C) NCRP Report #91. **dose equivalent limits, radiation protection, personnel monitoring (Carlton, Bushong, Noz, Selman)**

31. (B) A nurse is classified as a non-occupational worker as long as there are no regular duties assigned with radiation-producing equipment. Therefore, the limit for non-occupational infrequent exposure applies, which is 0.5 rem per year. **NCRP Report #91, dose equivalent limit, radiation protection (Carlton, Bushong, Noz)**

32. (C) Exposure dose estimates are calculated from an mR/mAs chart by multiplying the mAs by the mR/mAs for the kVp used. In this example because 100 kVp produces 6.8 mR/mAs, the answer is found as 15 mAs x 6.8 mR = 102.0 mR. **radiation units, mR/mAs (Carlton, Bushong)**

33. (B) The negative end is the cathode, the positive end is the anode. **x-ray tubes (Carlton, Bushong, Selman, Curry)**

34. (D) More than 99% of the incident high-speed electron energy from the cathode is converted to heat upon impact at the anode. **x-ray production, bremstrahlung, characteristic (Bushong, Selman, Curry, Carlton)**

35. (D) The timer, kVp meter, and line voltage compensator are all controls that must be low voltage to protect operators when they adjust the controls. **basic x-ray circuit, step-up transformers (Bushong, Selman, Carlton, Curry)**

36. (B) The high-tension transformer is the main step-up transformer in the x-ray circuit. It converts the low, incoming line voltage into the kilovoltage range needed to produce x-rays. **basic x-ray circuit, step-up transformers (Bushong, Selman, Carlton, Curry)**

37. (B) HU = 800 mA x 0.12 s x 80 kVp x 1.41 constant, which is 10,829 HU per exposure. 100,000 HU/10,820 = 9.2, so only 9 exposures may be made. **tube rating charts, heat units (Bushong, Selman, Carlton, Cullinan)**

38. (C) The ampere (A) is the unit of electrical current. **ampere, current, electricity (Bushong, Selman, Carlton)**

39. (C) Sodium-activated cesium iodide is the most common image intensifying tube input screen phosphor. **image intensification tube, cesium iodide (Bushong, Cullinan, Selman, Carlton)**

40. (B) Because a three-phase, six-pulse generator produces more energy than a single-phase unit, it will cause 35% more heat. **heat units (Bushong, Curry, Cullinan, Carlton)**

41. (D) It is called a sine wave because it depends on the mathematical sine between the plane of the armature and a plane perpendicular to the lines of force creating it. **sine wave, generator (Carlton, Bushong, Selman)**

42. (D) Bremstrahlung radiation produces approximately 90% of the primary beam with the remainder coming from characteristic photons. **target interactions, bremstrahlung, characteristic (Bushong, Selman, Cullinan, Carlton)**

43. (B) This is the definition of the minimum reaction time. **automatic exposure control, phototiming, minimum reaction time (Cullinan, Carlton, Bushong)**

44. (A) Increasing strength, speed, angle, and number of coil turns will all increase the voltage produced by an electrical generator. **electromagnetism, generators (Carlton, Bushong, Selman)**

45. (A) Smaller anode angles and smaller actual focal spot sizes will both reduce effective focal spot size. **focal spot, anode angle, target angle (Carlton, Bushong, Selman, Cullinan, Curry)**

46. (D) X-ray tube filaments are made of tungsten. **x-ray tubes, filament (Carlton, Bushong, Curry, Cullinan, Selman)**

47. (C) Power ratings are determined by V x A = W. 120,000 V x 0.8 A = 96,000 watts. **power, generators (Carlton, Bushong, Curry, Selman)**

48. (D) A diode is a solid state rectifier semiconductor. **diode (Carlton, Bushong, Selman)**

49. (C) Standard video uses a 525-line raster scanning pattern. High-resolution video uses a 1,050-line pattern. **fluoroscopy, raster pattern (Carlton, Bushong, Selman, Curry)**

50. (A) The anode has a positive charge, the cathode a negative. The focal track part of the anode assembly. **x-ray tube, cathode (Carlton, Bushong, Selman, Curry)**

51. (C) High-speed rotating anodes usually spin at 10,000 to 12,000 revolutions per minute (rpm). **rotating anode, anode (Carlton, Bushong, Cullinan, Curry, Selman)**

52.	(A) This is a definition of mutual induction, which occurs only in alternating currents. **transformers, electromagnetism, mutual induction (Carlton, Bushong, Selman)**

53.	(A) Or 186,000 miles/second. **light, speed of light (Carlton, Selman, Bushong)**

54.	(D) Plastic does not have many free electrons and, therefore, inhibits the flow of electrons. It is one of the best insulating materials. **electricity, insulators (Carlton, Bushong, Selman)**

55.	(A) Because a linear parallel grid has lines that are perpendicular to the central ray but parallel to each other, the grid can be used with either side toward the tube. All focused grids have a tube side that must face the x-ray tube to assure that the grid lines are focused toward the tube. **grids (Cullinan, Carlton, Bushong, Selman)**

56.	(D) The terms phosphorescent, luminescence, afterglow, and screen lag all describe the emission of light photons after incident photons have ceased to activate intensifying screen phosphors. **intensifying screens, screen lag (Carlton, Cullinan, Bushong, Selman)**

57.	(C) A spinning top test is valid only with single-phase, two-pulse equipment. It is made by spinning a metal disk with a single hole on top of a cassette during an exposure. Because each Hz of full-wave rectified current has two points where no radiation is being emitted, each pulse will produce two dots on the film as it images the hole in the disk. Because 60 Hz current is being used, a full second of exposure will produce 120 dots (60 Hz x 2 pulses). 120 dots x 0.05 s = 6 dots. **quality control, spinning top, timer accuracy (Carlton, Bushong, Selman)**

58.	(B) Vibration of the bucky tray would produce motion by moving the cassette. Drifting of the overhead tube would produce motion as during tomography. Bumping of the control console would not affect the tube, patient, or image receptor. **quality control, motion (Carlton, Gray, Cullinan)**

59.	(B) mA stations should be within 10% of their stated values. **quality control, kVp accuracy (Gray, Carlton, Bushong)**

60.	(D) Black tree-like branching marks on a film usually are caused by static electricity discharges. **quality control, film, static discharge (Gray, Carlton, Bushong)**

61.	(C) This test is primarily for ion chamber sensitivity because it permits evaluation of each chamber individually. However, it also can be used for individual chamber accuracy through reproduceability tests. **quality control, automatic exposure control (Gray, Carlton, Bushong)**

62.	(B) Lead gloves and aprons should be periodically checked to rule out tears or holes. Lead walls are not normally checked unless significant rebuilding or damage has occurred. **quality control, radiation protection (Bushong, Gray, Selman, Carlton)**

63. (A) The prime factor that controls and regulates radiographic density is mAs. **density, prime factors (Carlton, Bushong, Cullinan, Selman, Carroll)**

64. (C) If film/screen speed is doubled (from 100 to 200), then mAs must be halved to maintain the same density. The 15% rule states that a decrease of 15% of the kVp will result in a halving of density. **15% rule, film/screen combinations (Carlton, Bushong, Cullinan, Selman, Carroll)**

65. (B) old mAs/X = old distance^2/new distance^2, which is 80 mAs/X = 40"^{2}/55"^{2}, which is 80 mAs/X = 1,600/3,025, which is 1,600 X = 242,000, which is X = 151 mAs. **inverse square law [to maintain density], density maintenance law (Carlton, Bushong, Cullinan, Selman)**

66. (A) The greatest recorded detail is always provided by the smallest focal spot. **focal spot size, recorded detail (Carlton, Bushong, Cullinan, Selman)**

67. (C) Large effective focal spot size, short FFD, and large OFD all contribute to decreased recorded detail. Short OFD improves recorded detail. **recorded detail, penumbra (Carlton, Cullinan)**

68. (C) Most densities below OD 0.25 appear clear on a radiograph; above the 2.50 to 3.00 range, they all appear black, although a densitometer can distinguish density differences above 4.00. **D log E curves, H & D curves, sensitometry (Carlton, Curry, Bushong, Selman, Cullinan, Carroll)**

69. (B) Decreasing the FOD will decrease the magnification and increase the recorded detail. **recorded detail, magnification (Carlton, Cullinan, Carroll, Bushong, Selman, Curry)**

70. (D) Changing from a 400 to a 200 relative speed film/screen combination requires a doubling of mAs to maintain the same density. Changing from 36 to 72 mAs accomplishes this compensation, thus maintaining the density. The film/screen combination has no effect on magnification. **film/screen combinations (Carlton, Cullinan, Carroll)**

71. (B) Increasing the size of the primary beam field will increase the amount of scattered radiation produced, thus decreasing contrast and increasing density. **beam restriction, collimation, contrast (Carlton, Cullinan, Carroll)**

72. (A) Increasing the grid ratio will absorb more secondary scattered radiation, thus decreasing density and increasing contrast. **grids, density, contrast (Carlton, Cullinan, Carroll)**

73. (A) Grid ratio is the height of the lead strip divided by the width of the interspace. **grids (Carlton, Bushong, Selman, Curry, Cullinan)**

74. (A) X-ray tube output, and, therefore, image density, is increased by a high vacuum inside the glass envelope, a smooth anode focal track, and decreased added filtration. **x-ray tubes (Carlton, Cullinan, Bushong, Selman, Carroll)**

75. (A) Low kVp reduces scatter production. Large part thickness increases scatter production. Film speed has no effect on scatter production. **scatter, kVp, contrast (Carlton, Cullinan)**

76. (B) Both the PA lumbar spine and lateral L5-S1 lumbar spot are concave in relationship to the primary beam coming from the x-ray tube. This permits the diverging photons to pass through the joint spaces. The PA thoracic spine has a convex relationship to the primary beam and superimposes the joint spaces. **alignment, distortion (Carlton, Cullinan)**

77. (B) Magnification is calculated as FFD/FOD, so 180/176 = 1.02. Therefore, a 10.2 cm image is 1.02 times larger than the heart or 10.0 cm wide (10.2 cm/1.02 magnification factor). **magnification, size distortion, distortion (Carlton, Cullinan, Curry, Bushong, Selman)**

78. (B) The cervical spine is normally imaged between 60 to 70 kVp. **kVp, contrast, technique factors, technical factors (Carlton, Cullinan)**

79. (C) Increasing part thickness decreases density and increases contrast. It has no effect on recorded detail or distortion. **anatomic part, part thickness, contrast, density, recorded detail, detail, distortion (Carlton, Cullinan)**

80. (C) Glutaraldehyde is the hardener in the developer, and potassium alum is the hardener in the fixer. Hydroquinone is a reducing agent. **processing, developer, fixer (Carlton, Bushong, Cullinan, Selman, Curry)**

81. (B) Average gradient is a measurement of the slope of the straight line portion of the D log E (H&D or characteristic) curve. High average gradient films typically exhibit high contrast, high speed, and narrow latitude. A typical high average gradient film is shown as film A in Figure 13. **D log E curves, sensitometry, characteristic curves, H&D curves (Carlton, Cullinan, Bushong, Selman, Curry)**

82. (D) The formula for converting from one grid ratio to another is mAs_1/mAs_2 = grid conversion factor$_1$/grid conversion factor$_2$. Therefore 14 mAs/mAs$_2$ = 4/5.5, which is 4 mAs$_2$ = 77, which is mAs$_2$ = 19 mAs. **grids, grid conversion, bucky factor (Carlton, Cullinan, Bushong)**

83. (A) Emaciation and atrophy decrease beam attenuation, thus requiring decreased technical factors. Abscesses increase beam attenuation, thus requiring increased technical factors. **pathology, tissue density, density (Carlton, Cullinan, Bushong)**

84. (C) Small effective focal spot size contributes to increased recorded detail. Short FFD and long OFD decrease recorded detail. **recorded detail, penumbra (Carlton, Cullinan)**

85. (D) When no other factors are considered, the highest kVp always produces the lowest, or longest, scale of contrast. **contrast, kVp (Carlton, Bushong, Cullinan, Selman)**

86. (C) Film fog increases density and decreases contrast. It has no effect on distortion and recorded detail. **fog, contrast, density, recorded detail, detail, distortion (Carlton, Cullinan, Bushong)**

87. (B) A slower film/screen combination requires an increase in primary beam quantity and/or quality. Increasing mAs and kVp and decreasing FFD would achieve this effect. **film/screen combinations (Carlton, Cullinan, Bushong, Selman, Curry)**

88. (D) Motion primarily affects recorded detail. It has a lesser effect on contrast and density and no effect on distortion. **motion, recorded detail, detail (Carlton, Bushong, Cullinan)**

89. (B) Low-resolution films tend to be high speed, low contrast, wide latitude, and have lower patient dose requirements. **film, sensitometry (Carlton, Cullinan, Bushong, Selman, Curry)**

90. (A) A focused grid has its grid lines directed toward the focal spot of the x-ray tube. **grids, focused grids (Carlton, Bushong, Selman, Curry, Cullinan)**

91. (A) Low contrast films have less-steep, straight-line portions. This produces a film that permits a wide range of exposures to be made within a specified range of density values. This is essentially the definition of a wide latitude film. **D log E curves, sensitometric curves, sensitometry, film latitude (Carlton,Cullinan, Carroll, Curry, Bushong)**

92. (B) Abdominal compression reduces the thickness of the part, thus increasing density and contrast. It has no appreciable effect on recorded detail. **compression, density, contrast (Carlton, Cullinan)**

93. (B) Magnification is calculated as FFD/FOD so 100/98.6 = 1.01. Therefore, a 2.1 cm image is 1.01 times larger than the cyst, or 2.1 cm wide (2.1 cm/1.01 magnification factor). **magnification, size distortion, distortion (Carlton, Cullinan, Curry, Bushong, Selman)**

94. (A) High kVp and large part thicknesses increase scatter production. A small OFD decreases the air-gap which permits most scattered radiation to reach the film. However, this has no effect on scatter production. **scatter, kVp, contrast (Carlton, Cullinan)**

95. (A) Both heat in a storage area and light from a cracked safelight filter will fog film. Excessively warm wash water may damage the surface of a film but would not add density to the image. **darkroom, base-plus-fog levels, sensitometry (Carlton, Cullinan, Bushong, Selman)**

96. (B) Flat storage of cassettes is recommended to prevent warping of the cassette and screens, thus producing poor film-screen contact. **cassettes (Carlton, Carroll, Bushong)**

97. (C) A sensitometer produces a sensitized optical wedge on a film. A dosimeter is a dose meter. A densitometer is a density meter. A galvanometer measures electrical current. **radiation measurement, dosimetry (Bushong, Selman, Carlton)**

98. (A) Rapid temperature changes can cause moisture from the air to condense on the film and leave spots. **film, film storage (Carlton, Selman, Cullinan)**

99. (B) The recirculation or circulation system of an automatic processor stabilizes solution temperatures, agitates the solutions, and mixes replenishment chemistry into the tanks. **automatic processing, film processing, processing (Selman, Carlton, Bushong, Cullinan)**

100. (A) Age fog occurs as a result of background radiation and heat to which film is subjected during storage. **film, film storage (Carlton, Cullinan)**

101. (B) A 90 second processor immerses the film for approximately 20 to 25 seconds in the developer solution. **automatic processing (Carlton, Selman, Bushong)**

102. (B) Permitting an automatic film processor to run for 15 to 20 minutes prior to developing the first films permits the developer solution to be properly mixed and to reach optimal temperature. **automatic processing, quality control (Selman, Carlton)**

103. (C) A dark-red filter will produce light that is outside the sensitivity range of yellow-green sensitive film. **darkroom, safelights (Carlton, Cullinan, Bushong, Selman)**

104. (C) Alternate right-side and left-side film feeding equalizes the wear on the transport rollers. Using the guides at the sides of the feed tray assures straight transport through the system, thus avoiding jamming. **automatic processors, processing, film processing (Carlton, Bushong, Cullinan, Selman)**

105. (A) Increasing grid ratio will increase contrast and decrease density. It has no effect on distortion. **grids, contrast, density (Carlton, Cullinan, Carroll)**

106. (B) According to the 15% rule, a 15% increase in kVp will approximately double the image density. **15% rule (Carlton, Cullinan, Carroll)**

107. (A) Areas with low-density anatomic structures will be the first to exhibit the effects of increased fog of any type. Loss of the ability to perceive the lightest densities will decrease information on the image. **fog, contrast (Cullinan, Carlton, Carroll)**

108. (B) An increase in kVp to increase density also will produce lower contrast and increased scatter production. kVp has no effect on recorded detail. **kVp, contrast (Carlton, Cullinan, Carroll)**

109.   (B) Increased FFD and decreased focal spot size both increase recorded detail. Higher intensifying screen speed will decrease recorded detail. **recorded detail, detail, penumbra (Carlton, Cullinan, Carroll)**

110.   (D) This is a definition of distortion. **distortion (Carlton, Cullinan, Bushong, Carroll)**

111.   (C) Anterior oblique projections would place the orbit closest to the image receptor, thus producing the best possible recorded detail. **recorded detail, detail (Carlton, Cullinan, Ballinger)**

112.   (B) Contrast can be decreased only by increasing the kVp. Of the two choices at more than the original 68 kVp, only 79 kVp at 0.7 mAs will maintain density according to the 15% rule. **15% rule, contrast (Carlton, Cullinan, Carroll)**

113.   (C) Both decreased kVp and decreased primary beam field size will reduce scatter and increase contrast. Changes in automatic exposure control density controls affect only density. **scatter, contrast (Carlton, Bushong, Selman, Cullinan, Carroll)**

114.   (C) Both increased OFD and decreased primary beam field size will reduce scattered radiation reaching the image receptor. Increased kVp will increase scatter production. **scatter (Bushong, Selman, Cullinan, Carlton, Carroll)**

115.   (B) mAs controls the number of the primary beam photons, which is considered the quantity factor. **mAs (Carlton, Bushong, Selman, Cullinan)**

116.   (D) The left hypochondriac abdominal region would have the most gas if it were in the stomach. This would produce the greatest density in that area because the gas would attenuate less of the primary beam. **part thickness, body regions (Carlton, Ballinger, Carroll, Cullinan)**

117.   (B) The coronal plane divides the body into anterior and posterior sections. **coronal plane (Ballinger, Bontrager, Eisenberg POSITIONING)**

118.   (C) This is a definition of cephalad. **cephalad (Ballinger, Bontrager, Eisenberg POSITIONING)**

119.   (C) This is a definition of plantar. **plantar (Ballinger, Bontrager, Eisenberg POSITIONING)**

120.   (B) A patient is lying on his or her back when he or she is supine. This places the posterior portion of the body on the x-ray table, closest to the image receptor. **supine (Ballinger, Bontrager, Eisenberg POSITIONING)**

121.   (D) This is a description of an AP lordotic chest. The AP axial chest is performed with the patient leaning toward the film holder. **lungs, chest (Ballinger, Bontrager, Eisenberg)**

122. (B) The central ray should be directed to the proximal interphalangeal joint for PA projections of the digits. **digit, finger (Ballinger, Bontrager, Eisenberg)**

123. (D) With a 15° to 20° cephalad angle for the AP oblique position, the 45° obliquity demonstrates the intervertebral foramina and pedicles farthest from the image receptor. **cervical vertebrae, cervical spine (Ballinger, Bontrager, Eisenberg)**

124. (B) The T12-L1 through L3-L4 intervertebral foramina are demonstrated by the lateral lumbar spine projection. The L4-L5 intervertebral foramina is best demonstrated on an oblique lumbar spine projection. **lumbar vertebrae, lumbar spine (Ballinger, Bontrager, Eisenberg)**

125. (C) Only the 11th and 12th pairs of ribs are not attached to the sternum and, therefore, are referred to as floating ribs. **thorax, ribs (Anthony, Hole)**

126. (D) The lateral cervical spine projections demonstrated the vertebral interspaces, inferior five articular facets, and the spinous processes. **cervical vertebrae, cervical spine (Ballinger, Bontrager, Eisenberg)**

127. (B) Both the radius and ulna have a styloid process at their distal ends. The humerus has no styloid process. **forearm, radius, ulna, humerus (Ballinger, Anthony, Hole)**

128. (C) The axillary portions of the ribs are best demonstrated by oblique positions. **bony thorax, ribs (Ballinger, Bontrager, Eisenberg)**

129. (C) Extension of the neck when radiographing the atlas and axis in a lateral position removes the mandibular rami from superimposition. **vertebral column, atlas and axis, cervical (Ballinger, Bontrager, Eisenberg)**

130. (D) The radius articulates with the navicular, which is also known as the scaphoid, and the lunate (semilunar). **wrist (Ballinger, Bontrager, Eisenberg, Anthony, Hole)**

131. (C) The atlas (C1) of the cervical spine is illustrated by #3 in Figure 23. **vertebral column, cervical spine (Ballinger, Hole, Anthony, Eisenberg, Bontrager)**

132. (A) The dens or odontoid process of the cervical spine is illustrated by #1 in Figure 23. **vertebral column, cervical spine (Ballinger, Hole, Anthony, Eisenberg, Bontrager)**

133. (B) The mastoid tip of the temporal bone is illustrated by #2 in Figure 23. **mastoid, sinuses, temporal bone (Ballinger, Hole, Anthony, Eisenberg, Bontrager)**

134. (B) The axiolateral position (Lysholm method) requires a 35° caudal central ray angle. **temporal bone, petrous portion (Ballinger, Bontrager, Eisenberg)**

135. (C) The central ray should be angled 35° caudally for an AP axial position for temporomandibular joints. **temporomandibular articulations, temporomandibular joints (Ballinger, Bontrager, Eisenberg)**

136. (B) The PA oblique axial position (Law method) requires a 25° to 30° cephalad central ray angle. **facial bones (Ballinger, Bontrager, Eisenberg)**

137. (A) The petrous ridges of the temporal bone should appear below the maxillae on a parietoacanthial position (Waters method). **skull, petrous ridges (Ballinger, Bontrager, Eisenberg)**

138. (A) The superior orbital fissure is located between the greater and lesser wings of the sphenoid bone. **skull (Ballinger, Bontrager, Eisenberg)**

139. (D) The temporomandibular joints are formed by the articulation of the condyloid processes of the mandible with the mandibular fossae of the temporal bones. **skull (Anthony, Hole, Ballinger, Bontrager, Eisenberg)**

140. (C) The central ray for a PA chest should be directed to the level of the 6th-7th thoracic vertebra. **chest (Ballinger, Bontrager, Eisenberg)**

141. (B) Shallow breathing during an RAO projection of the sternum is used to blur pulmonary markings. **bony thorax, sternum (Ballinger, Bontrager, Eisenberg)**

142. (D) The femoral neck is located by drawing a line between the anterior superior iliac spine and the superior margin of the symphysis pubis, marking the center of the line, and then drawing a line from this point to a point 1" distal to the lateral-most portion of the greater trochanter. **pelvis, hip, femur (Ballinger, Bontrager, Eisenberg)**

143. (A) Both the Merchant and Settegast methods demonstrate the patellofemoral joint. The Holmblad method demonstrates the intercondyloid fossa. **patella (Ballinger, Bontrager, Eisenberg)**

144. (A) This is a definition of spina bifida. **spina bifida (Eisenberg PATHOLOGY)**

145. (B) Because a PA projection places the clavicle closer to the image receptor, it provides improved resolution. **clavicle (Ballinger, Bontrager, Eisenberg)**

146. (A) The right lateral decubitus position will cause barium to fall and air to rise within the colon. If barium appears laterally within the ascending colon, it is toward the right side of the body. Therefore, the patient was positioned with the right side down, which is a right lateral decubitus position. **digestive system, colon (Ballinger, Bontrager, Eisenberg)**

147. (C) The elbow must be flexed 90° for the lateral projection. **elbow (Ballinger, Bontrager, Eisenberg)**

148. (D) The LPO produces the best image of the fundus of the stomach during a stomach examination. **stomach, digestive system, gastrointestinal (Ballinger, Bontrager, Eisenberg)**

149. (A) Percutaneous transhepatic cholangiography is an examination of the biliary tract that uses a needle inserted from the right lateral intercostal space toward the liver hilum as described in the question. **digestive system, biliary system, liver, gallbladder (Ballinger, Snopek, Tortorici)**

150. (B) On deep inhalation, the ribs move anteriorly, superiorly, and laterally. **bony thorax, ribs (Ballinger, Bontrager, Eisenberg)**

151. (C) The male pelvis is heavier, wider, and deeper, and the sacrum is more narrow than the female pelvis. **pelvis (Ballinger, Bontrager, Eisenberg, Anthony, Hole)**

152. (B) The radius and ulna articulate at both the wrist and elbow. **forearm, elbow, wrist (Ballinger, Bontrager, Eisenberg)**

153. (A) The central ray should be angled 15° caudally for an axiolateral position (Law method) of the mastoid process when the midsagittal plane is rotated 15° toward the image receptor from a true lateral position. **temporal bone, mastoid process (Ballinger, Bontrager, Eisenberg)**

154. (D) A properly performed AP axial projection of the skull by the Townes method should demonstrate the petrous pyramids of the temporal bone symmetrically, the dorsum sellae and posterior clinoid processes within the shadow of the foramen magnum, and the inion should be located near the center of the film. **skull (Ballinger, Bontrager, Eisenberg)**

155. (A) The mandible has two rami and a mental protuberance. The hyoid has two cornua. **skull (Anthony, Hole, Ballinger, Bontrager, Eisenberg)**

156. (C) The left kidney is slightly longer and narrower than the right kidney. The right kidney lies slightly more inferior because of the space occupied by the liver. **urinary system (Anthony, Hole, Ballinger, Bontrager, Eisenberg)**

157. (C) Peristalsis is the normal contractive waves of the digestive system that propel material from the pharynx through the rectum. **digestive system, gastrointestinal, peristalsis (Hole, Anthony, Ballinger, Eisenberg)**

158. (A) The left apophysial joints are well demonstrated on a LPO of the lumbar spine. The first 4 intervertebral foramina are best demonstrated on a lateral projection of the lumbar spine. **vertebral column, lumbar spine (Ballinger, Bontrager, Eisenberg)**

159. (A) Osteopetrosis (marble bone) is an increase in bone density resulting from failure of bone resorption. Osteoporosis is a decrease in bone density caused by accelerated resorption. Osteochondroma (exostosis) is a benign projection of normal bone. **osteopetrosis, osteoporosis (Eisenberg (PATHOLOGY))**

160. (A) The manubrium is illustrated by #1 in Figure 27. **bony thorax, sternum** **(Ballinger, Bontrager, Eisenberg, Anthony, Hole)**

161. (A) The medial epicondyle is illustrated by #6 in Figure 27. **upper extremity, humerus (Ballinger, Bontrager, Eisenberg, Anthony, Hole)**

162. (C) The acromion process of the scapula is illustrated by #15 in Figure 27. **shoulder girdle, scapula (Ballinger, Bontrager, Eisenberg, Anthony, Hole)**

163. (B) The 8th rib is illustrated by #10 in Figure 27. **bony thorax, rib** **(Ballinger, Bontrager, Eisenberg, Anthony, Hole)**

164. (B) The splenic flexure usually is higher than the left side because of the position of the liver. **digestive system, gastrointestinal, colon (Ballinger, Hole, Anthony)**

165. (B) The parotid glands are the largest salivary glands. **salivary glands (Ballinger, Bontrager, Eisenberg, Hole, Anthony)**

166. (A) The upper ribs are best demonstrated by full inhalation, which lowers the diaphragm to reveal the greatest number of upper ribs. **bony thorax, ribs (Ballinger, Bontrager, Eisenberg)**

167. (D) Both hip joints should be fully extended to avoid patients with lower-back pain assuming a protective position that could reduce the lumbosacral angle. **vertebral column, lumbosacral junction (Ballinger, Bontrager, Eisenberg)**

168. (B) The capitulum (capitellum) and greater tubercle are on the lateral side of the humerus. **humerus (Ballinger, Bontrager, Eisenberg, Anthony, Hole)**

169. (C) The axiolateral position (Schuller method) requires a 25° caudal central ray angle. **temporal bone, petrous portion (Ballinger, Bontrager, Eisenberg)**

170. (D) The acanthion is the centering point for a parietoacanthial projection (Waters method) of the paranasal sinuses. **paranasal sinuses, sinuses (Ballinger, Bontrager, Eisenberg)**

171. (C) The recommended preparation for a urographic examination includes a non-gas-forming laxative and NPO after midnight the day of the examination. The patient should be hydrated, not in a reduced hydration state. **urinary system (Anthony, Hole, Ballinger, Bontrager, Eisenberg)**

172. (D) An axial (Chassard-Lapine method) radiograph of the rectosigmoid region of the colon is achieved by having the patient sit on the side of the x-ray table with legs hanging down and then grasp the ankles for support while the central ray is centered perpendicularly through the lumbosacral region at the level of the greater trochanters. **colon (Ballinger, Bontrager, Eisenberg)**

173.   (B) When a patient denies knowledge of the possible effects of the use of contrast media, the effects should be explained and verification of understanding, preferably in writing, should be obtained from the patient. **consent (Ehrlich, Gurley, Torres)**

174.   (A) Angiography and cardiac catherization are complex procedures with significant risks to patient health that should have a signed informed consent form. Lung tomography does not normally require a signed form, although informed consent should always be obtained verbally. **informed consent (Ehrlich, Torres, Gurley)**

175.   (B) Sims' position places the patient on one side, the top arm flexed and the bottom arm extended behind the body, and the body obliqued with the top knee flexed level with the pelvis. **Sims' position (Ehrlich, Torres)**

176.   (A) Increasing physical distance and crossing arms or legs serve as barriers to communication. Using simple layman's terminology usually increases communication, unless the patient makes it obvious that complex terminology is understood. **communication (Torres, Ehrlich)**

177.   (C) It is permissible to let water run from the elbows when doing a surgical scrub. It is not permissible to touch the faucet handles, pick up anything from the sink, or letting water run from the hands. **washing, hand washing (Torres, Ehrlich)**

178.   (B) A lead apron must be worn under the surgical scrub gown but over the scrub suit. **surgical asepsis (Torres, Ehrlich)**

179.   (A) Only tuberculosis is bacterial in origin. Herpes simplex and AIDS are viral. **infection control (Torres, Ehrlich)**

180.   (D) Because fatigue, stress, and a low-grade fever all tend to diminish the body's immune system, a radiographer with these conditions is more likely to become a host to patient-borne infection. **infection control (Ehrlich, Torres)**

181.   (C) Sterile persons must pass back-to-back, not front-to-front. **asepsis, sterile technique (Torres, Ehrlich)**

182.   (B) Strict (protective or reverse) isolation procedures are designed to protect a patient who is at high risk of infection due to a debilitated state, for example, severe burn patients or radiation therapy patients whose immune systems have been suppressed by treatment. **infection control (Torres, Ehrlich)**

183.   (A) Pertussis (whooping cough) and influenzal meningitis require only simple respiratory isolation. Pneumonic plague requires strict (protective or reverse) isolation. **isolation (Torres, Ehrlich)**

184.   (C) Normal, adult systolic blood pressure ranges from 110 to 140 mm Hg. **vital signs (Torres, Ehrlich)**

185.   (A) Cyanosis often is observed in the nail beds, mouth, and gums, and in the earlobes. It is not seen in the conjunctiva of the eyes. **vital signs (Torres, Ehrlich)**

186.   (A) Contrast media toxicity is most significant at the cellular level. **contrast media, iodinated contrast agents (Snopek, Torres, Ehrlich)**

187.   (C) Lymphangiographic injectors deliver a slow flow rate while arteriographic injectors are used for faster and higher volume injections. **contrast media, iodinated contrast agents (Snopek, Torres, Ehrlich)**

188.   (C) Hyperosmolar solutions have an ionic concentration higher than normal body fluids. **contrast material (Snopek, Tortorici, Torres)**

189.   (A) Anaphylactic shock is the most likely type of shock that occurs during iodinated contrast media studies. **shock (Torres)**

190.   (D) Non-ionic contrast material causes fewer adverse reactions, does not disrupt homeostasis, and does not disassociate in solution. **contrast material, contrast agents (Torres)**

191.   (B) 15 to 20 drops/min is a safe infusion rate for intravenous fluids. **patient care (Torres, Ehrlich)**

192.   (D) Positive contrast materials increase x-ray absorption. They decrease image density, are liquid, and are radiopaque. **contrast material (Torres, Tortorici, Snopek)**

193.   (D) A soap suds enema solution produces a mild irritation of the bowel, thus promoting peristalsis and defecation. For an adult patient, 1,000 to 1,500 ml of fluid are usually needed for this type of enema. **enemas (Ehrlich, Torres)**

194.   (D) Common reactions to the first symptoms of a heart attack are to ignore them or attribute them to some other cause; have them occur suddenly without warning; and for them to subside and return later. **cardiopulmonary resuscitation (Torres, Ehrlich)**

195.   (C) A hand at the throat is a universal distress signal for an obstructed airway. **medical emergencies, choking (Torres, Ehrlich)**

196.   (C) The recommended rate of artificial ventilations for an adult is once every 5 seconds. **cardiopulmonary resuscitation (Torres, Ehrlich)**

197.   (A) Hyperglycemia is usually of slow onset, while both hypoglycemia and seizures may occur very rapidly without warning. **acute emergencies, medical emergencies (Ehrlich, Torres)**

198.   (B) Depending on the type of iodinated contrast medium used, between 0.1 and 5% of all patients may exhibit some type of reaction to the contrast medium. **iodinated contrast media (Ehrlich, Torres, Ballinger)**

199. (B) Syncope is a mild form of neurogenic shock, often referred to as fainting. **medical emergencies, acute emergencies (Ehrlich, Torres)**

200. (D) Nasogastric and nasointestinal tubes are used to maintain decompression of the gastrointestinal tract, to feed patients, and to treat gastrointestinal diseases. **drainage tubes, bedside radiography (Torres, Ehrlich)**

APPENDIX A: REFERENCES

Ballinger, Philip W., *Merrill's Atlas of Radiographic Positions and Radiologic Procedures*, St. Louis: C.V. Mosby Co., 7th edition, 1991.

Bontrager, Kenneth and Anthony, Barry, *Textbook of Radiographic Positioning and Related Anatomy*, St. Louis: C.V. Mosby Co., 2nd edition, 1987.

Bushong, Stewart, *Radiologic Science for Technologists: Physics, Biology and Protection*, St. Louis: C.V. Mosby Co., 5th edition, 1992.

Carlton, Richard and Adler, Arlene McKenna, *Principles of Radiographic Imaging: An Art And a Science*, Albany: Delmar Publishers, 1992.

Carroll, Quinn, *Fuch's Principles of Radiographic Exposure, Processing and Quality Control*, Springfield, Illinois: Charles C. Thomas Publishers, 3rd edition, 1985.

Curry, Thomas S., Dowdey, James E., and Murray, Robert C., *Christensen's Physics of Diagnostic Radiology*, Philadelphia: Lea & Febiger, 4th edition, 1990.

Cullinan, Angeline M., *Producing Quality Radiographs*, Philadelphia: J.B. Lippincott, 1987.

Donohue, Daniel P., *An Analysis of Radiographic Quality: Lab Manual and Workbook*, Rockville, MD: Aspen Publishers, Inc., 2nd edition, 1984.

Eisenberg, Ronald L., Dennis, Cynthia A., and May, Chris R., *Radiographic Positioning*, Boston: Little, Brown & Company, 1989.

Eisenberg, Ronald L. and Dennis, Cynthia A., *Comprehensive Radiographic Pathology*, St. Louis: C.V. Mosby Co., 1990.

Ehrlich, Ruth A. and McCloskey, Ellen D., *Patient Care in Radiography*, St. Louis: C.V. Mosby Co., 3rd edition, 1989.

Gray, Joel E., Winkler, Norlin T., Stears, John, and Frank, Eugene D., *Quality Control in Diagnostic Imaging*, Baltimore: University Park Press, 1983.

Gurley, LaVerne and Callaway, William, *Introduction to Radiologic Technology*, St. Louis: C.V. Mosby Co., 2nd edition, 1986.

Hall, Eric J., *Radiobiology for the Radiologist*, Philadelphia: J.B. Lippincott, 3rd edition, 1988.

Hole, John W., Jr., *Human Anatomy and Physiology*, Dubuque, IA: William C. Brown Publishers, 2nd edition, 1981.

Jenkins, David, *Radiographic Photography and Imaging Processes*, Lancaster, England: MTP Press Ltd., 1980.

National Council on Radiation Protection and Measurements, *NCRP Report #39: Basic Radiation Protection Criteria*, Washington, D.C.: NCRP, 1971.

National Council on Radiation Protection and Measurements, *NCRP Report #49: Structural Shielding Design and Evaluation for Medical Use of X-Rays and Gamma-Rays of Energies Up to 10 MeV*, Washington, D.C.: NCRP, 1976.

National Council on Radiation Protection and Measurements, *NCRP Report #54: Medical Exposure of Pregnant and Potentially Pregnant Women*, Washington, D.C.: NCRP, 1977.

National Council on Radiation Protection and Measurements, *NCRP Report #91: Recommendations on Limits for Exposure to Ionizing Radiation*, Washington, D.C.: NCRP, 1987.

National Council on Radiation Protection and Measurements, *NCRP Report #102: Medical X-Ray, Electron Beam, and Gamma-Ray Protection for Energies Up to 50 MeV (Equipment Design, Performance, and Use)*, Washington, D.C.: NCRP, 1989.

Noz, Marilyn E. and Maguire, Gerald Q., *Radiation Protection in the Radiologic and Health Sciences*, Philadelphia: Lea & Febiger, 2nd edition, 1985.

Selman, Joseph, *X-Ray and Radium Physics*, Springfield, IL: Charles C. Thomas Publisher, 7th edition, 1987.

Seeram, Euclid, *X-Ray Imaging Equipment*, Springfield, IL: Charles C. Thomas Publishers, 1985.

Snopek, Albert, *Fundamentals of Special Radiographic Procedures*, Philadelphia: W.B. Saunders Co., 2nd edition, 1984.

Thibodeau, G.A., *Anthony's Textbook of Anatomy and Physiology*, St. Louis: C.V. Mosby Co., 13th edition, 1990.

Torres, Lillian, *Basic Medical Techniques and Patient Care for Radiologic Technologists*, Philadelphia: J.B. Lippincott Company, 3rd edition, 1989.

Tortorici, Marianne R., *Fundamentals of Angiography*, St. Louis: C.V. Mosby Co., 1982.

Travis, Elizabeth LaTorre, *Primer of Medical Radiobiology*, Chicago: Yearbook, 2nd edition, 1989.

APPENDIX B: DOSE EQUIVALENT LIMITS AND MAXIMUM PERMISSIBLE DOSES

EFFECTIVE DOSE EQUIVALENT LIMIT RECOMMENDATIONS

	SI	Conventional
Annual Occupational		
effective dose equivalent limit		
(whole body)	50 mSv	5 rem
lens of eye	150 mSv	15 rem
all others (red bone marrow,		
breast, lung, skin, extremities)	500 mSv	50 rem
cumulative exposure guide	10 mSv x age	1 rem x age
Annual Public		
continuous or frequent exposure	1 mSv	0.1 rem
infrequent	5 mSv	0.5 rem
lens of eye, skin, extremities	50 mSv	5 rem
Embryo-Fetus		
total limit	5 mSv	0.5 rem
monthly limit	0.5 mSv	0.05 rem
Educational		
effective dose equivalent limit		
(whole body)	1 mSv	0.1 rem
lens of eye, skin, extremities	50 mSv	5 rem

Adapted by permission from NCRP Report No. 91: Recommendations on Limits for Exposure to Ionizing Radiation (Table 22.i), 1987.

MAXIMUM PERMISSIBLE DOSE RECOMMENDATIONS
and non-occupational absorbed dose limit recommendations

	SI	Annual Conventional SI		Quarterly Conventional
Occupational MPDs				
combined whole body	50 mSv	5 rem	12.5 mSv	1.25 rem
long-term accumulation				
(N = age in years)	50(N-18)	mSv5		(N-18) rem
skin	150 mSv	15 rem		
hands	750 mSv	75 rem	250 mSv	25 rem
forearms	300 mSv	30 rem	100 mSv	10 rem
other tissues, organs,				
organ systems	150 mSv	15 rem	50 mSv	5 rem
pregnancy (for entire				
gestational period)	5 mSv	0.5 rem		

Non-occupational absorbed dose limit recommendations

whole body	5 mSv	0.5 rem
students	1 mSv	0.1 rem

Adapted by permission from NCRP Report No. 39: Basic Radiation Protection Criteria, 1971.

APPENDIX C: SI RADIATION UNITS

COMPARISON BETWEEN SI AND CONVENTIONAL UNITS

Quantity	Symbol for Quantity	Expression in SI Units	Expression in Symbols for SI Units	Special Name for SI Unit	Symbol Using Special Name	Conventional Unit	Symbol for Conventional Unit	Value of Conventional Unit in SI Units
Activity	A	1 per second	s^{-1}	becquerel	Bq	curie	Ci	3.7×10^{10}Bq
Absorbed Dose	D	joule per kilogram	J/kg^{-1}	gray	Gy	rad	rad	0.01 Gy
Dose Equivalent	H	joule per kilogram	J/kg^{-1}	sievert	Sv	rem	rem	0.01 Sv
Exposure	X	coulomb per kilogram	C/kg^{-1}			roentgen	R	2.58×10^{-4} C/kg^{-1}

Adapted by permission from NCRP Report No. 82: SI Units in Radiation Protection and Measurements.

APPENDIX D: TABLE OF COMMON ABBREVIATIONS AND SYMBOLS

ABBREVIATIONS

A	ampere
AP	anteroposterior
BaE	barium enema
b.i.d.	twice daily
BP	blood pressure
C	centigrade or Celsius
c	with
cc	cubic centimeter (equal to milliliter)
CHF	congestive heart failure
cm	centimeter
CT	computed tomography
D.C.	discontinue
DNR	do not resuscitate
ECG	electrocardiogram
ER	emergency room
FFD	focus-film distance
FOD	focus-object distance
G.B.	gall bladder
g	gram
gr	grain
gtt.	drop/s
GU	genitourinary
Gy	gray
Gyn	gynecology
hr/s	hour/s

ABBREVIATIONS cont.

H_2O	water
HVL	half value layer
Hz	Hertz (cycles per second)
ICU	intensive care unit
IM	intramuscular
IV	intravenous
keV	kilo electron volts
kg	kilogram
KUB	kidneys, ureters, bladder
kV	kilovolts, kilovoltage
kVp	kilovoltage peak
kW	kilowatts, kilowattage
L	left
LAO	left anterior oblique
LAT	lateral
LET	linear energy transfer
LLQ	left lower quadrant of the abdomen
LPO	left posterior oblique
LUQ	left upper quadrant of the abdomen
mA	milliampere/s
mAs	milliampere-seconds
meV	million electron volts
mg	milligram
MI	myocardial infarction
ml	milliliter (equal to cubic centimeter)
mm	millimeter

MPD	maximum permissible dose
mR	milliroentgen
mrad	millirad
mrem	millirem
mSv	millisievert
mμ	microgram
nm	nanometer
NPO	nothing by mouth
OFD	object-film distance
OR	operating room
PA	posteroanterior
pH	hydrogen ion concentration
prn	as necessary
q.d.	every day
q.h.	every hour
q.i.d.	4 times daily
q.2 h.	every 2 hours
q.4 h.	every 4 hours
R	right
R	roentgen
rad	radiation absorbed dose
RAO	right anterior oblique
RBC	red blood cell
RBE	relative biological effect
rem	radiation equivalency in man
RLQ	right lower quadrant of the abdomen

ABBREVIATIONS cont.

RPO	right posterior oblique
rpm	revolutions per minute
RUQ	right upper quadrant of the abdomen
Rx	therapy
s	second
s	without
stat	at once
Sv	sievert
t.i.d.	3 times daily
URI	upper respiratory infection
V	volt
W	watt
WBC	white blood cell
WC	wheelchair
x	times

GREEK ALPHABET

α	alpha	alpha particle
ß	beta	beta particle
τ	gamma	gamma ray
λ	lambda	wavelength
μ	mu	micro
υ	nu	frequency
Ω	omega	resistance

SYMBOLS

°	degree	
♂	male	
♀	female	
Δ	delta	change
φ	cosine	phase
↓	less, lower	
↑	greater, higher	
√	square root	

APPENDIX E: STATE LICENSING AGENCIES

As of this printing, 25 states and Puerto Rico had licensing laws for radiographers in effect. Although the laws and regulations vary widely from state to state, as of this printing, all states that require licenses would accept the Examination in Radiography of the American Registry of Radiologic Technologists (ARRT) to obtain a license to practice.

Students or radiographers desiring information should contact the appropriate agency for the particular state. Although addresses and phone numbers sometimes change, the most current for each of the licensing states and Puerto Rico are listed below.

ARIZONA
State of Arizona
Medical Radiologic Technology Board of Examiners
4814 South 40th Street
Phoenix, AZ 85040
602-255-4845

CALIFORNIA
State of California
Radiologic Health Branch
714 P Street
Sacramento, CA 95814
916-445-6695

DELAWARE
State of Delaware
Office of Radiation Control
Robbins Building
P.O. Box 637
Dover, DE 19903
302-736-4731

FLORIDA
State of Florida
Radiologic Health Program
1317 Winewood Boulevard
Tallahassee, FL 32399-0700
904-487-3451

HAWAII
State of Hawaii
Radiologic Technology Board
Department of Health
Noise and Radiation Branch
591 Ala Moana Boulevard
Honolulu, HI 96813-2498
808-548-4383

ILLINOIS

State of Illinois
Division of Radiologic Technologist Certification
Illinois Department of Nuclear Safety
1035 Outer Park Drive
Springfield, IL 62704
217-785-9915

INDIANA

State of Indiana
Radiological Health Section
P.O. Box 1964
Indianapolis, IN 46206-1964
317-633-0150

IOWA

State of Iowa
Department of Health
Lucas State Office Building
Des Moines, IA 50319-0075
515-281-3478

KENTUCKY

State of Kentucky
Radiation Control Branch
275 East Main Street
Frankfort, KY 40621
502-564-3700

LOUISIANA

Louisiana State Radiologic Technology Board of Examiners
3108 Cleary Avenue, Suite 207
Metairie, LA 70002
504-838-5231

MAINE

State of Maine
Radiologic Technology Board of Examiners
State House Station #35
Augusta, ME 04333
207-582-8723

MARYLAND

State of Maryland
Public Health Engineer
2500 Broening Highway
Baltimore, MD 21224
301-631-3300

MASSACHUSETTS

State of Massachusetts
Radiation Control Program
150 Tremont Street, 11th Floor
Boston, MA 02111
617-727-6214

MONTANA

State of Montana
Department of Commerce
Board of Radiologic Technologists
1424 Ninth Avenue
Helena, MT 59620
406-444-4288

NEBRASKA

State of Nebraska
Division of Radiological Health
301 Centennial Mall South
Lincoln, NE 68509
402-471-2168

NEW JERSEY

State of New Jersey
Department of Environmental Protection
Bureau of Radiological Health
CN 415
Trenton, NJ 08625-0415
609-987-2022

NEW MEXICO

State of New Mexico
Radiation Protection Bureau
P.O. Box 968
Santa Fe, NM 87504-0968
505-827-2773
505-827-2941

NEW YORK

Bureau of Environment Radiation Protection
New York State Department of Health - Room 325
2 University Place
Albany NY 12203
518-458-6482

OREGON

Health Licensing Boards
Oregon State Health Division
P.O. Box 231
Portland, OR 97207
503-229-5054

TENNESSEE

State of Tennessee
Board of Medical Examiners
283 Plus Park Boulevard
Nashville, TN 37217
615-367-6231

TEXAS

Texas Department of Health
Medical Radiologic Technology Program
1100 West 49th Street
Austin, TX 78756-3183
512-459-2960

VERMONT

State of Vermont
Board of Radiologic Technology
Division of Licensing and Registration
Office of the Secretary of State
Pavilion Office Building
Montpelier, VT 05609-1101
802-828-2886

WASHINGTON

Washington State Office of Radiation
Olympic Building S. 220
217 Pine Street
Seattle, WA 98101-1549
206-464-6840

WEST VIRGINIA

State of West Virginia
Room 303, Valley One Complex
3049 Robert C. Byrd Drive
Beckley, WV 25801
304-256-6985

WYOMING

State of Wyoming
Board of Radiologic Technologist Examiners
1312 Monroe Avenue
Cheyenne, WY 82001
307-778-7319

PUERTO RICO

University of Puerto Rico
Medical Sciences Campus
Department of Environmental Health
G.P.O. Box 5067
San Juan, PR 00936
809-758-2525, extension 1424